DATE DUE			

HUMAN MILK AND INFANT FORMULA

FOOD SCIENCE AND TECHNOLOGY

A SERIES OF MONOGRAPHS

Series Editors

George F. Stewart
University of California, Davis

Bernard S. Schweigert
University of California, Davis

John Hawthorn
University of Strathclyde, Glasgow

Advisory Board

A complete list of the books in this series appears at the end of the volume.

HUMAN MILK
AND INFANT FORMULA

Vernal S. Packard

Department of Food Science and Nutrition
University of Minnesota
St. Paul, Minnesota

1982

ACADEMIC PRESS

A Subsidiary of Harcourt Brace Jovanovich, Publishers
New York   London
Paris   San Diego   San Francisco   São Paulo   Sydney   Tokyo   Toronto

613.2

P12h

126692

Nov.1983

ACADEMIC PRESS, INC.
111 Fifth Avenue, New York, New York 10003

United Kingdom Edition published by
ACADEMIC PRESS, INC. (LONDON) LTD.
24/28 Oval Road, London NW1 7DX

Library of Congress Cataloging in Publication Data

Packard, Vernal S.
  Human milk and infant formula.

  (Food science and technology)
  Bibliography: p.
  Includes index.
  1. Milk, Human--Composition. 2. Infants--Nutrition.
3. Infant formulas. I. Title. II. Series. [DNLM:
1. Milk. 2. Infant food. 3. Milk, Human. WS 125
P119h]
QP246.P3 1982   613.2'0880542   82-8876
ISBN 0-12-543420-0   AACR2

PRINTED IN THE UNITED STATES OF AMERICA

82 83 84 85   9 8 7 6 5 4 3 2 1

Contents

Preface

This book is a "semitechnical" summary of the scientific literature on human milk and infant formula. I have sought to treat these two major sources of infant food in light of the needs of mothers both of the industrialized world and of developing nations, keeping in mind both the diversity and similarity of the conditions under which humanity survives.

I choose not to judge as "better" either infant formula or human milk. Both are clearly needed. Even if mother's milk is better under most conditions, it is not so under all conditions; and if a mother, of her own volition, and for whatever reason, elects not to breast-feed, infant formula remains the ideal substitute.

It should be kept in mind that formula is only as good as scientific knowledge and processing can make it. Because infant nutritional needs are most often based on the composition of mother's milk, a section of this book is devoted to human milk composition and to the significant causes of variation in macronutrients, vitamins, and minerals. Direct comparisons with bovine milk, the most common source of ingredients for infant formula, are also made. Where appropriate, the text indicates the present status of infant formula as it reflects the specific nutrient or nutritional need in question.

Human milk is more than food, however. It is also a source of immune agents which can, among other functions, hold intestinal disease in check—almost as important as nutrition itself. Thus, a chapter is devoted to the nature and function of the immune components of mother's milk. Research now suggests that these or similar immune factors can also be processed into infant formula. A discussion of this concept, the product itself, and the results of clinical trials on diarrhetic infants forms a section of this chapter.

Another chapter of the book considers mammary infections generally, but also concentrates on infections caused by *Staphylococcus aureus*. Along with a discussion of drug and environmental contaminants of breast milk, these topics are presented to make students, public health workers, and mothers aware of the scope of the problems. These considerations undergird a chapter devoted to sanitary expression, storage, and processing of human milk for infant feeding purposes.

The foregoing subject matter supports a realistic appraisal of the use and misuse of infant foods. Most of the information is also directly related to formulation and processing of infant formula. Both topics are reviewed, again with an eye to the needs of both developed and underdeveloped nations.

Since "feeding" goes on beyond infancy, I have concluded this work with an analysis of the role of lactose in the human diet. "Lactose intolerance" has been the subject of much debate. Some individuals and certain races seem more prone to this digestive upset than do others. Because lactose intolerance can affect children, food aid, in the form of milk or milk products, has even come under scrutiny. In light of these facts and the general shortage of food worldwide, it seems essential to re-examine the use of milk for growing children, especially among children of the Third World.

It has been my conviction, reinforced now by investigation of the scientific literature, that ignorance and poverty, not infant formula, are the two greatest deterrents to infant and child well-being. I sincerely hope, therefore, that the information presented herein will serve as a useful educational resource. To this end, I dedicate this book to the children of the world and to the servants of their health—public health workers, food scientists, and technologists, pediatricians, nurses, and nutritionists, students of these disciplines, and, of course, concerned mothers. Moreover, and solely because of my belief that poverty—even more than ignorance—controls the fate of our children, I pledge all royalties from this book to an international infant/child relief agency. And if, in the end, this amounts to no more than a seed, my hope is that it may bring forth good fruit.

Introduction

Mother's milk—it has been humankind's first food for as long as the human race has existed. For perhaps 2 million years, human milk has served to nurture life in its infancy. Yet only within the past 50 years has a mother, who is faced with loss of milk and lacking a wet nurse, had a reasonable substitute on which to rely. Although infant formula has not been used very long, much has happened during that period of time. Most importantly, the human population doubled, adding 2 billion persons to the planet. As a consequence, the need for weaning foods doubled, and the need for a human milk substitute for those mothers who either chose not to or were unable to breast-feed expanded to an unprecedented level.

In addition to rapid population growth, a scientific–industrial complex came into its own, creating a new world. Science discovered chemicals for controlling insects, weeds, or other pests; industry found ways of producing these chemicals in amounts needed to serve the entire farm community. Pesticides thus became a part of the environment, permitting the cultivation of ever-increasing quantities of food. Unfortunately, some of these same chemicals began to show up in the blood, fat, and tissues of the human and livestock population; some also began to appear in the milk of both animals and humans. You could consider these chemicals intentional contaminants of the environment. But literally thousands of other contaminants were being found at the same time, including pollutants like methyl mercury, lead, cadmium, polychlorinated biphenyls (PCB's), and radioactive (nuclear) isotopes (e.g., strontium-90 and iodine-131).

Those pollutants that found their way to milk supplies were often in such minute amounts as to require other scientific breakthroughs in detection methods sensitive enough to measure them. Contaminants of milk and food were soon to become measureable in parts per million, parts per billion, and even parts per trillion. This exquisite ability to detect and quantify results was used to measure the presence of tens of thousands of chemical compounds unknown or nonexistent less than 50 years ago. Among these compounds are not only the pollutants and contaminants already mentioned but also certain vitamins and minerals. To know needs, you must first be able to detect and measure amounts. Thus, the new measuring tools allowed scientists to determine the precise level of need for most nutrients. Scientists were also able to detect and measure poisons the world had not recognized before. For instance, aflatoxins, poisons produced by certain molds, were discovered and were found to be among the most potent cancer-causing compounds known to humankind. Some have been found in food and feed, and some small amounts, mostly of less toxic cousins, have shown up in the milk of humans and animals.

The scientific–industrial complex also combined in another area of great importance. The end result, as is usually the case, bore fruit and, at the same time, posed problems never before encountered. The following example illustrates this dilemma. In 1929, Sir Alexander Fleming first described the antibiotic penicillin. The drug had been discovered quite by chance when a culture of bacteria, of a type called staphylococci, was accidentally contaminated with a penicillin-producing mold. Within 50 years, penicillin and other antibiotics were administered to dairy cows at a rate of some 350 tons annually in the United States. It was the greatest boon to disease treatment ever. In the face of that benefit, a germ of cow's udders, staphylococci, replaced other germs as the most common infective agent of these milk-producing animals. Partly for the same reason, it became a common infective agent of the human breast. It is destructive of milk-making tissue, and certain strains produce toxins so potent that as little as 1 μg causes illness. We learned that infants could become ill on such small amounts, and on milk produced and fed directly from the mother's breast. But that was only one problem. Some infants have been found to react to antibiotics. The mother who has taken penicillin for some illness, as in the treatment of other milk-producing species, may find her milk contaminated with the drug. If not told otherwise, she feeds it unknowingly to her infant. This may only rarely be a serious problem. Nonetheless, the same industries that produce antibiotics by the tons have also come up with untold amounts of other drugs. In 50 years the developed world has become the largest user of drugs in history. Some of these chemicals have been taken for purely medical reasons. Still other drugs have been taken for "kicks." Today infants are born with the drug habits of the mother. Others are born deformed or otherwise mentally or physically afflicted. No matter what the drug or what the reason for taking (or giving) it, chances are that mother's milk is in some way tainted.

There has been another development, after 2 million years, that has finally come into widespread practice—pasteurization, a heat treatment of milk. It is a truly significant factor in the control of human disease. Pasteurization absolutely ensures the destruction of viruses and germs such as polio, diphtheria, tuberculosis, and typhoid. Pasteurized milk never contains live germs unless it is recontaminated. Although pasteurizaton achieved widespread adoption only during the past 50 years, a movement that shuns such protection for the "benefits" of raw milk has already formed. (However, this movement is found only in countries where the mother has a choice.) In poor nations, diseases spread by contaminated forumla have rallied world concern. A new emphasis has focused on the "immune factors" of human milk. The science of immunology, a science as much in its infancy as the human counterparts it seeks to help, has begun to produce a signficant literature. A new technology has developed and has issued its own challenge: Tell us what it is in human milk that provides immune responses, and we can put many of those same factors into infant formula with a consistency that human milk can never match.

Indeed, human milk is best seen within the context of 2 million years of evolution. No doubt additions to, or subtle changes in, factors known to fight infant disease have evolved, some in direct response to new or unusual bacterial, viral, or chemical attacking agents. Nutrient composition, too, has no doubt altered. Certainly the composition of milk of different mammalian species differs markedly. In the milk of whales there is little or no sugar. There is fat, though, to the level of light cream (19–20%). After all, the young whale, coping with frigid seas, needs a quick source of high-density energy. Fat, with twice the calories of sugar (carbohydrate), provides just that. For similar reasons, reindeer's milk is the equal of whale milk in level of fat, though with nominal amounts of sugar (2.6%) as well. Milk of mares is low in fat (1.6%) but, at least on the average, higher than cow's, goat's, or human milk in the level of sugar (carbohydrate). Can anyone doubt that nature evolved these differences for the special needs of the newborn mammal? If this is true for major milk ingredients, it must likewise be true for certain minor components, though perhaps for less obvious reasons. Thus, I propose in this volume to examine some of these differences and to try to identify weaknesses or potential shortcomings of both human milk and infant formulas. Neither are as good as they might be under a variety of conditions and for a number of reasons. Therefore, blind advocacy of breast feeding or formula feeding is ill-advised. Humanity needs both sources of food.

CURRENT INFANT FEEDING PRACTICES

Breast-feeding is on the rise in the United States. From 1973 to 1975, the percentage of breast-feeding American mothers rose from 25% to 35%. These figures, taken from a national health statistics survey, (U.S. Dept.

Health, Education and Welfare, 1979), represent the increase in breast feeding overall. Differentiating between Black and Caucasian women, the statistics show a decidedly higher rate of increase in breast feeding among whites (33% compared with 15%) for the years 1973–1975. There is an even more dramatic difference when education is considered. Given an education of 12 years or more, 48% of mothers chose breast feeding during the 2 years surveyed. Among those with less than 12 years of schooling, the percentage goes down by half, that is, to 24%.

The trend, therefore, seems clear and reflects the trend generally in developed nations around the world. Nevertheless, other considerations enter in. As the survey further showed, less than one-tenth of breast-feeding mothers continued to breast-feed beyond 3 months. If second births are considered, fractions in all categories move down. Thus, the report concludes that the overall impact of breast feeding on American society is yet relatively minor. Putting it differently, a large majority of American mothers still rely on bottle feeding, either of infant formula or some other substitute for breast milk.

Similarly, a Czechoslovakian survey (Salata, 1979) found 40% of infants being breast-fed for 28 days or less, or not at all. A 1975 study representative of the situation in England and Wales (Hide, 1979) showed 50% of mothers attempting to breast-feed. However, less than half of these women succeeded in holding lactation for more than 6 weeks. Diaries kept by 1000 women residing on the Isle of Wight showed that 50% were breast-feeding at the end of 1 week postpartum, but only 33% were still breast-feeding after 3 months. These data were taken for the year 1974. A somewhat earlier study, conducted in Canada during 1965–1971, showed 5% of Canadian mothers breast-feeding solely (Myeres, 1979). As many as 25% started the practice initially, but the majority (75%) of these women had resorted to bottle feeding by 3 months. In Sweden in 1975, as many as 46% of infants were still being breast-fed at 2 months of age, and the trend was up from earlier years.

Generally, it is the affluent segment of the developed world that appears to be turning to breast feeding. Reasons given for either bottle feeding or breast feeding are varied. Personal, social, cultural, and family factors enter into the decision. Often the choice has been made by early pregnancy. Not the least of determining factors, according to some studies, is the husbands' feelings in the matter.

In developing nations the situation appears to be quite different. A Canadian survey (North-South Institute, 1979) made in Bangladesh, Haiti, Honduras, India, and St. Vincent found breast feeding to be "very well established" and frequently undertaken for up to 2 years. A World Health Organization (WHO) analysis provides somewhat similar findings (Hofvander and Petros-Barvazian, 1978). Considering 24,000 mother–child pairs in Chile, Ethiopia, Guatemala, India, Nigeria, Philippines, Zaire, Sweden, and Hungary), breast feeding was noted to be declining among the urban elite but to be constant and prolonged among the rural poor. Other studies tend to confirm this picture. Taking the urban poor into account, a survey in India (Nath and Geervani, 1978) found 44% of mothers breast feeding up to 2 years. For those giving up earlier, the reason generally cited was inadequate amounts of milk. Taken as a whole, low-income mothers in India have been found to breast-feed an average of 19.8 months. Duration decreases generally with increasing affluence.

In rural Bangladesh 98% of the women were found to be breast-feeding 1 year after giving birth. Average duration was 30 months. These data, gathered in 1974, come from a study by American workers (Huffman *et al.*, 1980). Total suckling time in this instance was inversely related to level of education and infant nutritional status. In this respect women of developing nations appear to be following earlier trends of their counterparts in developed nations. New or different practices often take place first among the wealthier and more highly educated segments of society. This may be seen as the trend-setting class. But while this class of society in developing nations is still turning to bottle feeding, the same general class in the developed nations, having earlier initiated the practice of bottle feeding, is now turning back to breast feeding.

Still other factors obviously influence nursing practices. A Caribbean study (Gueri *et al.*, 1978) emphasizes two of them. Of 418 women interviewed, 98% indicated plans to breast-feed. In fact, only 64% did so. Early use of the bottle was seen as a significant factor in changing the minds of many. A reevaluation at 4 months after delivery found only 6% still breast-feeding. Most mothers had weaned their infants by this time, and the majority of the women who had done so were employed at a job away from home. Increasingly, the need to work is a consideration in infant-feeding practices.

Often the reason given for substituting the bottle is a lack of breast milk. Whether a lack in fact exists is another matter. Nonetheless, many women in both developed and Third World nations apparently become concerned. A study of Malaysian women (Kee, 1975) found the incidence of breast feeding to be 84%. About a third of those who fed infant formula claimed to do so because of a lack of milk. Another sizable group (25%) felt that their infants preferred the bottle. Breast-feeding mothers also cited infant preference as a reasons for holding to this practice. In addition, these women found breast feeding cheap and convenient. They were receptive also to traditional advice. Interestingly enough, advice from professional health workers had little influence on the decision of Malaysian women either to breast-feed or to use infant formula.

Informed sources suggest that 90% or more of all women should be able to breast-feed successfully. But this is the ideal. Realities of life often place the actual percentage of breast-feeding mothers at a much lower level. This is true presently in most developed nations of the world. It is often the case in the Third World, especially if duration of breast feeding beyond 2 to 3 months is considered. Even assuming that a maximum number of mothers accept and carry out the practice, there remains a very large number of women who for one or more reasons are unable to breast-feed. Environmental pollutants of mother's milk and drug and smoking habits of some women make the desirability of breast feeding questionable. Likewise, psychological factors take a heavy toll, if not initially, very early during lactation. The dietary needs of prematurely born infants and those of infants born with a number of different dietary afflictions preclude mother's milk as food. For these infants, there is every reason to improve the substitute food products on which the survival of the newborn depends. There are similar and equally pressing reasons to do so for the many who depend on a second source of food as a supplement or weaning food.

APPROACH

Because cow's milk* most often serves as the major source of ingredients in infant formula, and because the scientific literature is far more extensive on this than on any other mammalian species, a work of this nature perhaps best begins with a comparison of human milk and cow's milk; this approach is taken with an eye to the need to improve the nutrient composition of infant formula. At the same time, both human milk and infant formula are best considered in light of the latest scientific recommendations for infant nutrition. Thus, the first part of this book is devoted to these considerations.

The second section deals with the immune factors of mother's milk, that is, the disease-fighting potential of this food. Here certain advantages of human milk will become clear. Formula, too, can be processed with a certain level of built-in immune potency. The research proving the efficacy of such formulations is considered in this section, along with a discussion of breast infections, allergic responses, contaminants of breast milk, and issues of drug use.

In the third section I focus on the formulation and processing of infant formula. Both nutrient and immune factors are discussed. Advent of human milk banks makes appropriate further consideration of precautions in obtaining, storing, and pasteurizing human milk. Finally, because the feeding of breast-fed infants must be supplemented at some point in time, and often with lactose-containing food(s), a chapter of this book is devoted to lactose "intolerance" at weaning and beyond.

---

*Throughout this book, I shall refer to cow's milk meaning milk of dairy cows.

1

Macronutrients and Energy

Though many similarities exist, human and cow's milk are not one and the same in gross composition or nutrient content. Cow's milk does not fulfill an infant's nutritional needs. This is the reason why infant formula, even one based on cow's milk components, is a quite different food from the milk from which it is prepared. Infant formula has been changing in composition, even in recent times. United States surveys show dramatic differences in the nutrient intake of infants in the years 1977–1978, compared with 1965. Most of these differences reflect changes in infant formula, which is now manufactured to be more similar to mother's milk, especially in gross composition (see Table 1). Keep in mind that values given in the table are averages. Differences among individuals of either groups can be very great.

Cow's milk shown in Table 1 is milk as produced in the United States. It is richer in fat content than most commercial whole milk, which, by federal regulation, need not contain more than 3.25% fat. In either case, human milk averages somewhat higher. Cow's milk is appreciably higher in protein and mineral matter. It is primarily these latter two components that must be modified in cow's milk if it is to be used as a substitute for mother's milk.

CARBOHYDRATES

More commonly referred to as milk sugar, lactose is the major carbohydrate of the milk of mammals. Human milk contains nearly 7% lactose (about 38% of caloric content), exceeding cow's milk by about 2% and averaging nearly the highest level of any mammalian species. Possibly this

7

TABLE 1

Gross Composition of Human and Cow's Milk (Grams per 100 Grams of Fluid Product)[a]

Component	Human milk[b]	Cow's milk[c]
Fat	4.4	3.7
Protein	1.03[d]	3.3
Milk sugar (lactose)	6.9	4.7
Mineral matter (as ash)	0.2	0.7
Water	87.5	87.8

[a]From U.S. Department of Agriculture (1976).

[b]Average of 591 samples.

[c]This is milk as produced in the U.S. The level of fat is reduced for most commercial uses.

[d]This value is reported as given in the source cited. It represents the average of 591 different samples, but of varying stages of lactation. Protein content of human milk falls off significantly after the sixth month of lactation. Average level of protein of mature human milk (excluding colostrum milk) as given in the scientific literature more frequently ranges from 1.2 to 1.8%. However, these values, and to some extent the value given in this table, may reflect a measurement of total nitrogen, which, in human milk, includes a large percentage of nonprotein nitrogen (approximately 25%). Taking this fact into account, "true" protein content of human milk may run nearly one-fourth lower than reported values.

implies a greater need for milk sugar for human offspring than for other mammals. Energy needs per unit of body weight are indeed the highest during infancy than at any other time. Carbohydrates, a ready source of energy, are obviously important in infant nutrition.

Lactose is a two-unit molecule (disaccharide) consisting of glucose and galactose. The latter component may serve a unique purpose. Along with certain lipids (fat and fatlike compounds), galactose forms a large part of brain matter. This being the case, lactose could well be present at high levels in human milk to aid in growth and development of the brain. Certainly there could be no better reason for ensuring that the infant receives ample amounts. Lactose intolerance (the inability to digest lactose readily) is another matter to be discussed later (see Chapter 9). For now it need only be said that human milk substitutes can be formulated as readily with 7% as 5% (or less) milk sugar. Lactose of cow's milk (or of other mammals) is identical to lactose of human milk. Between mammals, only amounts differ.

Healthy, full-term infants have no trouble digesting lactose. Preterm or low-weight (under 2500 g) infants may have some difficulty in this respect. For this reason, formula prepared for preterm, underweight infants is specially designed with one-third to one-half less lactose than might normally be used. The difference is made up with simple sugars (such as the glucose of corn syrup solids).

The presence of an enzyme called *lactase* facilitates lactose digestion.

Healthy infants have somewhat higher levels of lactase activity than adults. Infants are able to generate maltase and sucrase at comparable levels with adults. Thus common disaccharides are readily digested by full-term infants. Simple sugars (monosaccharides) are also well absorbed. On the other hand, starch, a complex carbohydrate, is not quite so readily digested because of the comparative lack of the enzyme, α amylase, required to break it down. Exposure to starch, however, results in an increase in α amylase activity in infants through 6 months of age.

No matter what the role of lactose in infant diets, the American Academy of Pediatrics (AAP) Committee on Nutrition gives its approval for the use of carbohydrates other than milk sugar in infant formula. The AAP further notes that carbohydrate can also be supplied from food sources other than formula (such as strained baby foods), sources that do not contain lactose. To an extent, the basis for such approval stems from the necessity to avoid diarrhea. Diet in which carbohydrates are supplied primarily as simple sugars may give rise to this malady.

Though the lactose content of mammalian milks is one of the most constant of properties, levels do vary. Again, averages deceive. Infections of the udder or breast tend to cause a decrease in lactose, which, to maintain proper osmotic balance, is compensated for by an increase in chlorides. The variations are slight, however, even in this case. Among individuals, variations in milk lactose content run much higher, from a low of perhaps 4% to as high as 8.9%. Thus, even breast-milk does not contain a common level of this nutrient. Variations also occur in other nutrients, of course, and these are documented elsewhere in this text.

Both human and cow's milk contain low levels of carbohydrates other than lactose. Probably as residuals of various metabolic processes, both milks contain the two monosaccharides, glucose and galactose, that comprise lactose. In addition, some human milk samples have been found to contain minor amounts of fructose (Sheibak et al., 1978). Glucosamines are found in the nonprotein nitrogen fraction of milk and perhaps arise again as residuals, this time from protein-bound carbohydrates. For example, human secretory immunoglobulin A of colostrum consists, by one estimate, of 2.5% glucosamine and 0.2% galactosamine. In addition, the protein/carbohydrate complex carries fucose (0.7%), mannose (2.6%), galactose (1.6%), and sialic acid (1.1%) (Tomana et al., 1972).

FAT

Fat is generally considered the most variable of all milk components, both in chemical composition and amount. The level in human milk has been reported to range all the way from 0.4% to 10%. Most values fall between

1.0% and 5.0%. Separate researches by different investigators around the world give the following average levels of fat in human milk: 2.02, 3.1, 3.2, 3.27, 3.7, 3.95, 4.5, and 5.3%. Values were ordered in ascending amounts for ease of review. Data in Table 1, taken from a United States Department of Agriculture (USDA) survey (1976), put the average at 4.4%. Remember, of course, that these are averages. There is always the question of individual differences, which can be very great. In fact, fat is the most variable component of human milk, both within an individual woman and between women. Even in cows, where years of genetic control has focused on increasing levels of fat production, herd averages (i.e., pooled, herd milk) range from 2.5 to 7.0%. Lacking genetic manipulation, some mother's milk may very well yield levels of fat of 0.4%, as already suggested. Some supplies might climb close to 10%.

Another factor should be considered. Reported values may reflect differences in sampling methods, especially when fat content is concerned. Foremilk is low in fat, hardly richer than skim milk. Last milk from the same breast will show about a threefold higher content of fat. Unless the milk sample is representative of all milk taken during a single milking, values will be distorted in one way or the other. Human milk is also known to vary in composition during the same day; it even varies from one breast to the other. Stage of lactation may also have a bearing on fat level. Colostrum (first milk after delivery) is generally low in both lactose and total lipids (fat). Some investigators find the level of milk fat increasing in milk throughout the duration of lactation. Others find no apparent trend.

Cow's colostrum is high in milk fat content; it declines gradually over the first 2 or 3 months, then rises slowly through late lactation. Cows also react to seasonal changes, attributed soley to changes in temperature. The milk fat level increases during fall and winter, then drops during the warm summer months. The kind and amount of feed also influences both the amount and the composition of cow's milk fat. When cows lack roughage, their milk fat level drops precipitously. Feeding polyunsaturated fats yields a higher level of polyunsaturation of milk fat, at least to a point. In order to feed such fat and get it through the rumen unaltered by rumen bacteria, it is necessary to encapsulate or otherwise protect it.

The amount of fat in the diet of women does not appear to be reflected generally in the amount of fat in their milk. Poorly nourished women show losses in total milk yield. The percentage of protein, fat, and carbohydrates remains fairly stable. However, the fact content of milk of severely underfed women may decline and may become a limiting nutrient to the breast-fed infant (Crawford et al., 1977). Studies in India (Belavady, 1978) show a generally lower level of milk fat of women of low socioeconomic status. Consider also that two women on the very same diet may show wide variations in milk composition. In such instances, genetic influences would seem significant. Also, frequency of milk output, stress, and lack of mammary gland stimulation prior to feeding are possible factors causing either lower levels of fat or milk yield.

Fatty Acid Composition

The most striking difference in fatty acid composition of human and cow's milk is the generally low level of short chain fatty acids in the former, along with a somewhat higher amount of polyunsaturated acids. Although data vary among different researchers, human milk fat appears to be made up of about 3.1% palmitoleic acid, 35–36% oleic acid, 8–10% linoleic acid, and about 1.2% linolenic acid. Only small to trace amounts of C_{20}–C_{22} unsaturated fatty acids are present. Chief among saturated fatty acids in human milk is palmitic acid, which is present in levels of 20–25%. In cow's milk, palmitoleic acid makes up about 2.5% of the fatty acids present. Oleic, linoleic, and linolenic acids are found at levels of 25–26, 2.5, and 1.6%, respectively. It should be noted that both cow's and goat's milk contain adequate amounts of linoleic and arachidonic acids to meet the infant's need for essential fatty acids. Either milk furnishes linoleic acid to near 1% of total calories.

As in human milk, palmitic acid is the major (28%) saturated fatty acid of cow's milk. Although C_4–C_8 fatty acids make up scarcely 1.5% of human milk fat, they are found at between 6% and 9% in cow's milk fat.

Another feature of human milk fatty acid content also stands out. The proportion of saturated to unsaturated acids is about equal. In cow's milk, the ratio is more nearly 65:35. It is at least in part due to these differences that unsaturated vegetable fats are now built into infant formulas. See Table 2 for a general comparison of the fatty acid content of human and cow's milk.

Fatty acid composition of mother's milk varies to some extent with diet. A diet high in carbohydrate content yields an increase in saturated fatty acids, especially lauric and myristic. Linoleic acid level drops. Vegetarian mothers produce milk fat with generally higher levels of linoleic and linolenic acids and less palmitic and stearic acids than nonvegetarians. Diets generally higher in polyunsaturated fats provide for milk fat high in unsaturated fatty acids. An abrupt change in the ratio of polyunsaturated to saturated fatty acids in the diet has been found reflected in milk fat composition within 12 hours. Corn oil with a polyunsaturated–saturated (P/S) ratio of 1.3 causes milk fat to increase in linoleic acid and to decrease in lauric and myristic acids, at least in comparison to milk fat produced on a more highly saturated diet. A similar change in fatty acid composition apparently occurs on those

TABLE 2

Fatty Acid Composition of Human and Cow's Milk Fat (Percentage by Weight)[a]

Fatty acids[b]	Human	Cow
Saturated		
Butyric (4:0)	—[c]	3.5
Caproic (6:0)	—[c]	1.9
Caprylic (8:0)	—[c]	1.3
Capric (10:0)	1.4	2.5
Lauric (12:0)	6.2	2.8
Myristic (14:0)	7.8	10.7
Palmitic (16:0)	22.1	27.8
Stearic (18:0)	6.7	12.6
Total	48.2	65.6
Monounsaturated		
Palmitoleic (16:1)	3.1	2.5
Oleic (18:1)	35.5	26.5
Gadoleic (20:1)	0.96	trace
Cetoleic (22:1)	trace	trace
Total	39.8	30.3
Polyunsaturated		
Linoleic (18:2)	8.9	2.5
Linolenic (18:3)	1.2	1.6
Parinaric (18:4)	—[c]	trace
Arachidonic (20:4)	0.72	trace
Eicosapentenoic (20:5)	trace	trace
Docosapentenoic (22:5)	trace	trace
Docosahexnenoic (22:6)	trace	trace
Total	12.0	4.1

[a]From U.S. Department of Agriculture (1976).

[b]Numbers in parentheses following the fatty acid name indicate the number of carbon atoms and number of double bonds, in that order. Common or scientific names are given for ease of discussion in the text. However, unsaturated fatty acids include both positional and geometric isomers.

[c]Presence of this fatty acid is uncertain.

diets considered appropriate for heart ailments provoked by high levels of blood serum cholesterol. However, a limit to the amount of polyunsaturated fats is suggested by the parallel need for higher levels of vitamin E, which serves as an antioxidant. Whether or not human milk of high unsaturated fatty acid content is proportionately higher in content of vitamin E is not known. As will be seen, this consideration becomes important as well in the formulation of infant formula. First, however, it is perhaps well to note that 98% of lipids of human milk fat are triglycerides, with less than 1% each of diglycerides, free fatty acids, and sterols. It is likewise noteworthy that the composition of lipids varies significantly over lactation. Colostrum milk fat differs chemically from transitional and mature milk fat, and there is reason to believe that these differences relate to specific physiological needs of the infant.

Infant formula, whether milk or soy in basic composition, comes generally formulated of vegetable fat. The net result is a fat more nearly the composition of human milk in fatty acid content. Soybean oil, oleo oil, and safflower oil are all polyunsaturated fats now used in formula products. Coconut oil, a relatively hard fat, provides a source of saturated fatty acids needed to balance the polyunsaturates. Cow's milk fat could serve the same purpose, with possibly even better results because of its better digestability. In general, however, formula fats are absorbed quite well by most infants and generally better than cow's milk fat alone. All premature infants absorb fat poorly, especially saturated fats. However, a diet high in polyunsaturated fats can lead to vitamin E deficiency and hemolytic anemia. Preterm infants are somewhat unique, then, in their dietary needs. Those born at full term generally utilize fats found in most present-day formula products. However, a factor related to fat resorption in the infant intestines should be mentioned. Fats are triglycerides; that is, a molecule of fat is made up of glycerol and three fatty acids. For ease of understanding, a molecule—a single unit—of fat can be considered to look like a block *E*. The three arms, then, become fatty acids. Best fat resorption tends to come in fats whose middle arm (2 position) is either palmitic or stearic acid. Both are saturated fatty acids, and both appear to be better absorbed when the outer arms of the fat have both been stripped away. The resulting compound is called a monoglyceride (a one-armed glyceride). For best absorption, this fatty acid arm (consisting preferably of palmitic acid) must hold down the middle position. Most vegetable fat contains only low levels of palmitic acid in the middle position. Milk fat of both the cow and the goat carry this fatty acid distributed fairly evenly throughout all three positions and, therefore, a modicum of molecules with palmitic acid in the 2 position. Thus, these sources of fat can serve a useful purpose in infant formula. In any event, the fat of infant formula should contain more than essential fatty acids alone. Nonetheless, it is important to note that cow's milk fat is relatively low in the essential linoleic acid. Skin lesions have been found to develop in infants fed milk-based formulas of low linoleic acid content. Present formulas meet needs in this respect, as does human milk.

Evidence also suggests that fats made up of medium-length fatty acids not only are more readily absorbed but may help in the control of certain disorders of fat absorption. To avoid ketosis, diets must not be overly high in fat and low in carbohydrates. Placing a maximum of 6g fat/100 kcal (54% of calories) provides for adequate amounts of both carbohydrates and

protein, while acting to prevent either ketosis or acidosis. Such is the
assertion of the American Academy of Pediatrics (1976). The Nutrition
Committee of this scientific body suggests the need for 3.3 g fat/100 kcal
infant formula. This would put fat at 30% of calories. Further recommendations call for a minimum of 300 mg/100 kcal (3.0% of calories)
linoleic acid. The 1971 Food and Drug Administration (FDA) regulations
demand a minimum of 15% of calories as fat and 2% as linoleic acid.

Digestion of fat takes place mainly in the infant's small intestines. It is here
that pancreatic lipase activity is at a high plane. Bile acids are also present,
but to a level below that found in the adult (Bongiovanni, 1965; Holt, 1972;
Norman et al., 1972). In full-term infants, the bile acid content of duodenal
fluid averages near 5 mg/ml. In children and adolescents, the level may
exceed 15 mg/ml. Note, too, that specific forms and proportion of bile
compounds differ in infants. There is no deoxycholate; the ratio of glycine to
taurine conjugates varies from the adult (see Anderson et al., 1980). Both
glycine and taurine are amino acids. Human milk contains much higher levels
of taurine than cow's milk. In infants, taurine is the compound most
frequently combined with bile acid. Later on, taurine is replaced mainly by
glycine in this respect. This change appears to occur earlier in bottle-fed than
breast-fed infants. The true significance of this fact is not yet known. Some
authorities speculate that the change plays a role in the management of
cholesterol (see Cholesterol, p. 15).

As components of bile, glycine and taurine enter digestive functions as
glyocholic and taurocholic acids. British scientists (Naismith and Cashel,
1979) found a marked increase in the activity of pancreatic lipase (the fat-
splitting enzyme) in the presence of taurocholic acid, even at very low levels.
Glyocholic acid also boosts the activity of lipase, but only at significantly
higher levels. The research in this case was done on infant formula. It was
concluded that bile composition was indeed an important determinant in fat
utilization by the human infant.

Human and cow's milk (thus milk-based formulas) also contain carnitine
(γ-trimethyl-β-hydroxybutyrobetaine), a compound found elsewhere in
muscle and liver tissue, and thought possibly to aid in the digestion of fat.
Evidence appears to be mounting of the need for supplementation of some
formula products with this compound. Human milk contains about 59
nmol/ml. Formula products based on milk or beef have been found to contain
50–656 nmol/ml. Those prepared of soy isolate (and specialized formulations from casein and also egg white) carry an amount equal to, or less than, 4
nmol/ml. Some formulas, therefore, appear deficient in carnitine and might
well be improved by its addition (Borum et al., 1979).

The formulator of infant formula should therefore consider as important
(1) amount of fat, (2) chemical composition of the fat, (3) configuration of the

triglyceride, (4) vitamin needs, and (5) minor constituents that might aid in fat digestion.

Fat, like lactose, serves an infant's need for energy. It finds its way into certain functions of the human brain; it becomes a significant contributor to the activity of the central nervous system. At excessive levels in the diet, fat can interfere with calcium absorption and absorption of certain fat-soluble vitamins. Evidence also exists indicating that the infant adjusts intake of milk in relation to fat content of the milk (Konishi and Goodpasture, 1981).

Cholesterol

Human milk contains cholesterol at about the same level as that found in the milk of cows, that is, 14 mg/100g fluid milk. At this level it exceeds (on the average) the amount found in goat's milk (11 mg/100 g), but is lower than that usually found in buffalo's milk (19 mg/100 g). Cholesterol level follows generally the amount of fat in milk, which explains why foremilk shows a lower content than last milk of any given extraction period. However, some evidence gives reasons to believe that the cholesterol content of milk increases during the day at a rate exceeding fat. There is also evidence to suggest some decrease in human milk cholesterol in women in the United States over the past 25 years, possibly due to dietary changes (Picciano *et al.*, 1978). Yet other research findings show no difference in the level of cholesterol in human milk with mothers ingesting diets high in polyunsaturated fat and relatively low in cholesterol versus diets low in polyunsaturated fat (relatively high in saturated fat) and high in cholesterol content (Mellies *et al.*, 1978). No doubt these facts express a difference in the long- versus short-term effects of dietary factors.

Most infant formula is prepared with vegetable (plant) fat and is very low or devoid of animal fat and cholesterol. Infants feeding on formulas of this type show lower blood serum cholesterol levels than breast-fed infants or infants fed cow's milk. In a comparison of 6-month-old Canadian infants (Vobecky *et al.*, 1979) showing high (200 mg/100 ml or above) versus low (less than 200 mg/ml) levels of blood serum cholesterol, more of the former (43%) than the latter (34%) were breast-fed initially. Those infants rated high in serum cholesterol were also noted to have received higher caloric intake, higher protein intake, and higher overall levels of milk intake. These infants were also introduced to solid foods at an earlier age.

Australian scientists (Nestel *et al.*, 1979) found higher serum cholesterol levels in infants fed milk-based formula, compared with infants fed soy-based formula. The latter also produced a significantly higher secretion of bile acids. These and other investigators believe that the magnitude of response to cholesterol becomes established early in life. Future ability to handle the compound may depend on early exposure to it.

Some scientists note that those animal species that exclusively combine bile acids with the amino acid taurine do not appear to develop atherosclerosis, even on high cholesterol diets. Early in life, the human infant utilizes taurine to a very large extent in the bile acid reaction. Later, glycine replaces taurine in this respect. Indeed, bottle-fed infants seem to make the conversion sooner than breast-fed infants. However, if the bile reaction provides resistance to cholesterol deposit in humans, such resistance would have to manifest itself long after the body has made the change from taurine to glycine in bile components. At least a small body of evidence indicates a tendency to lower blood cholesterol levels in adults who, as infants, were breast-fed exclusively the first 2 months of life.

Assuming a possible beneficial role of dietary cholesterol in the infant body, some researchers would recommend simulating in infant formula the level of cholesterol found in human milk. However, evidence of the specific function of dietary cholesterol in infant nutrition is far from clear. Some authorities suggest that it plays a role in the synthesis of bile salts or nerve tissue. Production of certain enzymes might also be stimulated, and these may later serve some function in cholesterol metabolism. Lacking more definitive evidence, however, recommendations on cholesterol content of infant formula seem ill-advised.

PROTEIN

Before considering the significance of the protein of milk and infant formula, some basic concepts need explanation. First, milk contains not one but several different major and a number of minor (in terms of amount) proteins. The protein found in highest concentration is casein. Casein is the protein that coagulates and falls out as curd in the presence of acid. But whey, the fluid remaining after casein is removed, also contains proteins. Collectively, they are referred to as whey proteins. Certain whey proteins, generally those found in the largest amounts, serve a nutritional significance. Others—immune proteins—are of importance mainly as a defense against disease. These latter will be considered in Chapter 4.

Proteins consist largely of some 20 amino acids arranged in various sequences, chainlike and coiled in rather specific configurations. Because amino acids contain nitrogen, the reference method for measuring the protein content of foodstuffs focuses on an analysis for nitrogen. Depending upon the amino acid composition of the protein(s) in question, a factor serves to convert nitrogen to protein. For milk proteins, this factor is 6.38. That figure times the amount of nitrogen yields protein content. But there is a complicating factor—that is, not all nitrogen in milk has its source in protein; there exist, in fact, nitrogenous compounds other than amino acids of protein. As a group, these constituents are termed nonprotein nitrogen (NPN). Some free amino acids form a part of NPN and can obviously serve the same nutritional function as their protein-bound counterparts. Other amino acids of NPN may be linked in small units called peptides; however, NPN consists of more than amino acids. A number of organic and trace amounts of inorganic nitrogen-containing components go to make up this fraction of milk constituents. Together, they constitute a significant source of nitrogen.

Distribution of nitrogen in milk gives rise to a kind of classification system. Those fractions pertinent to the discussion are outlined and defined as follows.

1. Total nitrogen: all nitrogen in milk, including protein and NPN.
2. True protein nitrogen: total nitrogen minus NPN.
3. Casein nitrogen: nitrogen originating in amino acids of casein.
4. Whey protein nitrogen: nitrogen originating in protein components of whey, that is, protein exclusive of casein.
5. Nonprotein nitrogen: all nitrogen-containing compounds not defined as protein. Free amino acids are classified as NPN, and also various organic and inorganic nitrogenous components.
6. Free amino acids: amino acids existing singly as such, that is, unlinked either to each other or to proteins. These amino acids may be identical to or different from those that comprise protein. Of particular importance in the latter category is taurine.

Proteins of human milk differ somewhat from proteins of cow's milk, both in kind and amount. The significance of these differences is still very much under study. As for their similarities, both protein sources are of high biological value. Both consist of a full complement of amino acids (see Table 3). However, the ratio of individual protein components varies. Human milk carries about 60% whey proteins and 40% casein. In cow's milk those percentages are, respectively, 20% and 80%. However, these figures include NPN, and this distorts their true meaning. As percentage of total nitrogen, which is a more precise way of evaluating content of these constituents, human milk harbors casein nitrogen, whey protein nitrogen, and NPN to levels of about 35%, 40%, and 25%, respectively. For cow's milk, the same values run more nearly 78%, 17%, and 5%. There are qualitative differences between the two milks in each of these fractions. One implication already is clear: Because whey proteins carry a higher level of sulfur-containing amino acids, human milk can be seen to bear a different ratio of these amino acids (to other amino acids) than cow's milk protein. Both this fact and the

TABLE 3
Amino Acid Content of Human and Cow's Milk[a]

Amino acid	Human milk[b]		Cow's milk[c]	
	% of protein	mg/100 g fluid milk	% of protein	mg/100 g fluid milk
Tryptophan	1.7	17	1.4	46
Threonine	4.5	46	4.5	148
Isoleucine	5.4	56	6.0	198
Leucine	9.2	95	9.7	321
Lysine	6.6	68	7.9	260
Phenylalanine	4.5	46	4.8	158
Tyrosine	5.1	53	4.8	158
Valine	6.1	63	6.7	220
Methionine	2.0	21	2.5	82
Cystine	1.8	19	0.9	30
Histidine	2.2	23	2.7	89
Arginine	4.2	43	3.6	119
Alanine	3.5	36	3.4	113
Aspartic acid	8.0	82	7.5	249
Glutamic acid	16.3	168	20.8	687
Glycine	2.5	26	2.1	69
Proline	8.0	82	9.7	318
Serine	4.2	43	5.4	178

[a]From U.S. Department of Agriculture (1976).
[b]Based upon 1.03% protein.
[c]Based upon 3.3% protein.

presence of certain polyunsaturated fatty acids have been cited as important in the development of the human brain. For infants born prematurely, the presence of ample amounts of dietary cystine could decrease stress on the immature liver, where difficulty might otherwise be encountered in converting methionine to cystine. The problem here is lack of an enzyme, cystathionase, produced by the liver and needed to make this particular amino acid conversion. Unable to perform this function adequately, the infant fails to produce enough body proteins. Weight gain stalls, and a variety of body functions throttle down. With formula, the problem is more or less resolved by maintaining an appropriate balance between lactalbumin and casein (see Table 19). At 0.9% of the former and 0.6% of the latter, a formula provides 1.5% protein, with a 60:40 ratio between the two protein sources. This comes close to the protein makeup of human milk. Not all products are so formulated, however. Nonetheless, growth studies in which protein hydrolysates, soy protein products, or meat-based protein products are substituted for human milk protein all indicate a response that is the equal of breast milk.

The protein content of human milk, like milk of other species, falls off rapidly over the first few days of lactation and reflects a relatively higher loss of those proteins important to immune functions. Colostrum averages about 2.0% protein; transitional and mature milk average 1.5% and 1.0%, respectively. Last milk of any one milking may show about a 1.3-fold increase in protein level. Neither quality nor quantity of protein in human milk appears related to the protein intake of the mother, except in instances of severely insufficient consumption of protein of poor biological quality, that is, poor essential amino acid content. Under the latter conditions, the level of essential amino acids in the milk may become a limiting factor to the breast-feeding infant. This has been the finding of recent research done on Guatemalan women in whose diets corn is the primary source of protein.

Casein can be considered a protein of mammalian milk that precipitates at a pH of between 4.0 and 5.0. Thus far, this type of protein has been found in milk of every species tested (Jenness and Sloan, 1970). In amino acid composition, with some few exceptions, casein of all species is quite similar (Woodward, 1976). Merely as a source of amino acids, therefore, one casein will serve nearly as well as another.

Casein is a complex protein, however. That is, casein consists of several unique protein fractions distinguished by certain analytical methods (electrophoresis, sedimentation, electron microscopy, immunological assay, etc.). In fractional composition, the casein of human milk does vary from that found in cow's milk. Given the three major casein fractions (α_s, β, and κ), cow's milk yields about 45% α_s-casein. Human milk has little or none of this component. Rather, human milk casein consists mainly of the β fraction, though some κ-casein appears to be somewhat similar to the α_{s1}-casein of cow's milk (Woodward, 1976). Goat's milk, too, apparently carries no α_{s1} fraction of casein.

A certain amount and kind of carbohydrate also comes associated with various casein fractions, and this too distinguishes to some extent the casein of one species from another. For example, α_{s1}-and β-caseins of cow's milk contain no hexose, hexosamine, or sialic acid. All three components are found in the κ-casein fragments of this species. On the other hand, human milk β-casein carries both hexoses and hexosamines, but no sialic acid, the latter of which, as in cow's milk, is found in the κ fragment (see Woodward, 1976).

Serological techniques also find application in differentiating protein components. Put to this kind of testing, antisera of a mixture of cow's milk α_{s1}-and κ-caseins precipitates bovine, goat's, and sheep's whole casein, but not human milk casein. Antisera to whole cow's milk casein causes precipitation of goat's milk, but not, again, whole casein of human milk (Glass, 1956).

Both human milk β-casein and cow's milk α_{s1}-casein are insoluble in dilute calcium chloride. The κ-caseins of milk of these species are both soluble in this chemical compound. Chymosin (rennin), the active protease of rennet, which is used to coagulate cow's milk in the cheese-making process, does not coagulate the casein of fresh human milk, even in presence of calcium chloride (Oosthuizen 1962). This last fact is thought to be due to the naturally high pH of human milk, that is, pH 7.0 as compared to pH 6.6 for cow's milk. Slight acidification of human milk in presence of chymosin does result in coagulation of casein (see Woodward, 1976). Upon acid precipitation alone, human milk produces a finer protein floc than cow's milk, perhaps indicative of somewhat better digestability potential. And whole casein of milk of these two species, if separated by high-speed centrifugation, shows differing amounts of inorganic ions (calcium, phosphorus, sodium, potassium, and chloride) and citrate. Thus the major protein of cow's and human milk does exhibit certain measureable differences. These should not be construed as major considerations necessarily in food value for infant feeding. In this regard, presence of α_s-casein of cow's milk possibly represents one of the more significant factors, and mainly as a potential allergen.

In whey protein components, human milk and cow's milk also differ, and possibly in at least one meaningful way. First, cow's milk contains some true globulins (immunoglobulins, euglobulins, and others) as well as an albumin-like protein generally called β-lactoglobulin. Globulins are distinguished from albumins by the need for some small amount of salt for solublization. Albumins are soluble in pure water. The two major serum (whey) proteins of cow's milk are α-lactalbumin and β-lactoglobulin. Until very recently, human milk was thought to contain none of the latter. Now, however, a protein identified as β-lactoglobulin has been isolated from this source. The amount present would have to be considered very slight indeed. The major protein of the albumin fraction of whey of mature human milk is α-lactalbumin; although other proteins, particularly lactoferrin, are also found in significant amounts. As a percentage of the total protein, α-lactalbumin, lactoferrin, serum albumin, and lysozyme have been found to account for 17.5%, 17.6%, 5.2%, and 5.1%, respectively (Lonnerdal et al., 1976). Both lactoferrin and lysozyme carry come immune potency, that is, inhibitory effect against certain microbial diseases. Immunoglobulins, however, the major immune components of milk, are also found in whey, with colostrum by far the richest source.

Important, perhaps, to nutritional considerations is the fact that human milk contains scarcely any β-lactoglobulin. If cow's milk is used as source of protein in infant formula, then casein and α-lactalbumin, in proper proportion, best simulate human milk protein. Indeed certain fractions of both gel-filtered and ultra-filtered cow's milk whey proteins have been found to compare very favorably in nutritional value to human milk protein (Forsum,

1973). Even fractions containing β-lactoglobulin compare favorably. However, protein components of foods are often implicated as allergens, and for this reason absence or near absence of β-lactoglobulin in human milk (thus infant formula) is given some significance. But other proteins are allergenic, too. Some proteins ingested by the mother reach breast milk in as yet allergenically active form. In such cases, breast milk itself may cause an allergic response (Kulangara, 1980). Allergenicity of cow's milk is considered in Chapter 4.

Nonprotein Nitrogen

Compared with cow's milk, human milk is a much larger reservoir of nitrogen components other than protein. Nonprotein nitrogen (NPN) consists of a variety of organic and trace amounts of inorganic compounds shed into the milk supply—some for nutritional purposes, others perhaps as debris of sorts. Among these compounds are peptides and free amino acids. The latter average higher amounts in human milk (30.8 versus 7.8 mg/100 ml) and no doubt are a nutritional advantage to the infant. Also found in NPN are urea, creatinine, and sugar amines (mainly glucosamine). A Japanese study (Nishikawa et al., 1976) puts the content of these three components at 27.4, 20.9, 111.1 mg/100 ml, respectively, in human milk. By comparison, cow's milk yields 31.7, 12.7, and 39.2 mg/100 ml. It is possible that one or more compounds of NPN promotes growth of *Lactobacillus bifidus* (see The Bifidus Factor, Chapter 4).

The total amount of NPN in human milk, averaging near 25% of all nitrogen, is significantly higher than in cow's milk, in which it averages about 5%. According to the literature, as analytical variants or as real differences, NPN in human milk ranges from 18 to 30 % of total nitrogen. Higher levels appear associated with colostrum milk. The level of NPN drops significantly within 1–15 days postpartum and appears to remain fairly constant throughout the remainder of lactation. In cow's milk, NPN varies to some extent by breed and feed. The range goes from 4.9 to 7.5% of total nitrogen.

Each species of mammal seems to carry a characteristic pattern of free amino acids in NPN. Scientists tend to give this fact come nutritional significance. Of late, emphasis has centered on taurine. Taurine is aminoethylsulfonic acid, a compound chemically related to the amino acids cystine and cysteine. The milk of various species differs greatly in the content of taurine. It is the most abundant free amino acid in the milk of the rhesus monkey, gerbil, mouse, cat, and dog. It is the second most abundant free amino acid in human milk. The same is true for the milk of the chimpanzee, baboon, rat, sheep, and Java monkey. Taurine is not a major contituent in the milk of the guinea pig, rabbit, mouse, or cow. The level of taurine has been found to average 41.3, 33.7, and 26.6 μmoles/100 ml in colostrum, transitional, and mature human milk, respectively. The four most abundant free amino acids in human milk are glutamate (146.7 μmoles/100 ml), glutamine (58.4), taurine (26.6), and alanine (20.6). In cow's milk, in the same units of measure, the predominant free amino acids are ethanolamine (17.6), glutamate (11.7), glycine (8.8), and serine (2.3). Taurine is present in cow's milk only to a level of 1.0 μmoles/100 ml during midlactation. The amount of taurine in colostrum averages near 30.5 μmoles/100 ml; the highest level overall comes about 1 week after calving. This pattern of high initial taurine content followed by a rather rapid decline in level is characteristic of several species of mammals.

These observations and others presented in the preceding discussion are the findings of scientists of the Department of Human Development and Genetics of the New York State Institute for Basic Research in Mental Retardation (Rassin et al., 1978). In a massive study by researchers of this same institute, the plasma level of taurine in infants was found to decline steadily (and ultimately to a lower level than those fed human milk) when feeding on formulas containing either 1.5 or 3.0% cow's milk protein with a casein–whey protein ratio similar to that found naturally in cow's milk, that is 82:18. The implications of this and other work remain unresolved. Nonetheless, it is known that taurine is found at particularly high levels in fetal brain tissue, giving rise to circumstantial evidence that taurine plays a role in the development of the brain. But taurine is also associated with bile acid, a compound similar to cholesterol in chemical structure. Bile acids and bile salts have an important function in aiding the absorption of nutrients from the intestines. Taurine-containing bile components are thought also to play a role in the management of cholesterol in the body (see cholesterol, this chapter).

As already implied, taurine occurs in human milk at much higher levels than in cow's milk. In the milk of several species, including the cow, the level drops markedly and quickly as lactation progresses. The highest amounts of taurine in cow's milk are noted about 1 week after calving.

Evidence of the kind indicated above led some scientists (Lindblad et al., 1978) to recommend that infant formula be formulated to contain 1.0–1.2 g of cow's milk protein per 100 ml; however, they further recommended that it be made consistent with mother's milk in the ratio of α-lactalbumin (as major or sole whey protein ingredient) to casein, and also in level of both taurine and cystine. Because whey proteins generally are low in content of phenylalanine, some authorities recommend this source of protein for infants suffering the nutritional disease hyperphenylalanemia (an oversensitivity to phenylalanine).

General Recommendations for Protein Intake

The Committee on Nutrition of the American Academy of Pediatrics does not specify the need to duplicate precisely in infant formula the amino acid composition of human milk. Rather, this scientific body sets forth amounts of protein needed for good health, along with general guidelines of quality. Quality here means biological value. Current recommendations for milk formulas for healthy infants call for a mimimum of 1.8 g protein/kcal food. The upper level is 4.5 g/kcal, but this is true only when the protein is of equal biological value to the casein of cow's milk. Any protein of poorer quality should be provided at correspondingly higher amounts. However, no protein whose biological quality is less than 70% the equal of casein is satisfactory. The National Academy of Science/National Research Council recommendations put essential amino acid requirements of infants at 35% of dietary protein.

Foman (1974), an authority on infant nutrition, suggests two levels of protein intake, one for birth through 4 months, a second for infants aged 4 months to 1 year. Respectively, these amounts are 1.6 g/kcal and 1.4 g/kcal.

You will note that the preceding recommendations are based on protein intake as related to total caloric intake. This is the preferred method of expressing requirements of infants because much of the protein consumed is used for growth. From birth through 4 months, proteins account for about 12% of the total weight gain, which averages about 3.5 kg for the normal infant. This same weight gain is achieved during the period 4 months to 1 year. But at this point protein accounts for 20% of that increase in weight. From this fact alone, protein needs would be assumed to differ for these two age periods.

Protein needs are also expressed, perhaps less meaningfully so, in terms of body weight. NAS/NRC recommendations are given in this manner. The recommended daily allowance (RDA), unchanged for the 1980 revision of these guidelines, remains 2.2 times the kilograms of body weight for infants from birth through 6 months. For an infant weighing 6 kg, the RDA becomes $6 \times 2.2 = 13.2$ g of protein (of suitable biological quality). For infants aged 6–12 months, the RDA is 2.0 times kilograms of body weight. To convert pounds to kilograms, divide pounds by 2.2.

In recent years protein has become entwined with calories in the nutritional disease state that has come to be known as protein–calorie malnutrition. Evidence has been presented that seems to imply a greater than normal need for protein for persons under stress of insufficient calories. Such evidence has usually originated in studies done on healthy subjects, that is, people who were not previously, nor at the time the research was initiated, either undernourished or malnourished. More recent evidence (Heqsted, 1978) obtained from research on baby monkeys maintained at low protein intake (sufficient only for holding weight, but not increase in weight) shows a quite different response. Rather than raising the need for protein, a lack of calories seemed in fact to protect to some extent against protein deficiency. This can possibly be viewed as hopeful news. It would suggest that protein needs of infants (generally healthy infants) could be met through a variety of sources, including those of most of the plant kingdom, and this would hold true even for those infants stressed to an extent by low caloric intake. Cereal gruels of local preparation take on somewhat better character as weaning foods in Third World countries in light of such evidence. But in no way does this fact detract from the obvious advantage of supplementing plant sources of protein with protein of mother's milk, infant formula, or other animal and/or marine sources. Rather, the critical consideration shifts from the amount of available protein to the infant's general health. If protein intake is adequate, though marginal, the child holds its own mainly if it is not jeopardized by illness. Any illness that is accompanied by fever or any illness that lowers the appetite, can rapidly draw the child into a deficiency state. Food sufficiency is thus directly linked to public health services. Where success has been achieved in improving nutritional health among the very poor, it has come perhaps less from increasing food supplies and more through emphasis on literacy and improved medical services. Note, however, that protein deficiency diseases do occur, though rarely, in the developed world. Four cases of kwashiorkor were recently diagnosed in California (Sinatra and Merritt, 1981). The cause was given as a substitution of nondairy creamer (with 190 kcal of protein) for infant formula.

Both too much and too little protein intake pose problems for the developing infant. For most, the latter must be seen as the more common threat. When protein intake drops to less than 6% of caloric intake, poor growth and poor brain development appear likely possibilities. Rarely should this be a problem for healthy (nondiseased) infants feeding solely on mother's milk during the first 3 months of life—even though the mother suffers from moderate undernourishment. The protein content of human milk tends to hold quite steady and uninfluenced by the state of nutrition of the mother during the earliest months of lactation. Only when the infant is 3–4 months of age, with the infant's need for protein increasing with increasing size, does the protein of human milk possibly become limiting if no supplemental supplies are present. Some researchers suggest that energy, not protein, is more often the limiting factor, and they propose supplemental feeding to begin at 2–3 months rather than 4–6 months. Not all authorities agree, however.

Most scientific data show the level of protein of human milk to run significantly higher during the first 6 months of lactation, compared to the second 6 months. After the first year, the protein content continues to fall and may reach as low as 0.6% during the second year of lactation. The range of protein may run from 0.58 to 2.2%; solids-not-fat (SNF) range from 4.0 to as high as 17%. Lactose follows a rather similar pattern as protein. Indeed, where infants fail to thrive on mother's milk, and more or less directly as a result of the mother's poor state of nutrition, it is a lack of fat (lipids) in the milk that appears to bode ill. While protein and lactose apparently hold at reasonably adequate levels, lipid content may fall to 1% or possibly lower. Furthermore, the total yield of milk suffers. Infant formula offers consistency in this respect. If protein intake of more than 10% of calories is considered unnecessary (though possibly not harmful), then a fabricated formula can ensure amounts never exceeding that. More importantly, it can ensure an amount never falling below need.

Protein and Preterm Infants

A debate rages over what should be considered the most appropriate food for preterm infants. Protein needs—greater than normal for these infants—lie at the heart of the issue. Past practices have centered chiefly on the use of infant formula, and protein levels have been adjusted to meet current recommendations. Now, however, a group of knowledgeable scientists and pediatricians are leaning toward recommending mother's milk for these infants and, moreover, recommending the milk of those very mothers who give birth prematurely. At this writing, the controversy is far from resolved, but some pertinent facts seem worthy of mention.

First, milk is indeed available in women giving birth 25–26 weeks into gestation. Although the infant may lack strength to suckle, the mother's milk supply, expressed either by hand or by the use of appropriate mechanical methods, can be utilized. Up to 1.8 liters per day may be available. However, some authorities are of the opinion that such milk is simply inadequate in both protein and mineral content. Others (Atkinson, et al., 1979, 1980) however, present data showing the protein level of such milk to be naturally higher than the level in milk of women delivering at full term. Comparing samples of preterm and full-term milk composited over the entire 24 hours and for the first month of lactation shows a higher level of protein nitrogen in preterm milk and a linear, parallel decline in protein nitrogen in full-term milk. Preterm milk was also found significantly higher in caloric content, due mainly to higher amounts of fat. Both protein nitrogen and NPN seemed qualitatively similar in the two supplies of milk. In addition, milk of preterm mothers yields a generally higher content of sodium, chloride, potassium, and calcium early in lactation. These levels decline over the first 4 weeks. In general, the content of sodium, potassium, chloride, magnesium, phosphorus, and calcium are equivalent in the two kinds of milk. Considering these facts, the researchers regard milk of preterm mothers to be adequate in protein, sodium, chloride, potassium, and magnesium. A higher energy level is also seen as desirable. A question remains, though, about the adequacy of calcium and phosphorus at the low level of intake of preterm infants, (see Calcium and Phosphorus, Chapter 3). Nevertheless, these and other scientists would suggest the use of the mother's own milk in preference either to formula or banked human milk. Not all authorities agree, and after many years of observation and experiences, some very much disagree. Thus, the controversy continues.

ENERGY NEEDS AND SUPPLY

Precise energy needs of the infant are poorly understood. During the first year there are requirements for basal metabolism, growth, and activity. Activity, a significant "unknown," can account for as much as 35% of total calorie expenditure to 2 months of age, and up to 48% at 6 or 7 months of age. In calories per se, this adds up to 150 to 300, respectively, for those two age periods. For this reason, any standard of daily need must be viewed with caution. Still, such standards are set, and Table 4 summarizes those recommended by the Food and Agriculture Organization and the World Health Organization (FAO/WHO). It is helpful to understand further that caloric needs of infancy, in terms of overall weight, surpass those of any other age. Given the average composition of mother's milk shown in Table 1, this food provides about 67–68 kcal/100 ml. This is the level (670/liter) recommended for infant formulas. It would take a daily production rate of about 800 ml of milk of "average" composition for a mother to provide 540 cal of food energy, the daily requirement recommended by FAO/WHO for the 3-month-old infant. Such a rate would appear to be a somewhat above average output of most women. Some scientists assert that energy needs at 2–3 months warrant supplementation at this early date. Again, disagreement exists. Nonetheless, the figures cited in the preceeding discussion suggest some value in occasional supplemental feeding. Moreover, they give evidence of the rather thin margin upon which most breast-fed infants are asked to survive. Nature, it would seem, provides just about enough food, with little room for complications brought on by any factor(s) that lowers milk or nutrient yield, which is what one would expect from the harsh clash of evolutionary process working against the natural limitations of the human body.

TABLE 4
Energy Requirements of Infants and Children[a]

Age	Body weight (kg)[b]	kcal/kg body weight	kcal/day
<3 months	4.5	120	540
3–5 months	6.4	115	735
6–8 months	7.9	110	870
9–11 months	9.3	105	980
Average, first year	7.3	112	820
1–3 years	13.4	101	1360
4–6 years	20.2	91	1830

[a]From FAO/WHO ad hoc Expert Committee (1973).
[b]To convert kilograms to pounds, multiply by 2.2.

GENERAL DIETARY CONSIDERATIONS

This section presents some facts that relate to infant dietary needs generally. First, only about 26% of calories are required for "growth" of the infant during the first 2 months. Growth here should be considered as more than simply an increase in body weight. It should also imply a differentiation of cells, that is, of cell maturation. Some cells go to make up muscles, some brain tissue, others nerve endings. Likewise, the ability of the body to produce essential enzymes to carry out the myriad life processes is a "growth" function. All these growth activities are in a constant state of dynamic change. Neurons, for example, begin to proliferate in profusion during the tenth week of pregnancy and continue on to the sixth month. Just after birth, glial cells of the brain begin to form in large numbers. Then neurons start to distinguish themselves as either axons or dendrites. From 3 months on through 5 years of age, the fatty sheath (myelin) that surrounds certain of the nerve fibers slowly grows into place. Brain and nerve development is a gradual, ever-changing condition of growth.

Body composition is also changing. Often this fact is overlooked in the setting of daily nutritional requirements of the infant. Through the first 4 months of life, the infant body consists mostly of water and fat. Proteins account for only about 12% of the infant's gain in weight at this time. If a mother feeds regular cow's milk, weight gain may be seen to increase at a higher rate. This is not a good sign for premature infants, because the weight comes from greater retention of water in response to the high level of mineral salts in cow's milk. It is the same kind of response noted in many adults who consume too much salt. If mineral intake is held constant (at an appropriate level) and caloric intake increased over needs, the infant tends to put on more weight as fat (lipids). If one lowers protein intake *below* need, more of the weight of a 3-month-old infant will be water; less (than usual) will be fat.

From 4 months to 1 year, an infant averages a weight increase of about 3.5 kg (7.7 lb). But unlike the first 4 months, in which protein accounts for 12% of this gain, protein now totals 20%. Thus, protein intake should be geared to these changing needs. Through 3 months, the infant's gastric secretions are limited. Enzymes, like pepsin and trypsin, which break down protein (proteolysis), are not present at levels high enough to digest excessive amounts of protein. At the same time, the overintake of protein stresses the kidneys. Each gram of protein contributes about 4 milliosmols (mOsm) of dissolved substances to the kidney fluid, and this load must be handled along with a variety of mineral elements. Any food (like normal cow's milk) that provides an overload both of protein and minerals is doubly taxing. Although this may not be a serious problem for many infants, it can be for the premature and underweight child. If normal weight at birth is taken as something over 3.0 kg (6.6 lb), then 7–12% of births in the developed world are underweight. In developing nations that figure can reach 40% due mainly to poor maternal nutrition. If the infant is not too small to suckle, the mother in many cases will breast-feed. She may do so adequately for perhaps 3 months. At that point supplemental feeding becomes more or less essential, depending upon the extent of mother's undernourishment—that is, if the child is to develop to full potential. At 5 months, the situation is even more critical.

At the other end of the spectrum lies the question of infant obesity. Here the research of scientists of the Department of Nutrition and Food Science of the University of Toronto, Canada (Dubois *et al.* 1979) challenges a long-held stereotype. Under study were 42 normal and 47 overweight infants, all 4–9 months of age. Common belief would say that the obese child is overfed, given solids at an early age, more than likely not breast-fed, and indulged by a mother who knowingly or unknowingly fails to read signs of satiety. Yet a comparison of the feeding practices of mothers of the two groups of infants involved in this study revealed no characteristic differences. The pattern of feeding was similar in both instances. Breast feeding, considered alone, was not shown to prevent the onset of obesity. In the feeding of infants, apparently even common sense must be put to the test.

2

Vitamins

Vitamins are among the most variable components of milk. Indeed, vitamin content of most foods varies widely. Whereas the emphasis in this discussion focuses on the differences found in the milk of various mammalian species, it is understood that the magnitude of variations in vitamin content of other foods may well exceed those found in milk.

Small though significant differences exist in the vitamin content of the milk of humans and of those mammals whose milk most frequently serves as a supplement or substitute for mother's milk. Unaccounted for, such differences can cause deficiency diseases in feeding infants. Deficiency states also arise in breast-fed infants, though usually under rather specific circumstances. Infant formula usually comes fortified with all the vitamins (and at appropriate levels) needed for good health of normal infants.

Several factors influence the level of vitamins in milk. These factors are not necessarily the same for different mammals, nor of equivalent impact. For mothers breast-feeding their infants, the two most important considerations are diet and drug intake. Practices both during pregnancy (or before) and during lactation are relevant.

Vitamins are usually distinguished as soluble either in water or fat. For ease of study, this division is used in the following discussion.

WATER-SOLUBLE VITAMINS

Vitamin C

One of the most important differences between the milk of humans and cows is the relative level of vitamin C. The milk of cows can be so lacking in this vitamin that infants feeding solely on this source may develop the scurvy.

29

This would not be the case if the milk of mares, donkeys, or camels was used. All three species provide ascorbic acid at levels in milk in excess of that found in human milk. In at least one area of the world (Somaliland), camel milk serves as a lifelong source of this vitamin. In general, breast milk is adequate to meet an infant's needs of vitamin C during early months. However, a word of caution seems advised; if there are nutrient differences between the milks of different species, differences between two individuals within the same species can be far greater.

That last statement is important enough to repeat: Individual differences in the vitamin content of milk within a species may vary more widely than differences between species. Taken on the average, the vitamin content of the milk of two women may well be found to differ by a greater magnitude than the milk of cows and women. Several reasons may account for this fact. Genetic differences no doubt are significant. Then, too, vitamin intake in food or feed causes variations. This latter is especially significant as related to the content of fat-soluble vitamins (vitamins A, D, K, and E) in the milk of cows. In this species these vitamins vary to a greater extent, generally speaking, than water-soluble vitamins. In human milk, variations occur in all vitamins, and the differences can be marked. Table 5 gives evidence of some of these variations for both water-soluble and fat-soluble vitamins.

Note that the average vitamin C content of human milk is given as 5.2 mg/100 ml. For cow's milk this value ranges between 1 and 2 mg (in the pasteurized product). Nevertheless, the range of vitamin C content in human milk runs from 0 through 11.2 mg/100 ml. Milk of some women would appear therefore to be deficient. On the average, though, such milk would serve an infant's needs. (See Tables 6 and 7 for the recommended daily allowances, or estimated safe and adequate levels, of vitamins for infants and children.) It is interesting to note that much of the difficulty in determining infant needs arises from the confusing lack of consistency of vitamin content of human milk. Either some infants can survive well on lesser amounts of certain vitamins, or mother's milk has to be seen as deficient in some instances. In any event, one cannot look at the vitamin content of human milk, in all its variations, and come up with very specific recommendations for infants. Nevertheless, most studies suggest the vitamin C level in human milk to be adequate for the newborn infant. This level varies seasonally, but seasonal differences appear due to differences in the intake of vitamin C in food. For this reason, you can find some researchers asserting vitamin C content of human milk to be lowest in the fall and highest in the spring. Others find just the opposite. The explanation for the variations is usually the same: The season of peak content of vitamin C in milk corresponds to the peak intake of vitamin C in food.

Consumption of fruits and vegetables most often accounts for increased

TABLE 5
Vitamin Content of Milk of Well-Nourished American Women (Amount per 100 ml)[a]

Vitamin	Number of samples	Average amount	Range Minimum	Maximum
Water-soluble				
Ascorbic acid (mg)	233	5.2	0	11.2
Thiamine (μg)	279	14	8	23
Riboflavin (μg)	275	37.5	19.8	79
Niacin (μg)	271	183	66	330
Vitamin B_6 (μg)	88	11.4	3.6	22
Pantothenic acid (μg)	416	230	86	584
Biotin (μg)	266	0.8	trace	4.2
Folacin (μg)	7	5.2	?	?
Vitamin B_{12} (μg)	32	0.046	0.02	0.06
Choline (mg)	29	9	5	14
Inositol (mg)	7	45	39	56
Fat-soluble				
Vitamin A				
Retinol equivalents	309	64	15	226
(mcg of retinol) IU	309	241	50	753
Vitamin D (IU)	—	0.42	—	—
Vitamin E (mg)	—	0.56	—	—
Vitamin K (μg)	—	1.5	—	—

[a]From U.S. Department of Agriculture (1976) and Causeret (1977).

levels of this vitamin in human milk. Find the season, whatever it is, in which the intake of these foods goes up, and the level of vitamin C in milk will likewise be found to go up. However, excessive intake of citrus fruits may cause diarrhea. Orange juice and tomatoes consumed by the mother can lead to colic in the breast-feeding infant. Thus, vitamin C levels in the body (and thereby the milk) must be maintained on a moderate intake of citrus fruits and from other sources. This should not be a problem in food-rich nations. The use of vitamin C supplements offers another convenient method of ensuring the adequacy of this vitamin in the diet. Recent studies done on low-income women in Texas (Sneed et al., 1979) show supplementation to be of advantage in raising vitamin C levels in milk, especially in those women whose diets were less than adequate. Over 50% of the test subjects were receiving less than ⅔ of the recommended level. The effect of supplementation on the content of vitamin C, vitamin B_{12}, vitamin B_6, and folacin in milk depended on the initial nutrient status. Thus, supplementation has been found to provide no significant change in the level of vitamin C, thiamine, riboflavin, vitamin B_6, vitamin B_{12}, or folacin in the milk of well-nourished

TABLE 6

Recommended Daily Allowance (RDA) of Vitamins for Infants and Children[a,b]

Vitamin	Infants (months)		Children (years)		
	0–6	6–12	1–3	4–6	7–10
Fat-soluble					
Vitamin A (R.E.)[c]	420	400	400	500	700
Vitamin D (μg)[d]	10	10	10	10	10
Vitamin E (mg α T.E.)[e]	3	4	5	6	7
Water-soluble					
Vitamin C (mg)	35	35	45	45	45
Thiamine (mg)	0.3	0.5	0.7	0.9	1.2
Riboflavin (mg)	0.4	0.6	0.8	1.0	1.4
Niacin (mg N.E.)[f]	6	8	9	11	16
Vitamin B_6 (mg)	0.3	0.6	0.9	1.3	1.6
Folacin (μg)	30	45	100	200	300
Vitamin B_{12} (μg)	0.5[g]	1.5	2.0	2.5	3.0

[a] Adapted from National Academy of Sciences/National Research Council (1979).

[b] Needs vary somewhat by size of infant or child. The values in this table are based on the average size of Americans of the age range given.

[c] Retinol equivalents. In this case, 1 retinol equivalent equals 1 μg retinol or 6 μg β-carotene.

[d] To convert micrograms to IU, assume 10 μg of vitamin D (cholecalciferol) to equal 400 IU.

[e] Alpha tocopherol equivalents. In this case, 1 mg d-α-tocopherol equals 1 α T.E.

[f] Niacin equivalents. In this case 1 N.E. is equal to 1 mg of niacin or 60 mg of dietary tryptophan.

[g] The RDA for vitamin B_{12} for infants is based on the average level of the vitamin found in human milk. Allowances after weaning are based on energy intake (as recommended by the American Academy of Pediatrics).

TABLE 7

Estimated Safe and Adequate Daily Dietary Intake of Selected Vitamins[a,b]

Vitamin	Infants (months)		Children (years)		
	0–6	6–12	1–3	4–6	7–10
Fat-soluble					
Vitamin K (μg)	12	10–20	15–30	20–40	30–60
Water-soluble					
Biotin (μg)	35	50	65	85	120
Pantothenic acid (mg)	2	3	3	3–4	4–5

[a] Adapted from National Academy of Sciences/National Research Council (1979).

[b] Information needed for the setting of precise allowances is lacking for the vitamins listed in this table. For this reason, ranges are presented in certain instances. Needs might also be expected to vary somewhat by body size. Values given are based on the average size of Americans for the age range given.

women at 6 months of lactation (Thomas *et al.*, 1979). The emphasis here falls directly on relative state of nutrition.

Cow's milk varies little in the content of vitamin C and most other water-soluble vitamins. Feed supply is not an important factor in this instance. This can be said to be true for all water-soluble vitamins, except possibly niacin and pyridoxine. In the winter these two vitamins are generally found in lower amounts than in the summer, when cows are consuming green feed. Other water-soluble vitamins remain generally uninfluenced by feed. Thus, cows can actually produce most of these vitamins even though their feed is lacking. Either the body synthesizes the vitamins, or rumen bacteria do it for the body.

NAS/NRC (1980) notes that breast-fed infants taking in 7–12 mg/day and bottle-fed infants consuming 7 mg/day of vitamin C are protected from scurvy, the disease state associated with deficiency of this vitamin.

B Vitamins

B vitamins vary significantly in human milk also, as the data in Table 5 attest. This group of vitamins includes thiamine (vitamin B_1), riboflavin (vitamin B_2), niacin (nicotinic acid or nicotinamide), vitamin B_6 (pyridoxine, pyridoxal, and pyridoxamine), biotin, pantothenic acid, folic acid (pteroylglutamic acid and related chemical structures), and vitamin B_{12}.

Of all the B vitamins, thiamine poses a somewhat unique problem. Both dietary intake and a variety of drugs influence level in breast milk. An infant suffering thiamine deficiency may emit a weak, high-pitched, squealing cry. Sometimes death occurs from heart failure (NAS/NRC, 1980). A deficiency state could arise in breast-fed infants if the mother's diet is seriously lacking in thiamine, if the mother is an alcoholic, or if the mother regulary takes certain drugs. Among drugs known to create a need for higher-than-average levels of B vitamins, are isoniazid (INH), hydralazine (Apresoline), penicillamine, and birth control pills (Brin, 1976). If thiamine stores become so low as to result in beriberi, the milk of the mother may become toxic to the breast-feeding infant. This is especially true, apparently, if the infant stores of this vitamin are also depleted. By one account, the toxic compound is suggested possibly to be methylglyoxal (see Cowie and Swinburne, 1977). Thus, breast-feeding has its obvious complications to women in all walks of life.

Russian researchers (see Causeret, 1977) have found seasonal variations in both the thiamine and riboflavin content of human milk. Like vitamin C, differences could be accounted for by level of intake. In the milk supply, thiamine varied from 29.7 to 18.5 μg/100 ml from autumn to spring. Riboflavin averaged 47.2 to 26.7 μg/100 ml for the two seasons, respectively. NAS/NRC (1980) gave as average riboflavin content of human milk 40 μg/100 ml. This scientific body also records evidence of increased need for riboflavin in women using oral contraceptives. The effect, if any, on riboflavin content of milk is not reported.

In milk of cows, the riboflavin level varies by breed. Jersey and Guernsey cattle show 30–60% higher amounts than Holsteins, Brown Swiss, or Ayrshires (Causeret, 1977). This would suggest specific differences between breeds. Of the significance this might imply for human milk, nothing is known.

Data on infant requirements for thiamine and riboflavin are somewhat limited. Thiamine needs appear to be related to energy output; riboflavin needs do not have the same relationship. The amount of thiamine in human milk reflects a possible infant requirement of 0.03 mg/kg of body weight (0.27 mg/1000 kcal). For the first and second half-year of life, respectively, the recommended daily allowance is given as 0.3 and 0.5 mg. Infant formula is considered to provide a margin of safety at a level of 0.5 mg/1000 kcal.

At an average level of 40 μg (0.04 mg)/100 ml riboflavin, and 850 ml milk production daily, a woman provides for her infant some 0.34 mg of the vitamin. Taking this value as evidence of need, NAS/NRC sets the recommended daily allowance (RDA) of riboflavin for infants at 0.4 and 0.6 mg for the first and second 6 months of life, respectively. For infant formula, FAO/WHO (1976) recommends 40 μg thiamine and 60 μg riboflavin per 100 available kilocalories (see Appendix 2).

Requirements for niacin during infancy (and in older children) are not known. As with certain other vitamins, assumptions of need are based upon the content in mother's milk. However, the situation is complicated by the fact that the amino acid tryptophan can to some extent substitute for niacin. That is, a portion of tryptophan of protein can be converted by the body to niacin. In adults the rate of conversion is about 60:1. For every 60 mg tryptophan, 1 mg niacin forms. In other words, 60 mg tryptophan can be considered 1 niacin unit equivalent. At least this is how it works out for adults. The conversion rate during infancy, and particularly under stress of protein malnutrition or other forms of malnutrition, is unknown. There are also no data on the requirements for niacin in pregnant and lactating women. Thus, the deficiency—in science, at any rate—is apparent. Concern for the infant arises out of our current state of ignorance. Milk protein (and thus, tryptophan content) varies widely among women. Niacin level in human milk—even among well-nourished women—also varies widely (see Table 5). Because niacin functions in respiratory processes, need for this vitamin is tied to energy expenditure. Energy output of infants, as already noted, can account for up to 35–48% of total calories at different points in time. Activity, therefore, represents a significant variable in assessing niacin needs.

Knowing these facts, one is obviously left guessing. You can only look at the *average* composition of human milk and assume that this composition in an *average* output of milk fulfills the niacin needs of infancy. This is the approach taken by NAS/NRC (1980). Figures of this scientific body put niacin content of human milk at 0.17 mg/100 ml (or 70 kcal) of milk and tryptophan at 22 mg. Given the tryptophan–niacin conversion rate previously indicated and an average energy expenditure, requirements for niacin even out at 8 niacin equivalents/1000 kcal from 0 to 6 months of age, and 6.6 niacin equivalents/1000 kcal (but not less than 8 niacin equivalents daily) for infants aged 6 months through adolescence. This need is readily met by a milk production rate of 850 ml daily. To what extent lesser output and dietary status of the mother might jeopardize the infant, no one can say. It is known only that animal foods are richer sources of tryptophan than plant foods. Of the latter, corn products, of the major food grains, come off poorest in this respect. Corn (and also wheat) appear to contain niacin, at least in part, in forms not readily available to the body. Corn, of course, is a major staple in several Latin American countries. Protein–calorie malnutrition is the most common deficiency condition in that part of the world. Pellagra, the niacin deficiency state, is characterized by skin disease, diarrhea, and, at worst, dementia.

Vitamin B_6 can be considered a generic term referring to one or more of three compounds that serve in related ways within the body. These substances are pyridoxine, pyridoxal, and pyridoxamine. In infants, deficiency in vitamin B_6 leads to convulsions, weight loss, stomach cramps, vomiting, and excessive irritability. As is so often the case with vitamins, human milk appears to provide just about enough B_6, with little to spare. Pyridoxine content runs from negligible to 1–2 μg/100 ml during the first few days following parturition. Amounts climb to between 3.6 and 27 μg from the first through the seventh month of lactation. For the data being cited, the average was 10.5 μg/100 ml. These are findings of a French scientist (see Causeret, 1977). Older data of the United States National Research Council put the average pyridoxine level of human milk at 18 μg/100 ml. This represents reasonably good agreement. Of note, too, is that the vitamin B_6 content of human milk can be increased significantly by oral administration of large amounts of the vitamin. Increasing the dietary level two to five times results in significant but not proportional increases in milk (Atkinson, S., 1979). In women consuming less than 2.5 mg/day of vitamin B_6, the level of the vitamin in their milk has been found to be significantly lower than in women whose intake exceeds 2.5 mg/day; these results were found on the third day of lactation. By the fourteenth day, no difference was found (Roepke and Kirskey, 1979a). Of importance is the fact that lower levels of vitamin B_6 are found in the milk of women taking in less than the recommended daily allowance of this vitamin.

In general, then, the influence of dietary intake of vitamin B_6 on the level of the vitamin in milk depends on the nutritional status of the mother and, to some extent, stage of lactation. In addition, the researchers cited above found a lower level of vitamin B_6 in the milk of women in poor physical condition. Content of this vitamin in milk also varies throughout the day; peak levels appear betwen 3:00 and 5:00 P.M.. Of special note, however, long-term use of oral contraceptives causes a drop in the level of vitamin B_6 in milk (Roepke and Kirskey, 1979b). Where supplementation is available, neither this nor other factors should be serious problems. Nor is there cause for concern when vitamin-fortified formula is used. The needs for vitamin B_6, however, may hinge on more than body requirements for the vitamin per se. United States Department of Agriculture (USDA) scientists have found reason to believe that the presence of vitamin B_6 aids uptake of zinc, a mineral very much needed in trace amounts (see Zinc, Chapter 3).

Vitamin B_6 deficiency symptoms have been observed in breast-fed infants when mother's milk contained the vitamin to a level of 6–8 $\mu g/100$ ml. A level of 260 μg per day has been found to protect convulsing infants. Admittedly based on limited information, NAS/NRC (1980) suggests as adequate a daily intake of 300 μg(0.3 mg) vitamin B_6 for the infant up to 6 months old. For infants in the 6 to 12 month age group, the necessary intake is placed at 600 μg(0.6 mg) per day. With vitamin B_6 consumption of less than 2.5 mg per day, the ratio of the vitamin to protein in human milk has been found to be 13 $\mu g/g$. At an intake of 2.5–5mg/day, the milk level goes up to about 23 $\mu g/g$. Data of this kind lead NAS/NRC (1980) to recommend an additional (over normal) 0.5 mg of vitamin B_6 per day for lactating women in order to provide for needs of the breast-feeding infant. Food sources of vitamin B_6 are not necessarily all that plentiful. Animals, poultry and fish products, and wheat germ are considered among the few important sources; thus, one is reminded of the nutritional risk under which much of humanity exists.

Cow's milk runs generally higher than human milk in content of vitamin B_6, that is, between 23 and 60 $\mu g/100$ ml. Infant formulas have been found adequate at B_6 levels of 15 $\mu g/g$ protein (or 40 $\mu g/100$ kcal).

Table 8 shows the average amounts of pantothenic acid, biotin, and vitamin B_{12} in human and cow's milk. Cow's milk is the richer source in all three instances. It is also important to note that the same analytical techniques were applied to both types of milk. For this reason, methodology should not have contributed greatly to analytical error. The amount of pantothenic acid shows an average of 140 and 490 $\mu g/100$ ml, respectively, in human and cow's milk. NAS/NRC (1980) cite these averages as, respectively, 200 and 350 $\mu g/100$ ml. Pantothenic acid is available in a number of vegetable and animal foods, and inadequate intake is not con-

TABLE 8
Pantothenic Acid, Vitamin B_{12}, and Biotin Content of Human and Cow's Milk
$(\mu g/100 \text{ ml})^{a,b}$

Vitamin	Human milk		Cow's milk	
	Average	Range	Average	Range
Pantothenic acid	140	70–270	490	350–660
Vitamin B_{12}	0.04	0.02–0.06	0.46	0.37–0.63
Biotin	1.09	0.43–1.82	5.79	3.71–7.81

[a] Adapted from Causeret (1977).
[b] The same analytical techniques were applied to both types of milk.

sidered a serious problem. Evidence suggests a need, however, to supply a somewhat higher than normal intake during nursing. Though lack of information prevents the setting of precise daily requirements, estimates of this amount by NAS/NRC scientists would put it at 2 mg for infants 0–6 months of age, and at 3 mg for older infants. The amount of pantothenic acid in human milk will be seen to come close to meeting needs at average levels of milk consumption (600–800 ml per day).

Like pantothenic acid, biotin shows wide variations in the milk of different individuals. Data in Table 8 cite 1.09 $\mu g/100$ ml as average. NAS/NRC (1980), referring to 1977 data of the Department of Health and Social Security, make this value 10 $\mu g/1000$ kcal. Assuming 70 kcal/100 ml milk, this value becomes 0.7 $\mu g/$ml. The two averages, therefore, are not too different. Australian scientists (Hood and Johnson, 1980) found levels of biotin to increase rapidly over the first few days of lactation. The average amount the first day was found to be 0.29 $\mu g/100$ ml. By the seventh day, the level had risen to 0.68 $\mu g/100$ ml. At two months, the average was 1.3 $\mu g/100$ ml. Significantly, the feeding of 3 mg of biotin per mother per day caused the level of the vitamin to increase sharply in the milk supply in a matter of days; it rose from 1.59 $\mu g/100$ ml on the first day of supplementation to 48.4 $\mu g/100$ ml by the tenth day.

From data of the kind given above, NAS/NRC estimates biotin requirements to be 35 and 50 μg daily for infants 0–6 months, and 6–12 months, respectively. By these terms, human milk is obviously very much lacking, and deficiencies would be widespread were it not for the contribution of the infant's own intestinal microorganisms. A number of bacteria (and certain fungi) synthesize biotin. That this source adds significantly to the total available biotin seems clear. But again, no one can give precise estimates as to how much derives of this source. The amount no doubt varies greatly in terms of the numbers and kinds of bacteria making up the intestinal microflora. This variance, together with the dietary status of the nursing mother, is an issue of some import. Generally, biotin occurs in a variety of foods. Good sources include liver, kidney, egg yolk, and some vegetables. Cereal grains, fruit, and certain meat foods have been cited as generally poor sources (Hardinge and Crooks, 1961). Some biotin of food is bound to other components, making it generally unavailable to the body. Deficiencies, therefore, must be considered somewhat less than remote possibilities, especially for the many persons subsisting mainly on cereal grains.

The milk levels of biotin might well grow precariously low. An infant's needs might have to be met through its own intestinal pool of bacteria, a questionable supply at best, particularly in the newborn. Taking these and other facts into consideration, it is not surprising perhaps that Australian researchers (Johnson et al., 1980) have found reason to link "crib death"—a syndrome that takes many thousands of infant lives annually—in some way to biotin deficiency. Lacking this vitamin, the infant appears to be placed in a situation of extreme vulnerability. Even mild stress (such as infection, somewhat excessive heat or cold, a missed feeding) triggers death. The deficiency state, the researchers suggest, could be induced by a lack of biotin in mother's milk or commercial baby food. Ordinarily, cow's milk, which supplies about 5 μg/100 ml of biotin, is a good source. However, if the milk is not fortified, some loss might be expected to occur due to certain processing treatments. With a trend to membrane filtration technologies as methods of concentrating whey protein ingredients for use in infant formula, such loss could indeed reach significant amounts. These are implications, at least, coming out of the research by Hood and Johnson (1980). They found about 50% loss of biotin, presumably free (available) biotin, from cheese whey dialyzed through cellulose casing. Dialysis of whole milk and skim milk caused losses near 60%. Analysis of both liquid and powdered infant formulas showed a wide range of biotin content; the levels in skimmed milk formulations were generally lower than those made from whole milk. Products made from skim milk and demineralized whey also showed lower biotin content than whole milk formulations. A formula derived of modified casein also proved low in biotin level. Thus, concern over biotin content of infant formulas seems justified, and Hood and Johnson (1980) recommend addition of biotin to formula based on cow's milk. Goat's milk ranges considerably higher in level of biotin than cow's milk, and these authors found the amount in a goat's milk infant formula to be reasonably high (453 ng/g dry matter). Formulas based on soy protein showed a wide range in biotin content (146–1564 ng/g).

The content of biotin in mother's milk appears related primarily to dietary intake. However, it is possible that stress might induce some loss, and this may be a possibly significant loss for the feeding infant if the level in the milk is already marginal. At the present time, though, the latter possibility remains a scientific question mark. Nonetheless, evidence of the kind cited above would seem to suggest a need either to ensure the mother's intake (thus milk level) of biotin or to rely on occasional feeding (or supplementation) of the infant with fortified infant formula or baby food.

The content of pantothenic acid, biotin, and vitamin B_{12} in human milk varies seasonally, as Russian scientists note (see Causeret, 1977); no doubt this is a result of differences in food intake. The time of lowest amounts of these vitamins was found to occur between June and August. Different results could perhaps be expected in different parts of the world depending upon food availability and habits. Once again the importance of nutrient intake is stressed. The following example illustrates this point.

Cyanocobalamin is the name given to the stable form of vitamin B_{12} most commonly used as a source of the vitamin in fortified or enriched foods. This is the name most likely to be listed on the label of infant formula. This form of the vitamin provides vitamin B_{12} potency in the same way as methyl, hydroxy, and adenosyl forms of cobalamin. In commercial production, bacteria serve as major suppliers of the vitamin. They may even serve to some extent as a source of the vitamin in humans. The issue is of more than academic interest.

Generally speaking, vitamin B_{12} deficiency does not occur in breast-fed infants of women who are well nourished. This fact should be emphasized. Vitamin B_{12} deficiency is rare in breast-fed infants of well-nourished mothers. It is rare where nursing mothers have access to meat, poultry, fish, and milk and other dairy products. Deficiencies, therefore, are limited generally and, again possibly even rarely, to strict vegetarians, those who shun or are forced by circumstances to exclude from their diet foods of animal origin. Even ignoring for the moment the question of deficiency, there is good evidence that vegetarians reflect lower serum levels of vitamin B_{12} than nonvegetarians. It is also known that the amount of the vitamin in milk parallels serum levels. Among nonvegetarians, wide variations in the level of this vitamin in milk also occurs. Some such individuals might produce milk of lower vitamin B_{12} content than vegetarians, but not as a rule.

At question here is whether or not a vegetarian mother might produce milk of such low vitamin B_{12} content as to cause a deficiency state in her breast-feeding infant. Such a case has been reported by the Pediatrics Department of the University of California, San Diego (Nyahn, 1978). Symptoms included the presence of dark blotches on the skin, severe anemia, and drowsiness. Undetected and untreated, a child becomes comatose. Death can result. No one appears to doubt the diagnosis in the above instance. Some authorities have questioned whether the deficiency state came about as a result of a dietary lack or was instead a peculiar disorder in the metabolism of this particular child. It has been suggested that B_{12} produced by bacteria within the oral cavity would prevent vegetarians from slipping into a state of deficiency. Milk supplies would thereby be guaranteed some marginal, though likely adequate, amounts.

The importance of this hypothesis can be assessed if one keeps in mind those millions of mothers who, by necessity, survive as vegetarians. It further underscores the appropriateness of judicious use of vitamin–mineral-fortified infant formula and/or vitamin B_{12} supplementation of breast-feeding mothers. Research in Thailand (Areekul and Utiswannakul, 1978) found nonsupplemented women to provide 81% of the recommended daily allowance of vitamin B_{12} to breast-feeding infants. Supplementation three times daily with 50 or 100 μg of the vitamin raised the percentage to 113 and 119, respectively. Even the lowest of these three values (81%) should not be considered a serious hazard, but obviously the vitamin B_{12} level in milk responds to dietary intake; where any doubt of deficiency exists, as in the milk of strict vegetarians, supplementation seems more than justified.

Protein binding of vitamin B_{12} in mother's milk appears to withhold the vitamin from bacteria that might otherwise use it up. Therefore, most of whatever amount of vitamin B_{12} is present in milk should be available to the infant.

Data gathered prior to 1961 on folic acid content of milk may be in error (Çauseret, 1977). At that time, techniques for measuring the presence of this vitamin were apparently imprecise. More recent data obtained with improved methods indicate higher amounts of this vitamin in human milk than originally thought (Causeret, 1977). The content varies greatly over lactation. In the first few days after birth, the amount of folic acid in human milk averages about 0.5 μg/100 ml. During the sixth through tenth days, the level rises to around 0.84 μg. From the second through the ninth month of lactation, the level plateaus at 4–5 μg. During the eleventh and twelfth month, the amount drops to 1.4 and 0.8 μg/100 ml, respectively. In cow's milk, the folic acid level ranges higher initially; it is about 10.5 μg/100 ml during the first week following calving, and then it falls to about the same level as human milk (5 μg) after 2–3 months.

Daily needs of folacin (the group name given to several compounds showing vitamin potency) are set by NAS/NRC (1980) at 30 μg for infants up to a half year old and 45 μg for the age group 6 months to 1 year. Vitamin potency remains intact as long as the parent molecule consists, in combined chemical form, of pteridine, p-aminobenzoic acid, and glutamic acid. Chemically speaking, folic acid is pteroylglutamic acid, abbreviated PGA. The vitamin is quite sensitive to heat treatment and is destroyed by the boiling treatment often given cow's milk as a pasteurization process in the Third World. One researcher (Ghitis, 1966) suggested the need for supplying supplemental folacin to infants fed pasteurized, sterilized, or dried cow's milk. In addition, goat's milk, a widely used infant food around the world, has a low content of this vitamin (0.6 μg/100 ml), and the folic acid that is present in goat's milk shows poor availability (Jenness, 1980). Again, supplementation is called for.

In a comparison of three groups of full-term infants, Smith et al. (1981) found serum and red blood cell folate stores to decrease from 42.2 and 633 ng/ml at birth to 22.4 and 458 ng/ml, respectively, at 6 weeks of age. These latter levels remained constant through 3 months. By contrast, infants fed formula showed increases in folate stores by 6 weeks and further increases by 6 months. Supplementation with iron made no difference in folate status of the formula-fed infants. These scientists found a significant correlation between maternal level of folate and folate status of their breast-fed infants at both 6 weeks and 3 months. In all cases, the breast-fed infants showed significantly lower content of folate in serum and red blood cells than the formula-fed groups.

The vitamin contents of both human and cow's milk are compared in Table 9. Data on human milk express differences between level of vitamins early in lactation and in mature milk. Data for cow's milk are given at two dilutions, as might be appropriate for infant feeding if cow's milk alone had to suffice.

The vitamin content of human milk may be seen to change markedly in some instances over the first few days of lactation. Generally, the level of water-soluble vitamins goes up, and the level of fat-soluble vitamins declines. Exceptions exist, though. None of the normal variations poses any risk to the infant.

FAT-SOLUBLE VITAMINS

In several ways fat-soluble vitamins tell a quite different story from water-soluble vitamins. If feed has little influence on the latter in cow's milk, it greatly affects some of the former. The more cows receive of vitamins A and E in feed, the higher the levels in the milk. So important is this influence that vitamin A may range from one and one-half to two times as high in summer milk compared with winter milk. Differences are due almost entirely to change in feed. Summer pasture, or green feed, causes the level of vitamin A content of cow's milk to rise sharply. On the other hand, vitamin A content of milk drops markedly as cows are fed dry winter feed. To avoid drastic changes, green fodder can be fed in the winter. Using carrots, carotene, or fish liver oil as feed or supplement will help maintain the milk's vitamin A potency. In practice, milk products are often fortified with vitamin A. Not only are natural variations thus compensated for, but reductions in vitamin A

TABLE 9
Vitamin Content of Human Milk and Cow's Milk[a] (Amount per 100 ml)

	Human Milk			Cow's Milk[b]		
	Colostrum 1st–5th day	Colostrum 6th–10th day	Mature	Pure	Diluted ¾ + ¼ water	Diluted ½ + ½ water
Water-Soluble						
Ascorbic acid (mg)	4.4	5.4	4.3	1.6	1.2	0.8
Thiamine (mcg)	15	6	16	42	31	21
Riboflavin (mcg)	29.6	33.2	42.6	157	118	78
Niacin (mcg)	75	175	172	85	66	42
Pyridoxine (mcg)	—	—	11	48	36	24
Pantothenic acid (mcg)	183	288	196	350	260	175
Vitamin B_{12} (mcg)	0.045	0.036	trace	0.56	0.42	0.28
Biotin (mcg)	0.1	0.4	0.4	3.5	2.6	1.7
Choline (mg)	—	—	9	13	10	6.5
Inositol (mg)	—	—	39	13	10	6.5
Fat-Soluble						
Vitamin A (mcg)	89	88	53	34	25	17
Total carotenoids (mcg)	112	38	27	38	28	19
Vitamin D (IU)	—	—	0.42	2.36	1.80	1.18
Vitamin E (mg)	1.28	1.32	0.56	0.06	0.04	0.03
Vitamin K (mcg)	—	—	1.5	5.8	4.4	2.9

[a]Adapted from Causeret (1977).
[b]Two dilutions are shown because cow's milk, if fed to infants, should be diluted prior to use.

as a result of lowered fat levels in low-fat and skim milk products are thus negated. As stated before, fat-soluble vitamins are lost when fat is removed from milk. Fortification restores levels to desired amounts.

Human milk contains somewhat higher vitamin A content than cow's milk. This is true even though total carotenoids average somewhat lower. Today, vitamin A activity of food is expressed as retinol equivalents. One retinol equivalent equals 1 μg of retinol, 6 μg of β-carotene, or 12 μg of other provitamin A carotenoids. In relation to the former standard, one retinol equivalent has a value equal to 3.33 International Units (IU) of retinol or 10 IU of β-carotene. Since blindness is the ultimate outcome of severe restriction of vitamin A intake, the need for adequate amounts is crucial. Indeed vitamin A deficiencies account for a large proportion of nutrition-related diseases in developing nations. So prevalent and so perverse is the problem that great effort is being made to fortify appropriate foods or food ingredients. Both tea and monosodium glutamate (MSG), a flavor enhancer, find use in this regard. Both see wide use within certain nations. Also, as Lebanese researchers have confirmed, the vitamin A level in human milk can be raised by administering axerophthol palmitate in oily suspension (see Causeret, 1977).

The amount of vitamin A in human milk is influenced by the level in the diet both during pregnancy and lactation. The vitamin occurs as retinol esters and precursor carotenes. Well-nourished mothers appear to carry abundant reserves in the liver. Still, NAS/NRC urges added intake for nursing mothers of 400 retinol equivalents. By this standard, RDA becomes 1200 retinol equivalents in total. Infant needs, based on the amount of vitamin A and provitamin A in human milk, come to 429 μg of retinol. This assumes an average retinol level of 49 μg/100 ml milk and milk production at 850 ml daily. At 6 months, with the addition of solid food to the infant diet, the RDA drops slightly to 400 retinol equivalents (300 as retinol and 100 as β-carotene).

Both vitamin A and vitamin D are potentially toxic in overuse. Mothers with ready access to vitamin supplements should resist the temptation to consume more or feed the infant more vitamin A than amounts generally considered adequate for needs.

In human and cow's milk, vitamin D activity appears to be enhanced by the presence of a water-soluble form of the vitamin. Not all researchers agree to its presence in milk. That is, vitamin D sulfate was recently reported as a water-soluble form of vitamin D to be found in human milk. Other scientists, attempting to confirm this fact, found an hydoxycholecalciferol-like compound (25-OHD$_3$), (see Atkinson, 1979). This fact is significant; although the former is known to provide vitamin D activity, the latter likely does not.

Data thus far obtained on what is considered to be vitamin D sulfate have shown it to be less toxic than fat-soluble vitamin D. The level in pooled, raw (unpasteurized) cow's milk ranges from 1.9 to near 5.0 μg/liter. Thus far, evidence points to the possibility that the water-soluble form of the vitamin is sensitive to heat, quite unlike fat-soluble vitamin D, which is stable even after sterilization treatment.

Compared with mature milk, colostrum milk of cows shows significantly higher levels of the water-soluble form of vitamin D (Antila et al., 1979). The range runs from about 7–10 μg/liter. In addition, seasonal trends exist; there is as much as 50–65% more water-soluble vitamin D in summer milk as in winter milk.

Human milk appears to have a considerably higher level of water-soluble vitamin D than cow's milk. Pooled samples of mature milk average about 8.8 μg/liter and range from 6.8 to 12.0 μg/liter (Antila et al., 1979). Using 400 IU (10 μg) as the recommended daily intake, the level of water-soluble vitamin D in human milk, if in fact an active form exists, nearly fulfills the daily needs on the average. However, as in cow's milk, various factors influence level. Individual differences occur. Milk produced in summer months may average 43% higher than winter milk. Limited research suggests, however, that the stage of lactation has little effect on the level of the water-soluble form of vitamin D in human milk.

The preceding facts notwithstanding, fat-soluble vitamin D can still serve the nutritional needs of infants as a supplement in infant formula. Though it may be obvious, it is well to note that deficiency is readily overcome by the use of fat-soluble vitamin D as a supplement or an additive to food.

Ultraviolet radiation offers another way of increasing vitamin D levels. In fact, it is the cow's relative exposure to the ultraviolet light of the sun that most determines the level of vitamin D in milk in the first place. It is the reason why seasonal variations often occur, at least when cows are housed inside buildings during certain months of the year. The content of fat-soluble vitamin D varies by as much as two times; the highest amounts usually come in August or September, the lowest from November through March. In the end, though, such differences appear rather unimportant. Cow's milk simply is not a good source of vitamin D. This fact has resulted in the widespread practice of fortification of cow's milk and infant formulas with vitamin D (often vitamin D_2 and/or D_3). Most formulas contain vitamin D to levels of 400 IU per quart. This vitamin is also added to evaporated milk and, most commonly, to commercial whole milk. Low fat and skim milk products (not recommended for infant feeding) often contain added vitamin D as well. Where mothers lack access to fortified foods, or elect not to use them, supplementation of the infant diet certainly appears warranted. The American Academy of Pediatrics recommends 400 IU per day. This amount no doubt is adequate, though in fact, infants have some difficulty in absorbing fat-soluble vitamins generally.

It is well to note that rickets, the bone-deforming disease resulting from vitamin D deficiency, occurs to this day even in the United States. Two reports of such cases are of recent origin. Generally, the problem seems confined to breast-fed infants of dark-skinned mothers, and mainly in sunlight-poor periods during winter months. However, any nursing mother who for religious or cultural reasons regularly wears dark outer garments may anticipate a somewhat lowered level of vitamin D in her milk supply. One of the major sources of vitamin D in the body is that produced from 7-dehydrocholesterol, which is present in the skin and which is converted to vitamin D through the ultraviolet rays of sunlight. The lack of exposure to sunlight bears directly on the vitamin D content of mother's milk. Although regular exposure likely provides ample amounts of the vitamin to breast-fed infants, most authorities still recommend supplementation for all infants to 400 IU daily.

Vitamin E occurs in both plant and animal foods. The most active form of vitamin E is α-tocopherol. Compared with vitamins A and D, this vitamin is not very toxic. Human milk averages somewhat higher levels than cow's milk, to the extent that breast-fed infants show increases in blood serum levels of vitamin E during the first several days of feeding. No such increase occurs when cow's milk is fed. The level of vitamin E in human milk ranges between 2 and 5 IU (1.3–3.3 mg d-α-tocopherol equivalent) per liter, and this amount is assumed adequate for infant needs. Fortified infant formula should contain 0.7 IU of vitamin E (α-tocopherol) per 100 cal. At the same time, formula should provide 1.0 IU of the vitamin per gram of the essential fatty acid, linoleic. This level is deemed sufficient for the normal infant and, generally, the infant of low birth-weight (NAS/NRC, 1980). Nonetheless, an oral supplement of 5 IU of water-soluble α-tocopherol is also recommended for infants whose weight at birth is lower than normal. The problem in this case arises from the somewhat poorer ability of such infants to absorb fat. The net effect is impaired utilization of vitamin E.

Note lastly in Table 9 the level of vitamin K in human and cow's milk. The latter in this case shows significantly higher amounts, and at all stages of lactation. Human milk has scarcely enough vitamin K for infant needs, especially during the first few days of life. Both low content of the vitamin and the infant's inability to consume much milk at this early stage puts overall intake at a borderline level or below. For this reason, the American Public Health Association (1979) and other authorities recommend intramuscular administration of vitamin K to the neonate (newborn infant) fed exclusively on breast milk. Within a few days time, milk alone will suffice as a source of this vitamin.

Vitamin K, a compound active in the process by which blood coagulation takes place, is needed to prevent bleeding (hemorrhaging). Green, leafy vegetables are perhaps the most important food source of the vitamin, although it is also present in fruit, dairy products, and cereal grains. In addition, certain bacteria synthesize the vitamin. Perhaps it is more accurate to refer to vitamin K in the plural. Several compounds have vitamin K activity. The one found in green plants (phylloquinone) is referred to as vitamin K_1. The ones produced by bacteria and found in animals (the menaquinones) are known as vitamin K_2. Synthetic compounds, naphthoquinone derivatives, also provide vitamin K activity.

Both the American Academy of Pediatrics and FAO/WHO recommend vitamin K in infant formula at a level of 4 μg/100 cal. At normal intake, an infant weighing 6 kg (13.2 lb) would receive 4–5 μg vitamin K/kg of body weight. In healthy infants having a normal intestinal microflora, bacteria would be expected to add some small amount of this vitamin to that supplied either by formula or by mature mother's milk. The latter averages near 1.5

μg/100 ml. Though an RDA cannot be set, adequate and safe daily levels of intake are given as 12 μg and 10–20 μg, respectively, for the first and second 6 months of life (NAS/NRC, 1980). Both formula and breast milk, at these average levels of vitamin K content, will serve the infant's needs during early life.

PROCESSING LOSSES IN VITAMIN CONTENT

Thus far the discussion has centered on natural variations in the content of vitamins in milk. However, that is only part of the story. There are processing and other losses to consider where cow's milk is concerned. The extent of such losses is shown in Table 10. As a general rule, the higher the heat treatment used in processing, the higher the loss in certain vitamins. Other vitamins, like riboflavin, nicotinic acid, pyridoxine, biotin, vitamin A, and fat-soluble vitamin D are scarcely influenced by any of the common processing treatments. However, two of these—riboflavin and vitamin A—can be lost, at least in part, by simple exposure to light. In particular, the loss of riboflavin is significant. Exposure to direct sunlight (in glass or certain plastic containers) can cause a 20–40% loss in this vitamin within an hour and 40–70% loss in 2 hours. Wavelengths under 610 mμ are responsible; those of 490–520 mμ are most detrimental. Diffused light, too, can cause loss of riboflavin, and by as much as 10–30% in a few hours. The return to clear glass bottles and the use of certain transparent plastic containers has no doubt resulted in more loss of this vitamin in milk in recent times. Milk, of course, is a major source of riboflavin in the Western diet.

In addition to the loss of riboflavin and vitamin A, some loss in pyridoxine may occur through exposure to light. The presence of oxygen will decrease the levels of ascorbic acid (vitamin C). In this latter case, ascorbic acid is altered to dehydroascorbic acid. This form of the vitamin remains biologically active but is less stable in heat. Pasteurization or other heat processing then causes degradation to an inactive chemical compound. Thus, unless air is removed from milk, it is nearly impossible to prevent the loss of the small amount of this vitamin that is present in milk as it comes from the cow. Loss usually comes to about ¾ of the original amount. In infant formula, processing losses are compensated for by the addition of overages or by the addition of vitamins after heat treatment.

Despite processing losses, cow's milk remains generally richer than human milk in most vitamins. Those vitamins found in higher amounts include vitamin B_1 (thiamine), vitamin B_2 (riboflavin), panthotenic acid, vitamin B_{12}, biotin, choline, vitamin D, and vitamin K. Found in lesser amounts are ascorbic acid, niacin, vitamin A, vitamin E, and inositol. Value of the latter to infants remains undetermined.

TABLE 10

Effect of Various Processing Treatments on Vitamin Loss in Cow's Milk[a]

Treatment	Percentage loss[b]										
	Thiamine	Riboflavin	Nicotinic acid	Pantothenic acid	Pyridoxine	Biotin	Vitamin B_{12}	Ascorbic acid	Vitamin A	Vitamin D	Folic acid
Pasteurizing (low temperature) 145°F–30 minutes	10	0	0	0	20	0	10?	20	0	0	10
Pasteurizing (HTST) 161°F–15 seconds	10	0	0	0	0	0	10	10	0	0	10
Ultra-high temperature	10	10	0	?	20	0	20	10	0	0	<10
Sterilization in bottle	35	0	0	?	—[c]	0	90	50	0	0	50
Evaporation	40	0	?	?	—[c]	10	90	60	0	0	?
Evaporation, with sugar added	10	0	0	?	0	10	30	15	0	0	?
Roller drying	15	0	?	?	0	10	30	30	0	0	?
Spray drying	10	0	?	?	0	10	20	20	0	0	?

[a]From Causeret (1977).

[b]A question mark indicates the possibility of some loss by light-induced changes.

[c]There is a noticeable loss in the biological availability of this vitamin under this processing treatment.

Those vitamins found in excess in cow's milk as compared with human milk pose no particular problem. Most are easily shed by the body. Of the vitamins found in lesser amounts in cow's milk, perhaps vitamin C and vitamin A pose the most serious potential threats to health. Lack of vitamin A is of little consequence when the infant receives adequate amounts of lipids generally and is growing normally.

VITAMIN CONTENT OF THE MILK OF OTHER MAMMALS

Of course, the milk of other mammals may differ significantly in nutrient content from either human or cow's milk. As already mentioned, mare's, donkey's, and camel's milk range higher than human milk in ascorbic acid. Sheep's milk runs high in riboflavin and niacin. Mare's and donkey's milk average lower in riboflavin than cow's milk. Goat's milk runs lower than cow's milk in vitamins B_6 and B_{12}. Yet in vitamin B_{12} content, goat's milk may run two times higher than human milk. Still, the amount is very low, and this milk might not meet daily needs as the sole source of food in older infants. Generally, goat's milk appears adequate for infant needs of vitamin A and niacin. Vitamin B_1, B_2 and pantothenate are usually found in excess of infant needs. Goat's milk seems deficient, however, in vitamins C, D, and B_{12}; pyridoxine (vitamin B_6); and folic acid. Indeed, folate content of goat's milk runs much lower than cow's milk. The average level is given as 0.6 μg/100 ml, with a range of 0.2–1.1 μg/100 ml. Goat's milk colostrum carries significantly higher levels (20.5 μg/100 ml), but it falls off sharply over the first two weeks of lactation. Around the world, goat's milk perhaps serves a larger share of the population than cow's milk. For the future, it looms more important than ever. As infant food, goat's milk deserves as much study as cow's milk. For excellent reviews of goat's milk composition, see Parkash and Jenness, (1968) and Jenness (1980).

Buffalo's milk, too, is a most important food, though chiefly in India. Both goat's and buffalo's milk yield lesser amounts of carotenoids than cow's milk. Carotenoids are precursors to vitamin A. They lend to milk its yellowish color. However, despite lack of carotenoids, goat's and buffalo's milk provide about as much vitamin A as cow's milk. Vitamin content of these two milk sources is shown in Table 11.

In infant formulas, the vitamin comparison of various milk sources remains largely academic. Whether the formula is of cow or soy origin, the vitamin content can be, and most often is, standardized. Minimum amounts and— equally important for such potentially toxic vitamins as vitamins A and D— maximum amounts are thereby guaranteed. See Appendix 2 for a listing of vitamins and other nutrients and the amount of each recommended for infant

TABLE 11
Vitamin Content of Milk of Various Animals[a]

Vitamin	Goat's milk (per 100 g)	Buffalo's milk (per 100 g)	Sheep's milk (per 100 g)	Mare's milk (per 100 g)
Ascorbic acid (mg)	1.29	2.25	3	10
Thiamine (mcg)	48	52	70	30
Riboflavin (mcg)	138	135	500	20
Niacin (mcg)	277	91	500	50
Pantothenic acid (mcg)	310	192	350	300
Vitamin B_6 (mcg)	46	23	—	30
Folacin (mcg)	1.0	6.0	0.2	0.1
Biotin (mcg)	4.0	13.4	9	—
Vitamin B_{12} (mcg)	0.065	0.363	0.3	0.3
Vitamin A (IU)	185	178	200	45

[a] Adapted from U.S. Department of Agriculture (1976) and Causeret (1977).

formulas by FAO/WHO. Appendix 3 shows the chemical form(s) of each vitamin approved as additives by the same international agencies.

SUMMARY

The vitamin content of human milk is highly variable. The level of any one vitamin in milk depends on the interrelation of such factors as diet, stage of lactation, alcohol or drug use, and the general health of the mother. Of all the causes of variation, diet is perhaps the most significant and pervasive. On a cereal grain diet, a strict vegetarian diet, or a diet low in protein and calories, several water-soluble vitamins of mother's milk may reach such low levels as to pose some health risk to breast-feeding infants whose diets are not otherwise supplemented. Those vitamins most limited by inadequate diet include vitamin C, vitamin B_1, vitamin B_2, vitamin B_{12}, and the fat-soluble vitamin A. Diet also plays a role in the level of nicotinic acid, pantothenic acid, and folic acid. In addition, the vitamin K content of human milk falls below need, at least for the first few days of life. The amount of vitamin D in mother's milk may fall short if exposure to sunlight is limited, especially in dark-skinned persons. The level of fat-soluble vitamins in mother's milk generally reflects maternal stores, both during and after pregnancy. In cows, the content of water-soluble vitamins in milk is not greatly altered by variations in kind and quality of feed. As a general rule, infant needs of all vitamins are met in fortified infant formulas.

3

Minerals

The major difference in the content of minerals of human milk and milk of mammals commonly used as substituted for human milk is not so much in kind as amount. On an average, human milk contains about 0.2% ash, the mineral matter remaining after incineration. Cow's milk averages about 0.72%, milk of the Indian buffalo 0.79%. Depending upon breed, goat's milk may average from 0.71% to 0.88% ash. Although these may appear to be rather small differences, overall they represent major factors in the feeding of infants. Table 12 provides a listing of several minerals and their content in human, cow's, goat's and buffalo's milk.

CALCIUM AND PHOSPHORUS

Calcium, a major nutrient of mammalian milk, contributes to the development of bones, muscle contraction, the transmission of nerve impulses, and blood clotting. It is a most important mineral, but cannot be considered without reference to phosphorus and vitamin D. The latter aids absorption of calcium from the digestive tract. Phosphorus also influences calcium uptake and is the complementary element with which calcium combines in forming the rigid structure of bone.

A ratio of calcium to phosphorus of between 1:1 and 1:2 provides for the best utilization of calcium. NAS/NRC (1980) guidelines recommend a ratio of 1.5:1. Human milk averages about 32 mg calcium and 14 mg phosphorus/100g fluid milk. The ratio of the two elements is about 2:1. Cow's milk with 119 mg calcium and 93 mg phosphorus/100g fluid milk, has a calcium/phosphorus ratio more nearly 1.2:1. Goat's milk falls in the same range. An infant formula prepared to substitute more perfectly for human

TABLE 12
Mineral Composition of the Milk of the Human, Cow, Goat, and Buffalo[a]

Mineral	Human	Cow (mg/100 grams fluid product)	Goat	Buffalo
Calcium	32	119	134	169
Phosphorus	14	93	111	117
Magnesium	3.0	13	14	31
Iron	0.03	0.05	0.05	0.12
Potassium	51	152	204	178
Sodium	17	49	50	52
Zinc	0.17	0.38	0.30	0.22

[a]Adapted from U.S. Department of Agriculture (1976).

milk would average one-fourth to one-third the calcium level of cow's milk, but only if the form of calcium used in the formula was as readily absorbed by the infant. Few if any forms meet this requirement. Perhaps ⅔ of calcium of mother's milk is retained by the infant. Retention of calcium from formula may run as low as 25% of the amount present. For this reason, calcium levels in formula products usually exceed the calcium content of human milk. FAO/WHO (Codex Alimentarius Commission, 1976) recommend 50 mg of calcium per 100 kcal of infant formula.

Although the calcium content of cow's milk is fairly stable, statistically validated differences have been observed both on a seasonal basis (lowest in July and August) and on a regional basis (Campbell et al., 1961). Such facts should perhaps be considered in the formulation of infant formula.

On occasion, cow's milk formulas have been found to cause hypocalcemia (a calcium deficiency) even though cow's milk ranges substantially higher in calcium than human milk (Condon et al., 1970). Possible reasons for such occurrences include formula that is (1) too high in phosphate content (2) too high in insoluble salts of fatty acids, and (3) too low in lactose content. High phosphate levels may cause hypocalcemic tetany in newborn infants (Mizrahi et al., 1968; American Academy of Pediatrics, 1978a). It is important, therefore, that formulas be made with appropriate forms and amounts of both calcium and phosphorus.

A study of breast-fed infants (Calkins, et al., 1978) placed calcium intake at 29, 29.3, and 28.6 mg/100 ml milk consumed at 1, 2, and 3 months of age, respectively. Phosphorus intake averaged very nearly half those amounts. The volume of milk was just over 600 ml daily over the 3-month period. Evidence suggests that the calcium level of human milk may fall off significantly beyond the third month of lactation. Also, the amount of both calcium and phosphorus tends to vary widely in milk of different individuals.

Generally, the level of calcium and phosphorus is not greatly influenced by diet. Confronted with a lack, the human body simply extracts the elements from bone deposits and transfers them to the milk. Learned estimates suggest a potential to mobilize about 250 mg calcium daily in this manner. This represents a loss of about 0.022% femoral bone daily (Atkinson and West, 1970). The needs of full-term infants appear well met by the amount of calcium and phosphous in mother's milk. The needs of preterm infants may be less well met. Two very recent cases of rickets, a calcium deficiency disease, have been attributed to inadequate levels of phosphorus in human milk. The problem arises partly from increased need for phosphorus in the preterm infant, whose skeletal growth is less complete. Thus, rickets was observed in an infant fed exclusively on human milk from a milk bank in the United States (Rowe *et al.*, 1979). An Israeli infant also developed rickets from breast-feeding. Again, phosphate depletion was given as cause (Sagy *et al.*, 1980). The milk of the mother at 5 months, contained 5.8–6.2 mg phosphorus/100 ml. The needs of the preterm infant are unique for a number of nutrients. While mother's milk, even the milk from the mother who delivers prematurely, may provide adequate amounts of most nutrients, it may fall short of adequacy in all nutrients.

MAGNESIUM

Magnesium is a mineral found widely distributed in nature. Deficiency in this mineral should be rare. Yet it happens, and it is a complicating factor accompanying the protein deficiency state, kwashiorkor. Human milk contains 3–4 mg magnesium/100 ml. Cow's milk averages about 12 mg/100 ml. FAO/WHO suggests a magnesium level in infant formula of 6 mg/100 kcal. A level of intake of 40–50 mg magnesium per day is considered appropriate for the infant of up to 6 kg (13.2 lb) (NAS/NRC, 1980). Most formula products would be adequate to the needs of both normal and low birth-weight infants. For the ages 0–6 months and 6–12 months, the recommended daily allowance (RDA) is put at 50 and 70 mg, respectively. Evidence also suggests that the milk of mothers delivering preterm is adequate in magnesium for infants' needs.

IRON

Neither human milk nor the milk of those mammals commonly used as replacement is a particularly good source of iron. Iron deficiency anemia, in which the hemoglobin level is too low for good health, is considered to be the most common disease of infants in the United States, particularly in the age group of 6–24 months (American Academy of Pediatrics, 1976). But take special note of the age span. Even though human milk is low in the level of iron, much of it is bound to protein. The form in which it is bound appears to make it readily available. Most of it is absorbed by the infant, and for this reason, iron needs are generally well met from breast-milk alone at least through 3 months of age. Iron in formula milk may also be absorbed well due to certain processing techniques, to be discussed later. Iron can also be provided in supplement form. However, a word of caution is in order. Too much iron in a diet could lead to diarrhea or a similar intestinal disorder, and too much iron will help sustain a condition of diarrhea of bacterial origin (see Lactoferrin and Transferrin, Chapter 4). Needs of the infant, therefore, must be weighed against these factors.

The iron content of cow's milk averages near 0.05 mg/100 g fluid milk. The level ranges somewhat higher in colostrum than in milk but is generally uninfluenced by the amount in feed (Thomas, 1970).

The level of iron in human milk averages about 0.03 mg/100 ml. Higher amounts (0.04 mg/100 ml) occur early in lactation, and the level gradually falls over the first 6–8 weeks. Supplementation of the mother's diet with nominal amounts of iron appears unrelated to the amount in milk (Picciano and Guthrie, 1976). Iron content also does not seem influenced by long-term use of oral birth control agents (Kirksey, et al., 1979).

General recommendations of the Committee on Nutrition of the American Academy of Pediatrics suggest 1.0–1.5 mg iron/kg of body weight per day, assuming such feeding is begun at the right time "with respect to initial iron endowment." This vague phrase is a tacit admission within the scientific community of indecision as to when to begin iron supplementation of an infant's diet. Some authorities, perhaps most, would say the best time is at 4 to 6 months of age. However, in recent years there has been a growing tendency to introduce "solid" (beikost) food (along with the iron that may be in it) at an ever earlier age. Although the norm used to be 6 months of age for this practice, it now reaches to the first week of birth, at least for some. Most authorities agree that there is little nutritional need to introduce solid food during the first half year of life. It is important to note two considerations. First, solid food is itself a source of iron, but this iron is not as readily available as the iron in mother's milk. Second, if solid food is fed along with breast milk, strong evidence indicates that the iron in breast milk will not be as readily absorbed. The advantage of mother's milk as a ready source of iron is thereby lost. The most critical period appears to be ages 4–6 months. Some authorities even suggest the possibility that early introduction of solid foods to breast-fed infants could lead to iron deficiency (Saarinen and Siimes, 1979). For preterm infants, another issue arises. Fed high levels of both polyunsaturated fatty acids and iron (as may be present in fortified formula or solid foods), infants face the risk of developing vitamin E deficiency. This may come about as a result of the infant's limited ability to absorb fat-soluble vitamins. The problem is associated with a hemolytic form of anemia. One solution is to omit iron in infant formula. Nonetheless, for full-term infants, NAS/NRC (1980) recommends 10 mg daily intake of iron through the first 6 months. Needs for infants of low birth-weight (under 2500 g) are given as 2 mg/kg of body weight per day. This is notably higher than that required by infants of normal weight.

A number of studies prove the relatively better bioavailability of iron in mother's milk as compared to cow's milk or iron-fortified infant formulas. To some extent such figures must be interpreted with caution. Availability of iron in infant formula depends entirely upon the chemical nature of the source of iron. Some forms of iron are more readily absorbed than others. This point is considered in Chapter 6. At the same time, a variety of indicators of iron status show the needs of infants to be equally well met at 6 months of age with either mother's milk or iron-fortified formula (Picciano and Deering, 1980). Use of more available forms of iron may also be expected in infant formulas of the future.

ZINC

Zinc follows a pattern not unlike iron. Although present at half the amount in human as in cow's milk, it is more readily absorbed from human milk, possibly because of the presence of a zinc-binding compound(s). United States Department of Agriculture (USDA) researchers (Evans and Johnson, 1980) identify one binding agent as picolinic acid (pyridine-2-carboxylic acid). Other researchers (Jacobs et al., 1981) find no picolinate in raw human milk ultrafiltrate, but suggest that citrate may be a binding agent. In any event, for whatever reason, breast milk meets the needs of infant victims of acrodermatitis, a rare, genetically transmitted disease that inhibits zinc absorption. Once the disease has been diagnosed, treatment commonly involves feeding zinc sulfate in amounts of 2 to 3 times normal needs, often as oral supplement. Zinc sulfate is a common mineral additive of infant formula. However, zinc-supplemented formula does not necessarily provide the same high level of zinc uptake as human milk, which is also used in treatment of the disease state. Because human milk is a good source of readily available zinc, symptoms of the disease usually show up at the weaning time of breast-fed infants. Untreated, the disease may be fatal. Certainly, safeguards to adequate zinc intake are warranted. Symptoms of zinc deficiency include rash, loss of hair, and diarrhea.

Note also that the level of zinc in human milk drops significantly (to about

40% of its original level) by the end of 3 months of lactation (Vaughan, *et al.*, 1978). Such milk at that point is less adequate as a source of zinc both for healthy infants and also for those afflicted with acrodermatitis. Note, too, that the mother's intake of zinc has little effect on the level of zinc in milk (Vuori *et al.*, 1980). These are the findings of researchers studying normal subjects delivering at full-term and consuming supplemental zinc at moderate levels. However, recent medical literature cites evidence of alleviation of acrodermatitislike symptoms in two prematurely born, breast-feeding infants whose mothers were supplemented with zinc sulfate (Zimmerman and Hambidge, 1980). Prior to supplementation, breast milk of these mothers was so low (36 and 50 μg zinc/100 ml, respectively) as to infer defective secretion of zinc into the milk. There is evidence, too, of a difference in the zinc levels in the milk of low- versus high- income urban women in India. However, the average concentration of zinc in the milk of low-income Indian mothers has been found to differ little from the average level found in the milk of American mothers (Belavady, 1978). Thus, no serious problems seem reflected by level of income. Nor does long-term use of oral contraceptives appear to influence the amount of zinc in mother's milk (Kirksey *et al.*, 1979). However, USDA scientists found a relationship between the zinc uptake from the intestines and level of vitamin B_6 (Anonymous, 1980). The vitamin B_6 content of mother's milk is indeed lowered by long-term use of oral contraceptives. It is possible, therefore, that zinc uptake of breast-feeding infants might at some point be impaired, not from inadequate levels of zinc, but from inadequate levels of vitamin B_6. The interaction of nutrients has profound implications, and science is still scratching the surface of its nature and meaning.

Identification of possible zinc-binding compounds in human or cow's milk carries important implications, at least to the extent that their presence or addition to infant formula would enhance zinc uptake. Research on badly malnourished infants and children illustrates the point. Golden and Golden (1981, 1981) found dietary zinc in inadequate amounts necessary to achieve appropriate gain in weight of infants recovering from marasmus. Neither milk-based nor soy formula provided zinc in appropriate amounts. The soy formula not only contained 25% less zinc than the milk formula, it also contained phytic acid, a zinc-withholding agent. The researchers concluded that current formulas were inadequate suppliers of zinc to support growth of recovering, malnourished children, and especially those also suffering from zinc deficiency.

The level of zinc in cow's milk ranges from 200 to 600 μg/100 ml (Parkash and Jenness, 1967). The amount varies with the level in feed (Miller, 1970), and cows in India grazing on forage low in zinc content have been found to yield milk with as little as 0.8–1.8 ppm (Iyer, 1957). Essentially all the zinc of cow's milk is found in skim milk. Of the total, only about 12% is present in free, dissolved (ultrafilterable) form. The rest is associated with casein, in part loosely and in part tightly bound (Parkash and Jenness, 1967). All casein-bound zinc is released by acidification to pH 2.0, only about half given up by dialysis at pH 6.6 (Parkash and Jenness, 1967). Such facts are important in terms of the amount of zinc ultimately ending up as a base level in infant formulas. Obviously, the technologies plied in fractionating various milk components for use in formula will retain or deplete more or less of whatever amount of zinc may be present. Of course, the initial amount is anything but a stable, consistent quantity. Thus, it is not surprising to see a rather wide range (0.10–13.5 ppm) reported for zinc content in a survey of infant formulas (Lonnerdal et al., 1981).

Precise infant requirements for zinc are not known. It is known that the zinc level in infant tissues goes down after birth. Whether or not this store should be replenished is undetermined. There is also evidence of somewhat higher need for zinc in male infants (Walravens, 1980). If human milk content of zinc is an indication, then general infant need may be taken to be about 2 mg per day. Mature mother's milk contains 0.2–0.5 mg/100 ml. Colostrum may run as high as 2 mg/100 ml. From these facts, tentative RDAs are set at 3 and 5 mg of zinc for the ages 0–6 months and 6–12 months, respectively. An increase in the zinc content of infant formula, from 0.18 up to 0.58 mg/100 ml, has been found to enhance growth rates in male, but not female, infants nourished on formula (Walravens and Hambidge, 1976). Failure to grow, leading at worst to dwarfism, is one of the most significant aspects of zinc deficiency.

The issue of need is therefore critical. The availability of zinc in food also becomes critical. Appendix 4 lists forms of zinc approved for infant formulas. Of the compounds listed, zinc can be expected to be more or less readily available, assuming no zinc-complexing agents are present. Phytate of plant foods is perhaps the most significant naturally occurring complexing agent. FAO/WHO suggest a need for 0.5 mg zinc/100 kcal infant formula. This level is the equivalent of about 0.35 mg/100 ml. Because excessive intake of zinc can aggravate a condition of marginal copper deficiency, the level of these two mineral elements should be balanced in foods (and/or supplements) supplied to infants as well as adults (NAS/NRC, 1980).

SODIUM, POTASSIUM, AND CHLORIDE

One factor that makes cow's milk generally unsuitable as food for infants is its high level of sodium. Yet unknowing mothers continue to feed natural cow's milk, and occasionally an infant expires of excess plasma sodium (hypernatraemia). This is especially a problem in developed nations. In poor countries, excessive sodium intake more often than not arises from improper reconstitution of dry infant formula. This same error could as readily be made in developed nations of the world, but access to liquid formulas, especially of ready-to-use strength, lowers reliance on dry formulas. Only about 10% of formula used in the United States is of the dry form (Anderson *et al.*, 1980).

Mothers often prepare homemade baby foods, and researchers have found that such foods very often exceed maximum sodium levels set for commercial foods of this type. In one study, 64% of homemade baby food breached 100 mg sodium/100 g food. This is an amount in excess of the National Academy of Science recommendations. In addition, the scientific literature records evidence of infant dehydration from hypernatraemia induced by breast feeding (Clarke *et al.*, 1979). No doubt occurrences are rare, and apparently they are found only among infants who are readily satisfied by a very low intake of mother's milk. In such cases, supplementation with infant formula corrects the problem.

However, if high levels of sodium pose health hazards, low intake can lead to arrested growth, particularly of low-weight infants. At times, this malady stems from the low sodium content of the milk of breast-feeding mothers. It may happen despite adequate caloric intake. Though mineral content of milk is among that food's most stable components, considerable variations in the amount of individual minerals may occur.

In cow's milk, sodium content tends to fall to some extent as the result of feed deficient in sodium. On the other hand, sodium content does not tend to increase greatly with feeds high in the level of this mineral. However, one effect of mastitis (a disease state of the udder) is an increase in sodium and chlorides, to the extent that such milk actually tastes salty. To maintain proper osmotic balance, an increase in sodium and chloride is usually accompanied by a decrease in lactose.

In the milk of humans, the level of both sodium and potassium ranges higher in colostrum milk (first 5 days) than in milk a week or 10 days into lactation (Aperia *et al.*, 1979). A United States study of infants fed soley on breast milk showed an average sodium intake of 15, 12.2, and 12.8 mg/100 ml milk in the first, second, and third month of life, respectively. Potassium intake was, respectively, 47.2, 42.7, and 40.7 mg/100 ml. At 3 months of age, the infants were receiving 0.6 milliequivalents (mEq) sodium, 1.2 mEq potassium, and 1.4 mEq chloride/kg of body weight (Calkins, *et al.*, 1978). (A milliequivalent is defined as the atomic weight of the element in milligrams, divided by valence. One milliequivalent of sodium, therefore, equals 23 [atomic weight] divided by 1.0 or 23 mg. At 166 mg sodium/liter, human milk contains 7 mEq sodium/liter [$161 \div 23 = 7$]. The potassium content of human milk averages near 500 mg/liter, thus 12.8 mEq/liter

[500 ÷ 39.1]. The chloride level, at 390 mg/liter, provides 11 mEq/liter [390 ÷ 35.5].)

The preceding are important expressions because of the necessity to maintain an appropriate ratio of ions and electrolytes in the infant diet. Imbalance leads to improper acid–base relationships (i.e., alkalosis and acidosis) in the body, which in turn create serious disease states or lead ultimately to death. For this reason, the ratio of sodium to potassium and the ratio of sodium plus potassium to chloride become major considerations. These ratios are calculated on a milliequivalent basis. For example, human milk has a ratio of sodium to potassium of about 0.5 (i.e., 7 ÷ 12.8). The ratio of sodium plus potassium to chloride averages 1.8 ([7 + 12.8] ÷11). Ideally, infant formula will match these ratios rather closely. Safe levels of these three nutrients are bracketed within the following ranges (as recommend by the American Academy of Pediatrics, 1976): sodium, 6–17 mEq; potassium, 14–34 mEq; and chloride, 11–29 mEq. Again, human milk averages near 7, 13, and 11 mEq of these electrolytes, respectively. For cow's milk, the values are, respectively, 22, 35, and 29 mEq. Most infant formulas will range within recommendations of the American Academy of Pediatrics. The Committee on Nutrition of this professional body proposes minimal levels of sodium, potassium, and chloride of 20, 80, and 55 mg/100 kcal, respectively.

Although there is no proof that high concentrations of salt (sodium) in the infant diet lead to hypertension in later life, the salt content of formulas has been voluntarily reduced to essential levels by most infant formula manufacturers in the United States. For children over 6 months of age, major sources of salt are cow's milk and adult food items. The American Academy of Pediatrics has found no adverse reaction in infants through 6 months of age at a sodium intake of 3 mEq/kg per day. Likewise, there is no evidence that infants are predisposed to hypertension at an intake of sodium of up to 9 mEq/kg per day. Human milk provides sodium at a rate of about 1.0 mEq/kg per day.

The lack of chloride in the infant diet causes alkalosis, a condition in which tissue fluids are too alkaline. The infant fails to gain weight, suffers loss of appetite, and is lethargic. This condition was recently diagnosed in formula-fed infants in which the level of chloride in the formula was 1–2 mEq/liter (Roy and Arant, 1979). Other causes may also have played a part in onset of the condition. Reduction in chloride might have resulted from one factor or a combination of several factors, including (1) a tendency to prepare formula with less salt, (2) addition of salts other than sodium chloride (3) inadvertent removal of chloride during water treatment to remove fluoride, and (4) difference in chloride content of soy product used in the formula (see Anderson et al., 1980). To this date, the exact cause of the disease state and of the low chloride level remains unknown. However, the problem and the obvious necessity to ensure adequate chloride level is clear.

One of the major reasons for concern about the mineral level in infant formula is the potential to overload the kidneys. *Renal solute load* is the phrase used to express the relative level of electrolytes (ionized salts) and other waste products handled by the kidneys. Solute load, as such, refers to the amount of dissolved substances in a fluid and includes, as major components, various carbohydrates as well as mineral and other dissolved substances. Unfortunately, the total solute load of infant formula is not of much value in predicting renal solute load, mainly because of the high content of carbohydrates (which yield essentially no renal secretion) (see Anderson *et al.*, 1980). To this date, the exact cause of the disease state and electrolytes. Some are lost in perspiration, and some are discharged through the lungs and intestines. Some are used in building body tissues.

Possibly the best test of solute strength of infant formulas is a measure of the *osmolality*, that is, the extent to which the freezing point or vapor pressure is lowered. Though not interchangeable, another related term—*osmolarity*—is also used to indicate solute strength. In essence, osmolarity is an expression of the number of solute particles per liter. Osmolality expresses the number of solute particles per kilogram of water. Osmolarity cannot be measured directly, but it can be calculated from the osmolality value (which can be measured). In any event, formula solute strength is best kept at an osmolarity of no more than 400 milliosmoles (mOsm)/liter for healthy infants (the recommendation of the American Academy of Pediatrics 1976). Osmolality (not osmolarity) of breast milk is reported variously as 250 mOsm/kg water (187.5 mOsm/liter) and 286 mOsm/kg water (204 mOsm/liter). Cow's milk osmolality is about 263 mOsm/kg water (193.8 mOsm/liter). A study of various infant formulas showed osmolality to range from 223 to 319 mOsm/kg water. In osmolarity, this range is equivalent to 173–217 mOsm/liter. Osmolarity is calculated from osmolality by the expression

Osmolarity (mOsm/liter) equals osmolality (mOsm/kg H_2O) multiplied by kg H_2O/liter solution. For example, if osmolality equals 200, then,

$$\text{osmolarity} = 200 \times [(1000 - 200)/1000]$$

$$= 200 \times 0.8$$

$$= 160$$

TRACE MINERALS

Trace minerals include cobalt, manganese, molybdenum, aluminum, barium, chromium, nickel, copper, iodine, boron, fluorine, and other mineral elements. Their content in cow's milk varies significantly depending upon feed. In limited research on human milk, dietary intake of trace minerals appears not to correlate well with levels in breast milk (Vaughan *et al.*, 1978; Kirksey *et al.*, 1979). Nonetheless, very wide variations occur in milk of different women, and levels tend to alter as lactation continues. Generally, the trace mineral level is higher in colostrum than in mature human milk. Copper content may drop to 20% of its original amount by 3 months of lactation (Vaughan *et al.*, 1978).

Copper

Normal infant needs for copper range between 0.05 and 0.1 mg/kg of body weight per day. This amount satisfies the needs of the full-term infant with some to spare, but it may not meet the needs of the premature infant. The copper content of human milk appears not greatly influenced by the intake of copper in food or as added supplement. Neither is the level of the element in milk altered by long-term use of oral contraceptives (Kirksey *et al.*, 1979). In tests on animals, milk deficiencies in copper occur under conditions of elevated serum cholesterol and excessive intake of zinc. It is appropriate, therefore, to balance the amount of copper and zinc intake (NAS/NRC, 1980). Like other minerals, certain forms of copper are less readily absorbed by the body than others. Thus, the recommendation for infant formula is that the amount present be adequate to supply to the infant 100 μg/kg of body weight per day (NAS/NRC, 1980). Human milk provides around 105 μg/100 ml early in lactation and 15 μg/ml late in lactation. Cow's milk averages about 33 μg copper/100 ml, although values found in the literature vary. Some reports put the copper content of cow's milk as low as 15 μg/100 ml. It is also known that the level in milk varies with the level in feed.

Iodine

The recommended iodine intake, like that of most other minerals, is based on the amount consumed in mother's milk, in this case 30 μg or more per day. The RDAs are therefore set at 40 and 50 μg for the periods 0–6 months and 6–12 months, respectively (NAS/NRC, 1980). The iodine level in cow's milk depends upon the iodine content of the feed. Normal amounts range between 10 and 30 μg/100 ml. If the iodine content of the feed is very high, the iodine level of the milk may climb as high or higher than 100 μg/100 ml. Use of iodine medications in feed is a major source of iodine in cow's milk (Hemken, 1980). Formulated as organic iodine complexes, such medications are shed more readily into milk than inorganic forms. Widespread, indiscriminate use of these compounds can result in milk of such high iodine level as to pose some risk to health. On the other hand, prior to the current common practice of iodine fortification, soy formulas were once reported as a cause of goiter in infants (Ripp, 1961).

Manganese

Human milk has been reported to provide manganese at a rate of about 1.8–2.5 μg/100 ml. Finnish scientists, however, have reported a lower level; their figures go from 0.59 μg/100 ml during the second week of lactation to 0.4 μg/100 ml at 2 months (Vuori, 1979b). Level remained at 0.4 μg/100 ml through 6 months, then increased. Conflicting reports occur in the scientific literature on the influence of intake of manganese on the level in human milk. Generally, little or no change is noted either from intake in food or from intake of manganese in supplement form. However, Finnish scientists have reported a distinct correlation between intake and the level in milk during the second week of lactation. Using 1.8–2.5 μg manganese per 100 ml as an average, an infant receives about 15 μg per day at normal intake. Even so, the newborn loses manganese from its body during the first few weeks of life (NAS/NRC, 1980). Science is unable to say exactly what this means. Deficiency of manganese appears to be very rare, if it occurs at all. Safe and adequate daily requirements are estimated to be 0.5–0.7 mg for infants up to 6 months of age. Thereafter, through 1 year, the estimate is 0.7–1.0 mg. FAO/WHO standards call for 5 μg manganese per 100/kcal infant formula.

Literature values for level of manganese in cow's milk vary considerably. One source (Dairy Council Digest, 1971a) gives the average as about 5.8 μg/100 ml (6.0 μg/100 g). Thomas (1970) suggests the range to be from 1.0 to 5.0 μg/100 ml. It is likely that much of the confusion arises from the fact that manganese level in milk varies more or less with amount in feed. Colostrum carries significantly higher stores (13–16 μg/100 ml) than milk per se. In cow's milk, manganese occurs as an organo-metallic compound. Along with copper, iron, molybdenum, and magnesium, some manganese comes associated with the fat globule membrane (Thomas, 1970).

Molybdenum

Molybdenum, another trace mineral, apparently carries with it little if any risk of deficiency. Precise RDAs are unknown, but infant need is estimated at 30–60 μg per day for the first 6 months of life (NAS/NRC, 1980). The estimate is derived by extrapolation based on body weight. Estimated need, therefore, increases to 40–80 μg during the second 6 months of life. Because excessive amounts of the mineral prove toxic at least to adults, intake should not greatly exceed the recommended amount. No international standard exists for this mineral in infant formula, but cow's milk is thought to contain about 6 μg/100 ml. At this level, no danger of overintake exists for the infant fed on formula derived of cow's milk. Moreover, some molybdenum is associated with the fat globule membrane, and this amount would not be found in most formula, which excludes the fat of cow's milk.

Fluorine

Fluorine, as its fluoride ion, occurs in milk and is a generally healthful mineral element. However, the overall content of fluorine in the food supply depends in large part on the amount found in the soil used to grow the food. This is true likewise for other anionic mineral elements like iodine and selenium. Fluorine is also added to water supplies as a means of maintaining or improving dental health. The level is usually standardized at 1 mg/liter (1 ppm). The water used for drinking and cooking adds some small additional amount of fluorine to the body. In the United States the combined daily intake of this element from food and water may be as low as 1 mg or as high as 4 mg. This is not considered excessive for adults. On the other hand, high levels of fluoride intake in children is known to cause a graying of tooth enamel. Teeth may become permanently discolored. This has happened in areas where the natural level of fluorine in water supplies has reached 2 or more mg/liter. For children 4 years of age or older, therefore, NAS/NRC specifies a fluoride intake of no more than 2.5 mg per day. Safe and adequate levels for infants are based on amounts assumed to be ingested normally from mother's milk. During the first 6 months this level may average about 0.1 mg per day. The question arises, however, as to whether or not a mother's intake of fluoridated water might cause an increase in fluoride content of her milk supply. Research suggests that it does not. The level in milk has been found to be similar among mothers consuming fluoridated (1.0 ppm) versus un-fluoridated (0.1 ppm) water (Dirks et al., 1974). In addition, the fluoride content was observed to remain constant in milk of fasting, lactating women ingesting 300 ml water with 1.0 or 5.0 ppm fluoride (Erickson, 1969).

In its 1979 recommendations the Committee on Nutrition of the American Academy of Pediatrics suggested 0.25 mg per day as the level of need of fluoride for infants and children 2 weeks to 2 years of age. This scientific body indicates that there is no need to supplement the infant diet with fluoride when the amount in drinking water reaches 3 ppm. At 0.7 ppm fluoride in water, supplementation may, in fact, be called for. However, formula-fed (and often breast-fed) infants do not necessarily need an additional source of water over that supplied by the formula, at least not in the early months of life. In ready-to-use formulas, intake of fluoride may well depend on the level of fluoride in the formula. One study has found some formulas to provide about 1.2 mg fluoride per day (Wiatrowski *et al.*, 1975). As related specifically to incidence of dental caries, Walton and Messer (1981) found a direct relation to history of use of fluoridated water, but not of duration of breast-feeding of infants. Infants bottle-fed for over 12 months were noted to have a higher incidence of caries than those bottle-fed for shorter periods. It was the opinion of these reasearchers that, in areas where water supplies contained less than optimal levels of fluorine, fluoride supplements were needed for breast-fed but not bottle-fed infants.

Level of fluoride in cow's milk varies from region to region, and depends upon amount of industrial contamination in the vicinity. In a contaminated area, amount may range from near 4 to as high as 354 μg/100 ml (40–3650 ng/g). Average level for the data from which this range was obtained was 21.3 μg/100 ml (220 ng/g) (see Cowie and Swinburne, 1977). In relatively uncontaminated regions, cow's milk has been found to average about 3.8 μg/100 ml (40 ng/g). Still other researchers find cow's milk to average 10.3 μg/100 ml and human milk, presumably from the same area, to range from 4.6 to 5.2 μg/100 ml (see Cowie and Swinburne, 1977). Perhaps partially for reasons of variability and also because amount of fluoride in mother's milk may not be ideal, a liquid supplement of 0.25 mg daily has been recommended for infants feeding solely on breast milk (Foman and Wei, 1976).

Infant formulas have been found to vary quite widely in amount of fluoride both within and between various brands (manufacturers). Need to dilute products gives rise to additional amounts of fluoride as may be present in the water. This source alone may contribute 0.4–0.5 mg fluoride per liter of canned, milk-based formula (Tinanoff and Mueller, 1978). Surveys of formula products indicates levels of fluoride to be higher than necessary in some instances.

Selenium

Selenium is another mineral required by the body in trace amounts, yet with a potential at least for toxicity in overdose. Such toxicity—and deficiency disease—are common among various livestock species. Grain, for example, can vary considerably in selenium content depending upon the amount of mineral in the soil on which it is grown. This is the reason cited for nutritional disease of animals. Yet neither deficiency nor toxicity diseases have been demonstrated in humans, perhaps because of the broad distribution of selenium in foods generally (NAS/NRC, 1980).

German scientists (Lombeck *et al.*, 1978) have found the selenium content of human milk to average higher levels in colostrum than in the milk of more advanced lactation. The amount varies considerably among individuals. The average level for the mature milk of German women who underwent tests was found to be 232 μg/kg dry weight of milk (28.3 μg/liter). The level ranged from 90 to 432 μg. Pooled cow's milk showed a selenium content of about 200 μg/kg dry weight. In one study, 0.7% of 1 ppm of dietary selenium ultimately reached the milk, and of this amount, 60% ultimately was found incorporated into casein (Mathias *et al.*, 1967).

Ten different brands of infant formula gave selenium values ranging from 18 to 100 μg/kg, on a dry-weight basis. Thus, formula was delivering from one-third to one-half the amount of selenium found in either cow's or human milk.

A United States survey of the milk of 241 women in 17 different states provided a range of selenium of 70–600 μg/kg dry weight (Shearer and Hadjimarkos, 1975). The average was 180 μg/kg. Certain regional differences were noted.

Other Trace Minerals

Other trace minerals than those thus far mentioned are now thought to play some essential role in human life (Dairy Council Digest, 1971a). There is no doubt that chromium is needed. Animal studies also point to certain essential functions for vanadium, nickel, silicon, and tin. In cow's milk, the level of chromium appears to hover around 1.4 μg/100 g. Vanadium is thought to occur in amounts less than 0.1 part per billion. Nickel and silicon occur at levels of about 6.5, and 82 μg/100 g. Nickel is apparently present as a contaminant only (Jenness and Patton, 1959). The range in the level of tin runs from 19 to 68 μg/100 g. More research, however, is needed to assess the true role and true essentiality of these latter mineral elements.

A recent survey indicated some rather wide variations in the level of certain mineral and trace mineral components of infant formulas (Lonnerdal *et al.*, 1981). Both excessively low and high concentrations of given mineral elements were reported for some products. A number of factors could be responsible. In general, consistent standardization would have to take into account variations in initial concentration in formula ingredients and the influence in dairy-based formulas of feed, medications, and udder health. In addition, technologies of protein separation and refinement may add or deplete from these components more or less of a variety of minerals and trace minerals. Quality control would require a rather exact accounting prior to fortification, if indeed fortification is needed.

The recommended daily allowance (RDA) of minerals for infants is shown in Table 13. Table 14 lists the estimated safe and adequate levels of intake of certain trace minerals for infants and children. FAO/WHO recommendations may be found in Appendix 2. FAO/WHO also provides a

TABLE 13
Recommended Daily Allowance of Certain Minerals for Infants[a]

Mineral	Infants[b] (months)		Children (years)[c]		
	0–6	6–12	1–3	4–6	7–10
Calcium (mg)	360	540	800	800	800
Phosphorous (mg)	240	360	800	800	800
Magnesium (mg)	50	70	150	200	250
Iron (mg)	10	15	15	10	10
Zinc (mg)	3	5	10	10	10
Iodine (μg)	40	50	70	90	120

[a]Adapted from National Academy of Sciences/National Research Council (1979).

[b]Needs vary somewhat by size of infants. The average weight and height for infants 0–6 months of age is considered to be 6 kg (13 lb), height 60 cm (24 inches). For infants 6–12 months of age these values are, respectively, 9 kg (20 lb), 71 cm (28 inches).

[c]Needs vary somewhat by size of children. For the age groups shown, average weight and height are considered to be, respectively: (1) age 1–3: 13 kg (29 lb), 90 cm (35 inches); (2) age 4–6: 20 kg (44 lb), 112 cm (44 inches); (3) age 7–10: 28 kg (62 lb), 132 cm (52 inches).

TABLE 14
Estimated Safe and Adequate Daily Dietary Intakes of Trace Minerals and Selected Electrolytes and Trace Minerals for Infants and Children[a]

	Infants (months)		Children (years)		
	0–6	6–12	1–3	4–6	7–10
Trace mineral (mg)[b,c]					
Copper	0.5–0.7	0.7–1.0	1.0–1.5	1.5–2.0	2.0–2.5
Manganese	0.5–0.7	0.7–1.0	1.0–1.5	1.5–2.0	2.0–3.0
Fluoride	0.1–0.5	0.2–1.0	0.5–1.5	1.0–2.5	1.5–2.5
Chromium	0.01–0.04	0.02–0.06	0.02–0.08	0.03–0.12	0.05–0.2
Selenium	0.01–0.04	0.02–0.06	0.02–0.08	0.03–0.12	0.05–0.2
Molybdenum	0.03–0.06	0.04–0.08	0.05–0.1	0.06–0.15	0.1–0.3
Electrolytes (mg)					
Sodium	115–350	250–750	325–975	450–1350	600–1800
Potassium	350–925	425–1275	550–1650	775–2325	1000–3000
Chloride	275–700	400–1200	500–1500	700–2100	925–2775

[a]Adapted from National Academy of Sciences/National Research Council (1979).

[b]Information in this table is given as a range of values, since data for making more precise estimates are lacking.

[c]Toxic levels of several trace minerals may exceed recommended daily intake by only a small margin. The upper levels of ranges shown in the table should not be exceeded on a regular basis.

listing of mineral additives approved for use in infant formulas and other infant foods. This is shown in Appendix 4.

MINERAL CONTENT OF GOAT'S MILK

The level of a number of major minerals of goat's milk is shown in Table 12. Goat's milk is particularly rich in calcium and phosphorus; the ratio is similar to that of cow's milk. Both minerals are of a form readily absorbed by the infant. The iron content of this milk is also similar to that of cow's milk that is, both sources are deficient. However, the uptake of iron from goat's milk has not yet been studied. The level of iron is considerably higher in colostrum than mature goat's milk. The same is true for copper, manganese, zinc, and iodine. Moreover, certain minerals of goat's milk increase in level just preceding estrus. Sodium, chloride, and potassium exhibit this phenomenon. Fasting, on the other hand, causes a decrease in the level of potassium and an increase in sodium, chloride, and citrate (also fat and protein). In general, goat's milk contains more potassium and as much chloride as cow's milk. Chloride content is positively correlated to the amount of potassium. It must be stressed, however, that very wide variations are to be found among and within various breeds. More importantly, the amount of potassium and chloride in goat's milk is so high as to pose the risk of acidosis (excess acidity in the fluids of body tissue) in infants fed the raw, undiluted product. Osmolality of pooled herd milk has been reported as 297 mOsm/kg. (For a discussion of goat's milk composition, see Jenness, 1980.)

SUMMARY

The mineral content of cow's, goat's, and buffalo's milk—as it occurs in the undiluted, natural state—is too high to serve appropriately, and without risks, as infant food. An infant's uptake of minerals from mother's milk is generally superior to forms used in formula. To some extent, this problem is overcome by the use in formulas of proportionately higher amounts. Both too little and excessive amounts of minerals pose health hazards for the infant. For this reason, infant formulas must be carefully balanced in the amount and ratio of various minerals. This is true of both macro and trace minerals. Of particular importance is the ratio of sodium to potassium and sodium plus potassium to chloride. On occasion, for a number of reasons, mother's milk may not satisfy infant needs for mineral nutrients. Both the iron and zinc of mother's milk are more readily absorbed by the infant than chemical forms used as ingredients in formula. However, the iron absorption from mother's milk may be significantly reduced by the early introduction of solid food. Zinc absorption is generally good as a result of the presence of zinc-/binding compounds. Most minerals appear to be present at higher concentrations in human colostrum than in the milk of later lactation. Most trace minerals appear little influenced by the level of intake by the mother or by the long-term use of oral contraceptives. Milk of mothers giving birth prematurely seems to be adequate to the preterm infant's need for sodium, chloride, potassium, and magnesium. Such milk, however, may not prove sufficient in the level of calcium and phosphorus.

4

Immune Factors

Dietary needs are known to vary by age, sex, weight, and other factors. At every age except infancy however, such needs are expressed soley as demand for more or less of a given nutrient(s). Level of nutrient intake is, of course, important to infants, too. However, the fragile nature of human life in its earliest days, the immaturity of body organs, the incomplete development of defense against disease—all add a second dimension to nutritional needs. Food must provide not only nutrients but, to the extent possible, protection from disease; this latter function serving in the interim as the body gathers its strength and mobilizes its own defenses. Fortunately, the newborn is not entirely defenseless; in fact, as we shall see, human infants come into the world better protected than certain other mammals. Nonetheless, like any newborn, the human infant is particularly vulnerable. For this reason, the most useful food is that which can supply both nutrients and immune factors.

In breast milk, immune factors come preprocessed by the mother. In infant formulas, they must be processed into the product. Indeed, the potential for doing this is very real. If this potential is not being achieved, part of the blame is due to our ignorance of the immune processes generally. Much of what is known from studies *in vitro* (outside the body) remains unconfirmed *in vivo* (in the functioning human body). The entities themselves, the "immune factors," have neither been entirely elucidated nor their functions precisely mapped out.

Still, one point remains clear. Milk of any mammalian species is *the* food through which the female passes to her offspring a variety of disease-fighting agents. The functions of these substances range from the control of allergies through the prevention of viral or bacterial diseases. Indeed, the end result of immune processes is to (1) reject or destroy both living and nonliving foreign agents; (2) neutralize pathogenic viruses, bacteria, and other living matter

68

and/or toxins secreted by these entities; and (3) recognize and destroy cancerous cells. Eventually, the infant's own immune system must perform these duties. However, mother's milk or immune-fortified formula provides safeguards in the interim. They do so with a defense centered on achieving the most intimate knowledge of the enemy and its tactics. Here, too, is where we should begin.

COMMON INFECTIOUS AGENTS

The infant scarcely emerges from the womb when its intestinal tract, formerly "clean," is suddenly flooded with a large number of microbes. Among these, certain genera of bacteria tend to predominate. The most common are coliform, Streptococcus, Lactobacillus, and Clostridium (see Speck, 1976; Reiter, 1978). Some members of these genera are, at worse, neither harmful nor helpful. Others are very much beneficial. Still others cause disease. Of the latter, one family of bacteria is by far the most notorious. It is called Enterobacteriaceae. The prefix *entero* implies habitation within the intestinal tract. These organisms actually thrive best in this environment. Not all members of this family necessarily cause disease, however. But some do, and among them are the ones most frequently involved in the intestinal diseases of infants. Certainly the names of genera of this family should raise warning signals to those persons charged with the responsibility for infant health (Chordash and Insalata, 1978). They include *Escherichia, Klebsiella, Erwinia, Serratia, Proteus, Salmonella, Shigella, Edwardsiella, Citrobacter, Enterobacter, Hafnia,* and *Yersinia.* Outside of this family, the most common intestinal infective bacteria are various strains of toxin-producing staphylococci. *Clostridium perfringens* also rightfully belongs in this list. In poorer parts of the world, *Vibrio cholerae*, the cholera germ, still takes a heavy toll of victims (see Nestlé, 1975).

Most of those mentioned are spread by clothing and hands through contaminated water and/or food. The disease they cause is infectious diarrhea—infectious as distinguished from other causes of diarrhea that do not involve microbes, for example, nutritional diarrhea. Of course, infectious agents are not limited to bacteria. Viruses, too, are highly infectious. In fact, recent evidence shows rotaviruses to be shed in feces of 50–60% of diarrhetic infants (see Reiter, 1978). Such prevalence places them as one of the major causes of infant diarrhea. At this point little else can be said about them except that infant susceptibility appears to depend on level of serum, not intestinal immune agents (Flewett *et al.*, 1974). It is the one major immune agent (IgG) that crosses the placenta prior to birth that serves as chief defender. This may seem surprising, for another immune agent (sIgA) has long been seen as the most important protector against infant diarrhea caused by various infectious agents.

Statistics seem to suggest that the infectious form of diarrhea accounts for perhaps 50–75% of all cases of infant diarrhea (see Nestlé, 1975). Rotavirus leads the list, at least for viruses. It may in fact be the predominant cause. However, bacterial infections are also most common, and perhaps the chief offender is enteropathogenic *Escherichia coli*. Although *E. coli* often attack children under 2 years of age, they seem to center their deadly activity on infants at their most vulnerable first few months of life.

Some strains of *E. coli* can penetrate cells lining the intestinal tract, multiply, and carry out the disease function inside these cells (Jones and Rutter, 1972; Sakazaki *et al.*, 1974). Other strains produce toxins (Gorbach and Khurana, 1972; Guerrant *et al.*, 1975). Thus, two distinct forms of diarrhea may result—one a kind of dysentery, the other a choleralike disease state induced by toxin. Both types of *E. coli* have been implicated in outbreaks of disease stemming from contamination of food and water (Chordash and Insalata, 1978). Of the two, it is the toxin(s)-producing *E. coli* that is perhaps more often associated with infant diarrhea. Two different toxins may be involved. Both can cause symptoms of disease. One is a small molecule (low molecular weight), nonantigenic, and stable to heat. The other—a somewhat larger, heat-sensitive toxin—is antigenic and similar to the cholera enterotoxin (Chordash and Insalata, 1978). Incidentally, it is the toxin-producing type of *E. coli* that often causes "travelers' diarrhea" in adults.

E. coli apparently have no other natural habitat outside the intestines. Other coliform organisms do, however. This brings up an important consideration in testing food and water for potential contamination. Coliform organisms, as a general group, are members of the Enterobacteriaceae family that ferment lactose, with gas production, within 48 hours at 35° C. A positive test indicates presence of coliform generally, without pinpointing origin. Obviously, a more appropriate test would focus on those coliform known to reside in the intestinal tract. These are called *fecal coliform* and include all *E. coli*. Although their presence in food and/or water would not conclusively indicate presence of disease—not all *E. coli* or other coliform produce disease—a positive test would give evidence of contamination with fecal matter, a known potential source of disease. A test for fecal coliform now replaces to a great extent the older, less definitive test for coliform organisms generally (Chordash and Insalata, 1978). The principle of the two methods is similar, except that the temperature of incubation for fecal coliform is higher, ranging from 42 to 45.5° C. Gas production from lactose fermentation follows within 24–48 hours.

Several different disease-causing strains of *E. coli* are distinguishable by immune-typing methods. A dozen or more such *serotypes*, designated "O," have thus far been indentified (Ewing, 1963). All produce a B-type K antigen. The frequency with which any one or more types appear to be implicated in disease seems to vary from one place to another both within a country and around the world. Two serotypes often associated with infant diarrhea are O 119:K69(B14) and O 111:K58(B4) (see Nestlé, 1975).

As significant as the serotype itself, however, is the mode by which diarrhea is promoted. It is, indeed, a highly specialized function that first and foremost requires "colonization" of the intestinal wall. Colonization here means attachment to the lining of the upper intestines by significant numbers of the organism (Chordash and Insalata, 1978). Only when this is accomplished is toxin produced, and only then are certain tissue cells penetrated.

To attach themselves to the intestinal wall, *E. coli* use hairlike outgrowths called *fimbriae* or *pili*. An antigen, a specialized "sticky" protein, aids the cause. This antigen can actually be transferred, or more accurately, the ability to produce the antigen can be transferred from those *E. coli* that possess it to those that do not (see Nestlé, 1975). The transfer takes place via genetic processes. The carrier, a small piece of genetic material, is called a *plasmid*. The process occurs, simply enough, by direct conjugal contact between bacterial cells.

Overall, then, the defense against *E. coli* must take place on two fronts. The one protects against colonization in the first place, allowing *E. coli* to be washed away through peristalsis, that is, movement of fecal matter down the intestines. In the event that colonies are formed, the other must hold the line against the toxin that is produced.

Defense—the only foolproof defense—also takes two forms. The most important, perhaps, is the prevention of transfer of the disease in the first place. The most frequent carriers are food, clothing, and hands. The mother herself, as she gives birth, is a source. *E. coli* can also be airborne. It survives for days or months as a part of dust and dirt of the household. In hospitals, it walks the corridors in and on the staff professionals and visitors. Prevention, therefore, is the first line of defense. The second line leads through the intricate pattern by which immune factors are generated, and it is to this defense network that we now turn.

IMMUNE RESPONSES

Immune responses are either active or passive. Active immunity is the response put forth by the body itself in its own defense. It is literally an entire defense establishment—a system capable of screening friend from foe, able to contruct arms and equipment for defense, and with the ability to transport this defense armament to the field of battle. Active immunity ultimately pervades—must pervade—the whole body. It does so through *humoral* and *cellular* defense units. The former implies a presence in various body fluids—blood, bile, and lymph. These are systems originating in the humors of the body, consisting, by traditional definition, of antibodies and complement. The latter specifies an immune function stemming from various body cells, for example, white blood cells. Humoral and cellular immune processes interact and complement each other; they also serve independent functions.

The active immune system has two obvious advantages over its passive counterpart. First, it has the ability to recognize enemies specific to the body within which it is acting. It need not depend on another mechanism "diagnosing" its own ills. Second, active immunity also holds within its power a kind of memory. It is able to "recall" certain former enemies, and a preestablished counterattack is ready and waiting. For this reason, certain childhood diseases need be suffered only once; a single immunization serves a lifetime. It now appears that it is possible to transfer this "memory" from one person to another, that is, from a person exposed to many diseases to a relative newcomer to the scene. Think of the system as a miniaturized computer, one that sits in the body processing incoming disease information. Over a lifetime it gathers immense amounts of data. If one extracts the computer from one body and injects into another, much of that data is transferable. The recipient is "immunized" to many of the same diseases, and to some for which standard immunization methods fail. Scientists give to this computerlike particle the name *transfer factor*. It resides in white blood cells of the body. Lacking such defense, a living body must greet each new invasion, no matter how repetitive in kind, as though it were a new, unknown enemy.

Preparing an active immune system is the foremost aim of all new life. Mother's milk provides a steady flow of passive immunity through the intestinal tract, but is there any protecton offered beyond the confines of the intestines? Could an infant fight off a disease of the blood, for example? Is there, indeed, any humoral defense at all? Yes, there is, or there can be, at any rate. However, the way in which humoral immunity is achieved varies among different mammalian species. Three such classes are defined. (see Nestlé, 1975). Some mammals—cattle, goats, sheep, pigs, and horses—simply come into the world with little or no humoral protection at all. They must gain all of it from immune agents present in the milk of the mother, and most of this immunity derives from colostrum. It is this milk that is most rich in immune agents, and the very life of the offspring depends on the speed with which it is able to gather its strength and begin suckling. Even an hour's delay may be too long, for the environment into which the animal has been delivered literally seethes with germs and other would-be enemies. An intestinal and humoral defense is mounted only after milk is ingested. In these species, humoral immunity is acquired by direct transfer of the immune agents through the intestinal wall into the body proper.

Other mammals—mice, rats, hedgehogs, dogs, and cats—can transfer immune factors to the offspring both prior to birth (across fetal membranes) and also after birth (in the manner already described). In a certain sense, they perhaps have the best of both worlds. A third class—humans, monkeys, rabbits, guinea pigs—is able to transfer an immune factor(s) through the placenta prior to birth but is able to gain little or no such immunity from maternal milk. In these mammals, mother's milk seems destined to provide an immune response in the intestinal tract only. Nonetheless, the offspring does have a form of passive humoral defense as transferred to the blood-stream prior to birth. In humans a single immune agent (IgG) serves this immune function, but it survives the infant body for only about 4–6 weeks. Even at three weeks' time the potency has dropped by half (see Nestlé, 1975). Effective defense, therefore, is lost well before the infant body has activated its own immune system. With intestinal immunity also on the wane, at least in terms of the immune activity of mother's milk, the child's vulnerability is again underscored. Moreover, a third factor may also increase risk at this time. This brings up one last note of distinction, that is, that immunity to a disease agent may either be specific or nonspecific in action.

When a human immune factory builds an antibody—one kind of immune agent that defends against a specific disease—it is exhibiting a specific immune response. It is erecting a defense designed in some detail to war against the very agent that triggered the response. It is as though the body were able to call on anti-tank guns to fend off tanks and on ground-to-air missiles to pick off planes. Antibodies protect the mother herself and her infant through the milk supply. In that way nursing infants receive highly specific protection against disease agents common to their environment.

Of course, specific types of disease vary around the world. For example, a Guatemalan mother can confer an immune response to her nursing infant of the diseases common to her country. Diseases also vary between communities and even from location to location within a community. Thus, defense of this type can be of immense help because certain diseases tend to prevail in certain communities or households at any one time. Conversely, mothers may not necessarily be able to provide a specific defense to diseases that they do not routinely encounter. For example, a mother may activate an immune response for her newborn infant to an intestinal disease that causes diarrhea in her family. However, she may not confer an immune milk defense to an intestinal disease common primarily to the hospital environment where her child is born. In answer to this kind of special problem, "immune-fortified" infant formula, which will be discussed later, finds one of its most important usages.) This is not to say that an immune response cannot be mustered against a disease remote to the mother's environment. Perhaps the best example of this potential is the finding that North American and Guatemalan mothers apparently carry in their milk equal concentrations of antibodies against *Vibrio cholera* and *E. coli* (Stoliar *et al.*, 1976). The former is only rarely if ever encountered by women in northern latitudes of the Americas. The extent to which this kind of immune response occurs, especially among more uncommon disease agents (or serotypes), is not known.

As the name implies, nonspecific immune activity is a nonselective defense mechanism. An acid environment in the infant's intestine holds in check a wide variety of both infectious and noninfectious bacteria. It does so with impunity and without specificity, except for those few organisms that can survive the acidic condition.

THE DEFENDERS

Several substances in human milk provide resistance to infant disease, particularly disease of the intestinal tract. As a group, they may be termed "immune factors." They consist of five rather highly specialized antibodies, the complement system, certain enzymes, two or more iron-binding proteins, various cellular components, and a factor that encourages growth of a bifido bacterium. A listing of important factors includes immunoglobulin A (IgA), immunoglobulin G (IgG), immunoglobulin M (IgM), immunoglobulin D (IgD), immunoglobulin E (IgE), complement, lysozyme, lactoferrin, transferrin, interferons, leucocytes (macrophages and lymphocytes), lactoperoxidase, and the bifidus factor. Only the immunoglobulins, complement, and certain cellular systems act with specificity. The rest are nonspecific defenders.

Immunoglobulins

Immunoglobulins (Igs) are antibodies. As such, Igs (1) cause bacteria to come together in aggregates (to agglutinate) that are easily cleansed from the intestinal cavity; (2) interfere with the process by which bacteria adhere to and colonize the intestinal lining; (3) aid other immune agents in their defense capabilities (a process called opsonization); (4) further specialized antibody production, that is, to fix complement; (5) neutralize toxins; and (6) kill viruses.

Discovery of antibodies is credited to Emil von Behring, a German scientist who first observed the presence of protective substances in the blood serum of previously immunized animals. These compounds rendered the toxins produced by bacteria harmless, giving rise to the term, "antitoxins." Further studies proved these chemical entities to be protein in nature and to fall ultimately into a class of proteins called gamma globulins. Because gamma globulins carry out immune functions, they are also aptly named immunoglobulins.

Immunoglobulins have their origin in genes. Genes, of course, are the fundamental units by which components of the body are synthesized and ultimately reproduced. To form an antibody, a genetic base must first be present. It is this base that provides for the synthesis of a highly specific antibody configuration, a kind of opposing image of the toxin or antigen against which it must defend. The process can perhaps be likened to the manner in which a blind person creates a "visual" concept of an object by touching its surface features. Having "touched" the essence of an invading toxin, the body calls forth from its genetic base an exact opposite, or unlike, image. To understand more clearly how this is done, it helps to have a mental picture of the core structure of an antibody.

An antibody consists of two pairs of identical chains of amino acids. The length of the chains of one pair is quite long. They are designated "H," for heavy. The other two are shorter. Their designation is "L," meaning light. Like pieces of string, the two H chains may be visualized as lying side-by-side between the two shorter ones. But, in addition, each chain should be seen as divided into two distinct parts. Both H and L chains are so divided. The tail section consists of a rather unvarying sequence of amino acids. For this reason, it is referred to as the "constant" region. Exposed at the very end is the carboxyl group of the last amino acid in the chain, that is, the carboxy-terminal group. Constant regions differ only to the extent that there exist two classes of L chains and eight classes of H chains. As a result, however, different immune functions can be carried out in this part of the antibody.

Again, both H and L chains have a constant region. Each also has, at the other end, a "variable" region. This portion includes the final 100 amino acids (Yelton and Scharff, 1980). At the forefront lies the amino-terminal group. The amino acids that make up this section vary in number and kind, much more so than those of the constant region. Consider also that each region consists of genetic material. There are constant-region genes and variable-region genes. Through substitution and alternative sequencing of amino acids, variable-region genes make possible a vast number of unique molecular designs and shapes. Literally, a key can be constructed to fit a single lock, a lock unlike any other in the world. Likewise, a lock can be synthesized to fit exactly over a key of exceedingly complex and unique shape. In either case, the variable region of the chain (and, thereby, the antibody) is constructed with great care and attention to specific features of the antigen against which battle must be waged. The antigen may be a relatively simple molecule, one that elicits only one specially designed antibody. Or it may be, as many proteins are, a highly complex antigen carrying on its surface any number of reactive sites. To the extent that these sites differ from one another, a different antibody is called forth. It is perhaps indicative of the number and complexity of conceivable antigens, that amino acids of genes of antibody construction can be so scrambled as to make possible 10 million or more unique configurations (Yelton and Scharff, 1980). In the end, of course, it is proposed that a separate antibody be designed to bind to each individual antigen or antigenic site.

In the process by which an antibody is formed, one of many possible L chain variable-region genes aligns itself with a constant-region gene. A heavy-chain variable-region gene does likewise. Once this happens, other immune agents commit themselves, as in a assembly plant, to produce indentical L and H chain variable-region units. Coupled with constant regions, a single antibody comes on line. Of the right type, it may wind up in the milk of mothers.

Five different antibodies occur. These are IgA, IgG, IgM, IgD, and IgE. All carry the same basic structure: two identical L chains and two identical H chains joined together by disulfide bonds. In addition, though, one other common feature should be noted: the antibodies all break into two segments in the presence of reducing agents or certain proteolytic (protein-splitting) enzymes (see Nestlé, 1975; Hamburger, 1976). One segment is named Fc (c for crystalline), the other Fab. If you imagine an antibody shaped like the letter Y, the Fc fragment would form the base, the Fab the two protruding arms. The arms, consisting of two L chains and the uppermost (variable-region) section of the two H chains, carry the ability to grasp and bind to antigen.

With these similarities between the structure of antibodies, it would seem that they must all function similarly. Nonetheless, there are differences, which we shall examine at this point.

Immunoglobulin A

Of all Igs, the need for immunoglobulin A (IgA) seems most apparent. The infant indeed lacks this immune factor. Exposure to it soon after birth is essential to safeguard against certain bacterial and viral diseases. Though an infant may survive well without it (and other similar factors), the safeguard is well taken, even in the relatively sanitary surroundings of a well-kept hospital.

IgA is an antibody found in all mucous secretions, that is, tears, saliva, nasal and bronchial fluids, milk (both colostrum and "mature" milk), and secretions along the intestinal lining (mucous membrane). (see Nestlé, 1975). In adults, IgA is the major immune body of the intestinal tract. It is an antibody, therefore, designed to handle toxins or toxic agents at this particular site. It must be, and does indeed become, resistant to degradation by enzymes active in this area of the body. IgA is so important as a protective mechanism that it is sometimes referred to as "antiseptic paint." It seems, in fact, to function as a coating able to act as a barrier to a variety of antigens (toxin agents), whether of dietary, bacterial, or viral origin. Confronted by a poisonous agent, IgA complexes attach to it and detain it while other digestive forces literally tear it apart. IgA also has the ability to control autoimmune (self acting against self) disease; it can hold malignancies in check. Lacking IgA, infants are more prone to developing allergies. A small portion of IgA is even absorbed intact directly through the infant's stomach during the first 18–24 hours (Ogra *et al.*, 1977). Early exposure through early breast feeding is obviously desirable. Some researchers claim that tuberculin immunity can be transferred in this way. In the arsenal of protective deterrents, IgA is a superweapon.

IgA may be envisioned as a protein molecule consisting of the core group of four amino acid chains (two L and two H chains). These four chains of amino acids combine to form a single IgA unit, an IgA *monomer*. Two monomers, then, can join to form a *dimer*. The bridge holding them together is called a *J* (junction) *chain*. The J chain itself is attached to each of the monomers by means of disulfide (two sulfur units joined together) linkage (see Nestlé, 1975). It is as though a bridge connected two adjoining towns. The point where each actually links up the bridge is a specially designed fraction of the two protein units. The one is Fc, the second is Fab, the antigen-binding fragment.

Thus far, we have described a dimer consisting of two IgA molecules held together by a chain. The J chain itself is secreted by plasma cells (lymphocytes), the same cells that produce and secrete IgA monomers. However, there is one more very important addition that can be and often is made to the IgA dimer. This added component might be called a "key," a mechanism capable of unlocking and thereby disrupting an attacking disease agent. It is designed to fit specifically the disruptive trigger mechanism of common, rare, or even new types of warring antigens. Thus, a highly specialized IgA may be formed either by the mother's own, or her suckling infant's, contact with the specific disease agent (see Reiter, 1978). It is called a *secretory* component and designated by "s." The whole antibody then becomes, in abbreviated form, sIgA.

Monomeric IgA, dimeric IgA, and secretory IgA—these are the three faces of IgA. Each IgA differs in certain distinct ways. The dimer, for example, is about twice as hardy at resisting attack by trypsin, a major proteolytic (protein-splitting) enzyme of the stomach (see Nestlé, 1975). It is the J chain itself, not the secretory component, that protects the dimer. The secretory component (also joined to the Fc fragment) gives the antibody specificity. Suppose, for example, that a pregnant woman comes in contact with a rare serotype of *E. coli* that she has ingested in contaminated food. Her body now starts the process by which she herself would protect against the disease. She generates lymphocytes, cells able to produce sIgA. Some of these cells then home in on the mammary gland, there to provide sIgA specific to the rare form of *E. coli* to the breast-feeding child (See Reiter, 1978).

No doubt the IgA level of human colostrum varies considerably. Two investigations put the average at 410 and 457 mg/100 g of milk (Mata and Wyatt, 1971; Kuvaeva *et al.*, 1979). By 3–4 weeks, the level has dropped to near 35 mg/100 g. To some extent, increased intake of milk on the part of the infant compensates for the lower overall level of IgA. About 80% of IgA in human milk is present in the dimeric form. The infant is unable to produce sIgA until 2 months of age. Serum IgA, arising humorally, reaches only 20% of adult levels by the end of a year. (see Nestlé, 1975).

A certain amount of IgA in human milk appear to have some specificity for rotavirus (Otnaess and Orstavik, 1980). However, milk contains factors other than Igs that likewise seem to carry antiviral activity. IgA content of fecal matter is seen by some researchers as a way of determining the extent to which an infant has acquired immune protection. Infants fed either diluted cow's milk or infant formula before 1 month of age, are apt also to show higher blood serum titers of IgA than breast-fed infants (Saarinen and Siimes, 1979). This could be due to an IgA response to allergenic properties of milk protein or possibly to the presence of coliform in the milk products.

Thus far, IgA has been found in all vertebrates examined for its presence. The rate of production in milk, however, varies greatly. The human is literally a milk IgA factory. Cow's milk, on the other hand, carries only traces of the antibody. In this animal, IgA appears to be replaced with a very close kin, IgG. If cow's milk is to serve as a source of human antibodies in infant formula (as well it can), specialized forms of IgG will do the job.

Immunoglobulin G

IgA must come to the infant from a food source if it is to be provided at all. immunoglobulin G (IgG), however, is an antibody that crosses the placenta to lend immunity to the infant prior to birth; this is an immune activity that carries on for some few weeks or months. Authorities claim that the antibody has a half-life (the point at which the antibody titer, as compared to the level at birth, has been reduced by one-half) of 3 weeks (see Nestlé, 1975). The infant is born with about 60% of the IgG level of an adult. However, this level drops drastically before the infant is able to promote its own immune response. You will recall the initiation of that process to be between 2 and 3 months. Again, the vulnerability of the infant at that particular time in life is stressed.

IgG carries out a variety of functions similar to those of IgA. To an extent, the antibody patrols and acts as a defense in the intestinal tract. It is known to prevent adhesion (and, thereby, colonization) of various germs and to bind antigens. In this way, it aids the cleansing process of the bowels. It appears to be peculiarly effective in tying up bacterial toxins, like those of tetanus and diptheria. But IgG is also an antivirus in activity. It is serum IgG, not intestinal immunoglobulins, that fends off rotavirus attack (Stoliar et al., 1976). Moreover, IgG may help in neutralizing the polio virus. It seems to handle that part of the immune process by which foreign bodies (antigens) of all types are identified as such. Significantly, IgG provides an immune defense to the specific disease to which the mother is immune.

The structure of IgG and IgA are remarkably similar. Consisting of the basic two H and two L polypeptide chains linked by disulfide bonds, IgG has the same configuration as an IgA monomer. Like IgA, IgG can be considered a superweapon. Because the cow produces IgG in rather large quantities, this antibody promises to function for IgA in the infant formula of the future.

The cow does, in fact, produce IgA, IgM, and IgG; however, the latter predominates by far. Yet it is not manufactured in the mammary gland per se. Rather it arises in blood serum and simply filters into the milk supply. An immunization technique, in which cows are given a "shot" of human pathogens during pregancy, causes production of IgG with specific activity against the disease (see Nestlé, 1975).

Two subclasses of cow's milk IgG are known. They are designated IgG_1 and IgG_2. The former makes up 90% of the total. It differs from IgG_2 in its rather larger content of sialic acid. The IgG_1 serves mainly to increase the immune potency of infant formula (see Building Immune Factors into Infant Formula, this chapter).

IgM, IgD, and IgE

These immunoglobulins are found in far smaller quantities in human milk than either IgA or IgG. In human blood serum, for example, IgG and IgA average 10 mg and 1.5 mg/ml, respectively (Hamburger, 1976). By contrast, IgE is found in amounts measurable in nanograms (ng), that is, millionths of a milligram. The average level is 100 (ng)/ml (Hamburger, 1976). Still, each IgM, IgD, and IgE antibody carries the same basic configuration of the more prevalent IgG and IgA, and each carries out important immune functions. IgM shows a strong defense against gram-negative pathogens like *E. coli* and *Salmonella*. It differs in structure from IgG in two ways. Its H chain, given as μ-chain, shows a different composition. The presence of large amounts of the amino acid cystine provides for a circular configuration, one looking much like the hub of a wheel with five spokes. These pentameters consist of ten H and ten L chains (see Nestlé, 1975).

Like IgM, IgD and IgE resemble IgG except in the composition of their heavy chains. In a limited way, perhaps, both function within the intestinal tract as defenders against pathogens. However, IgE carries a special significance because it enters into allergic reactions (see The Problem of Allergies, this chapter). Rather than preventing disease, at least in this particular instance, it is a factor in causing an allergic response either to food or to air-borne allergens.

Research conducted by Bazaral *et al.*, (1971) confirms the presence of very small amounts of IgE (5 ng/ml) in the serum of some newborn infants. Other infants show no (or undetectably small) IgE. During the first 2 years of life, dramatic differences in the evolutionary pattern of this antibody exist between different infants. Some show scarcely any change in the IgE level, over that found at birth, through the entire first year. Within 6 to 9 months other infants have produced amounts exceeding that of most adults. This finding has some predictive value in assessing the likelihood of an infant to develop allergies (Hamburger, 1976). Once again it is important to stress the genetic base upon which all antibodies proliferate. Allergies are inheritable traits. There is convincing evidence that the 3-month-old infant, suffering relative deficiency in IgA, seems prone to premature activation of the IgE antibody system—at least when afflicted with an inborn susceptibility.

Activity Span of Milk Immunoglobulins

The major activity of immune globulins of milk is reserved for the first few days, perhaps even hours, of life. Their level in colostrum is high, but it falls off rapidly. IgG peaks the first day following birth, according to some researchers (Donat, 1976). By perhaps the sixth day it has reached its lowest level. IgA follows a similar pattern, but it shows two peaks—one the first day and a second (though lower) peak about the tenth day. By day twenty, IgA in milk has nearly dropped to its lowest point; it shows as much as a two- to tenfold (estimates vary) decrease in that period of time. IgM rises to its highest level within 1–2 days and falls to its lowest point within 6 days to 1 month. Two sources (Mata and Wyatt, 1971; Kuvaeva *et al.*, 1979) report the level of IgA, IgG, and IgM in colostrum as 410 and 451, 6 and 20, and

10 and 48 mg/100 ml, respectively. Apparently, nature intends to deliver its knockout punch quickly and decisively. By quickly withdrawing much of its immune globulin defense, nature forewarns the child of its personal responsibility to assert an immune response in its own behalf.

Complement

The ability of some antibodies to kill infectious agents depends upon the presence of an additional factor called *complement*. Some 11 different protein subunits (C1–C11) make up the classical pathway of complement fixation, the process by which antibodies bind complement and, in this way, become activated. Only intermediate pieces of the complement system exist in human and cow's milk. Early components are missing. Nonetheless, C3, C4, and C3 proactivator have been found. Presence of this latter compound leads some scientists to believe that an alternate to the classical complement fixation pathway may exist (see Nestlé, 1975). In any event, colostrum of cows, nonbactericidal because of its high level of IgG_1 (prozone effect), becomes a bacterial killer upon addition of fresh, mature (noncolostral) milk (see Reiter, 1978). The turnabout is explained by the presence in mature milk of a higher level of complement. As yet it is not known whether or not activity of C3 and C4 of human milk is dampened (prozone effect) by the presence of large amounts of sIgA. It is known that sIgA binds complement only in the presence of lysozyme (Hill and Porter, 1974). Activation of C3 by C3 proactivator in colostrum is essential to the process (opsinization) by which infectious bacteria are made vulnerable to attack by other immune agents (phagocytes). Because this process is in fact functional, an alternate pathway—one in which complement fixation is activated by IgA, IgG, or fragments thereof—has been suggested. In any event, the key role of complement is the enhancement of the activity of phagocytic cells (Watson, 1981).

Cellular Immune Factors

Leucocytes are white blood cells, large (comparatively speaking) cellular entities usually mobilized by the body as a result of infection. After some debate, consensus of scientific opinion indicates that leucocytes come to the infant in mother's milk in active ready-to-battle form. Most may be considered to be macrophages (monocytic phagocytes)—single cell components able to synthesize C3, C4, lysozyme, and lactoferrin (Nestlé, 1975). These predominate, by far. Remaining cellular factors divide between granulocytes and lymphocytes.

Leucocytes or macrophages serve as scavenger cells. They have the ability to process antigens and are known to provide regulatory functions. They inhibit the growth of tumors and appear particularly helpful in the control of ulcer-causing intestinal disease (necrotizing enteritis). Their importance to infant health may be judged by their numbers in human milk. Macrophages, which comprise the largest group of immune cells found there, make up 80–90% of the total. Daily secretion in milk ranges from 100 to 300 million (2000–4000/mm^3) (Nestlé, 1975), more than could be anticipated based upon human productive capacity alone. Wandering at random, trapped (after entering) in body tissue, macrophages act to kill bacteria, virus, or fungi by engulfment. They swallow their victim whole and then destroy it with lysozyme or lactoferrin, or with chemicals like hydrogen peroxide and superoxide. Coupled to lymphokines released by T-cells (see the following), macrophages grow in enzyme activity, in size, in anatomical complexity, *and* lethality (Watson and McMurray, 1979). Such cells no doubt contribute greatly to infant well-being.

Yet there is a situation in which leucocytes may actually cause an immunological problem. Evidence strongly suggests that this is one instance in which mother's milk should not be fed unless it has received one of two forms of processing. The problem relates mainly to preterm or low-weight infants. Leucocytes have been found to move across the intestinal wall, thus promoting an adverse immune response. It seems particularly essential not to feed susceptible infants milk of donors other than the mother. However, the problem is apparently resolved either by freezing or pasteurizing the milk prior to use. The latter treatment, of course, tends to be somewhat more destructive of the immune activity of the milk generally, and some potential benefits are thereby lost.

Lymphocytes come in two different forms. Those acted upon by the thymus are termed T-lymphocytes (T-cells). Activated by some invading chemical or germ, these cells mature as killer cells, helper cells, or suppressor cells. Killer cells react to neutralize foreign or transformed (cancer) cells. Helper cells provide an antibody response to any of a number of offending antigens. Suppressor cells act to bar production of a given antibody in a normal control process. Macrophages, antigen in their grasp, help stimulate T-cell functions. Body defense, in all ways, is a cooperative venture

Lymphocytes molded by the "bursa equivalent" (a factor originating in bone marrow and fetal liver and spleen), become B-lymphocytes (B-cells). These also go through a process of maturation that is only vaguely understood. Interacting with other cells of the immune system, more than likely triggered by some specific antigen, B-cells grow to plasma cells. These latter, in turn, have the ability to produce antibodies to some warring antigen. They are, in a sense, antibody factories. (For a review of this topic, see Archer, 1979.)

Both B-cells and T-cells are found in human milk. They are laden with lipids (fats). Though not found to produce IgG or IgM, some apparently are able to produce IgA.

NONSPECIFIC DEFENDERS

A number of human milk components seem to serve in one or more ways in the control of intestinal disease. Their various roles remain somewhat unclear. Their mode of action likewise still needs clarification in many instances, especially *in vivo*. Nevertheless, a brief coverage of these factors will at least highlight their presence and their potential.

Lysozyme

Lysozyme is an enzyme (organic catalyst) with the ability to lyse (split) cell walls of certain bacteria. It attacks *E. coli* and other disease-causing bacteria. Both gram-negative and gram-positive organisms appear susceptible to the activity of the lysozyme of milk (Vakil *et al.*, 1969). In particular, lysozyme is able to break apart those bacteria whose cell walls consist in large part of mucopeptide. The enzyme works alone or in concert with other defense agents (leucocytes or macrophages, complement, and IgA). Lysozyme is essential to the binding mechanism of complement to sIgA (Adinolfi *et al.*,1966; Hill and Porter, 1974). Along with IgA and complement, the enzyme acts strongly against *E. coli*.

In the body, lysozyme is synthesized in the parotid gland, the gastric mucosa, and, to a lesser degree, in the small intestine. It is resistant to digestion; it is recovered from the feces of breast fed, but not bottle fed, infants. Lysozymes of human milk, cow's milk, and egg albumen (a rich source) apparently differ in various ways. Certainly their ability to lyse different bacterial species varies; egg lysozyme displays a narrower spectrum of activity. Human and cow's milk lysozymes appear active against both gram-negative and gram-positive bacteria. Their activity in general more closely parallels each other than lysozyme of eggs, which appears not to lyse gram-negative bacteria except in the presence of EDTA. Still, there are some slight differences in the activity of human and cow's milk lysozymes. There are basic differences between them in antigenic and serological properties (see Reiter, 1978).

The lysozyme enzyme (*N*-acetylmuramyl hydrolase) attacks the mucopeptide content of bacterial cell walls. Generally, the more mucopeptide present, the more sensitive the organism to lysis. Even so, the most vulnerable bacteria, *Micrococcus lysodeikticus*, shows considerably greater resistance to egg, than to milk, lysozymes. Again, the difference is emphasized as it relates to practical considerations of usage.

Human milk lysozyme occurs to an average level of about 39 mg/100 ml; lysozyme of cow's milk ranges in level from 0 to 260 μg/100 ml (Vakil et al., 1969). On an average, lysozyme content of cow's milk runs much lower than that of human milk. Meyer et al. (1981) also found differences between breeds of cows. For five breeds investigated, lysozyme level varied from an average of 18 to 45 μg/100 ml. Milk from German Red and Jersey cows contained significantly higher amounts than other breeds tested. Lysozyme concentration was also found to increase, and to a maximum level within 34–48 hours, upon challenging the udder with *Staphylococcus aureus*. In a limited study of goat's milk, concentration of lysozyme has been found to average 25 μg/100 ml (see Jenness, 1980).

Lactoferrin and Transferrin

Lactoferrin and transferrin are two proteins with the ability to tie up iron. Both are found in human and cow's milk, though they also occur in other body secretions and fluids. Lactoferrin also is a part of the defense system of polymorphonuclear leucocytes (see Reiter, 1978), which likewise enter milk to add a degree of passive immune response.

These iron-binding proteins are properly considered aids to infants in resisting infection, particularly from certain strains of *E. coli* and *Candida albicans* and in fact, from any disease organism with a significant need for iron as a nutrient (Brock, 1980). Defense in this instance is thought to occur through the withholding of iron and the nutritional functions it serves in bacteria.

Lactoferrin seems to possess a somewhat higher level of iron-binding activity than transferrin. Under the right conditions, both interfere with the growth of disease bacteria by themselves. Certain antibodies may also lend assistance, thereby blocking the iron-binding mechanism of the bacteria, at least in part. Unable to chelate (bind) iron effectively, bacteria are at a loss to compete with lactoferrin and transferrin in this capacity. Conversely, if iron is added to milk and the two iron-binding proteins are saturated with it, they will indeed lose their power to prevent the growth of *E. coli* and other bacteria. Although the mode of action by which lactoferrin and transferrin actually inhibit growth remains somewhat unclear, it is possible that they deprive the organisms of a defense against one weapon—superoxide—of immune agents. An enzyme, dismutase, that might otherwise thwart effects of superoxide is lacking in coliform bacteria from which iron is withheld (Watson and McMurray, 1979). In general, gram-negative organisms have considerably greater need for iron than do lactobacilli (Reiter and Oram,

1968), a favorably important group of intestinal bacteria. Thus, lactoferrin and transferrin exert a kind of selective influence, doing away with disease bacteria without interfering greatly with the growth of desirable organisms.

Of course, these two proteins must also be resistant to the digestive forces of stomach and intestines. Lactoferrin (of cow's milk), particularly, has been found to be stubbornly intransigent to trypsin, pepsin, and chymotrypsin, but only in its noniron-bound (apoform) form. This is true *in vitro*; *in vivo* data remain yet to be obtained (see Reiter, 1978). Nevertheless, the evidence seems to indicate that the proteins possess a degree of resistance to breakdown.

Merely the presence of lactoferrin in the gastrointestinal tract is not sufficient. Other factors encourage or reduce its activity. For the protein to bind iron mole for mole (one each of protein and iron), bicarbonate is needed. Another buffer, citrate, a common constituent of milk, must be excluded, at least to an extent. This can readily be done and has been done *in vitro* for both cow's and human milk. The question is whether or not it might happen, similarly so, in the human body. Theory would say that it does (see Reiter, 1978). Assuming lactoferrin survives the acids and enzymes of the stomach, it should reach the intestines where bicarbonate floods the stomach juices and where, at this same time, citrate is absorbed out of the intestinal tract and into the body proper.

Human milk contains anywhere from 3 to possibly 100 times as much lactoferrin as cow's milk. The difference depends on the stage of lactation. Human milk seems to remain fairly high in its content of the iron-binding protein; although colostrum of cow's milk is flush (6 mg/ml) with it, later milk is less so (see Reiter, 1978). The content of lactoferrin in human milk has been reported to average 100 and 200 mg/100 ml by different sources (see Nestlé, 1975; Jenness, 1980). The level of transferrin is considered to be less than 5 mg/100 ml (see Jenness, 1980).

Importantly, lactoferrin of cow's milk shows strong inhibitory power to most *E. coli* found in infant feces (see Reiter, 1978). It can provide, therefore, a function in the infant similar to lactoferrin of human milk. Methods of concentrating cow's milk lactoferrin from cheese whey are being developed. In the future this protein will be present in infant formula to the extent needed or desirable. However, in formula fortified with iron, only that form of iron not readily taken up by lactoferrin would allow the protein its maximum effectiveness as a destroyer of disease bacteria. Moreover, a balance must be struck where iron-fortified formula is concerned. Iron deficiency anemia is a risk. Cow's milk contains more iron than human milk, though cow's milk is a poor source of this nutrient generally. At 0.2–0.3 μg/ml, iron in human milk is well absorbed by most infants. Breast milk alone generally satisfies an infant's need until the infant reaches three times its birth-weight (8–11 kg). To ensure as much with formula might well require the addition of iron to the product (but in a form not readily bound to lactoferrin, lest its bacteriostatic potency be diminished).

The addition of iron, however, must be weighed against the present health status of the infant. Where diarrhea already exists, supplemental iron, from whatever source, may simply worsen the situation. The problem may be particularly acute for the undernourished of the world. The evidence is mounting that infants who may survive a low intake of nutrients are taxed by intestinal disorders to either more serious nutritional deficiencies or death by starvation. Thus, control of coliform and/or other enteropathogenic diseases (and other ailments) comes second only to food itself. Infection accompanied by fever, for example, may raise the need for protein in an already protein-deficient child. Intestinal diseases may simply restrict the absorption of any of a number of essential nutrients. Control of diarrhea, possibly by limiting iron intake, becomes a valid way of attacking the problem. In any event, anemia is generally a problem reserved for the older infant, the infant who is not weaned by 1 year of age and the one fed commercial (unfortified with iron) market milk to the exclusion of other foods. The condition may be caused not just from lack of iron in food but from hemorrhaging brought about by excessive milk intake (1 liter or more a day). In any event, compared with normal cow's milk, formula better serves the needs of the infant weaned prior to 6 months of age.

Lactoperoxidase System

An enzyme of human and cow's milk, lactoperoxidase joins with two other chemical factors to produce a defense against a variety of human pathogens. The lactoperoxidase (LP) system is so potent that study is being made of its use as a cold sterilization technique (Reiter, 1978). Originally thought of chiefly as a defense against certain streptococci, it now appears that the LP system inhibits a variety of bacterial germs. It attacks gram-negative (and catalase-positive) bacteria. It is a nemesis of *E. coli*, *Pseudomonas flourescens*, *P. aeruginosa*, and *Salmonella typhimurium* (see Reiter, 1978). So far no human serotype of *E. coli* that has been pitted against it has survived. It is even active against strains of *Klebsiella aerogenes* (see Reiter, 1978) which are known to be resistant to the killing effect of various antibiotics.

The LP system works most effectively at pH levels below that of natural milk. Stomach acids (pH 2.0) help serve this function (see Reiter, 1978). Because the enzyme is active at relatively low pH, it likewise survives the acid, to be joined eventually be hydrogen peroxide and thiocyanate. Both these latter chemicals are necessary to activate the LP process fully.

Thiocyanate (SCN^-) originates either in milk (from liver and kidney functions) or the stomach. Hydrogen peroxide (H_2O_2) arises from the chemical reaction of glucose oxidase acting on glucose or from the activity of certain bacteria (see Reiter, 1978). Streptococci often produce H_2O_2 to which the bacteria themselves ultimately succumb. Like acid generated by bacteria, the end product (H_2O_2) limits streptococci from further growth and may even destroy them. Hydrogen peroxide combines first with lactoperoxidase. The two then oxidize SCN^- to an intermediate product. This intermediate product is poison to disease bacteria.

Lactobacilli also produce other bactericides like 2-deoxy-D-glucose. These too may help desirable intestinal bacteria compete more favorably with disease-producers. This thesis, however, has yet to be proven *in vivo*. Despite that fact, the LP system and lactobacilli are of proven worth. Lactobacilli are valuable both inherently and as H_2O_2 generators for LP and thiocyanate. Lactobacilli that can in fact "colonize" the intestinal tract are host-specific. That is, those lactobacilli that have come to hold the key that allows them to build colonies on the intestinal wall of the infant (just as disease bacteria must do to produce disease) do so only in the infant, not in other animal species. How these organisms come to be there in the first place requires further explanation.

The Bifidus Factor

It was the microscope that first brought lactobacilli to view. Culturing methods helped explain both their needs and their mode of action. Scientists probed, trying to link what was known of their presence in the vagina with what turned up in the intestines of the infant scarcely 24 hours after birth. In the meantime, humanity has learned how to kill these helpmates. We have done so, not necessarily willfully, but in the way of a bomb sent to destroy some enemies and which wipes out the good and the innocent as well. The bombs in this case may be called antibiotics. They have taught us something about ourselves and may point the way to construction of better infant formulas.

Lactic acid bacteria are found almost everywhere, and there are many different kinds and strains. They turn up in green plants and in the soil, in decay and ferment. Some such ferments (cheese, cultured milk, etc) are edible, and have been taken as nourishment. In any event, there is no way humanity can avoid these bacteria. They have become part of us, learning to survive in the wet mucous surfaces of the mouth, vagina, and lower intestines. They have thrived by aiding the survival of their host. Living within us, they wage a battle against certain other bacteria that would inhabit that same body but promote diarrhea, disease, and death. Their most potent weapon is acid.

Lactic acid bacteria are either round or rod-shaped. They are of the genera *Streptococcus* and *Lactobacillus*, of the family Lactobacteriaceae. These bacteria are able to break down lactose (milk sugar) and glucose to lactic acid. Some, typically the lactobacilli, do so extensively and then are able to survive this acid bath they have created. Other bacteria, including a number of enteropathogens (disease germs of the intestines) perish in that same medium. It is of possible advantage, then, particularly to the newborn vulnerable infant, to join forces with lactobacilli, especially a strain well equipped to flourish in the human intestinal tract. A strain of this type exists and shows up, usually without fail, in infants who are breast-fed. It has been called *Lactobacillus bifidus* for many years, but was recently renamed *Bifidobacterium bifidum*. Both names now appear in the scientific literature. Both a *Lactobacillus bifidus* (*Bifdobacterium bifidum*) type II and type IV have been isolated from the intestinal tract, though the latter apparently only from breast-fed infants. Within 3 to 4 days, the type IV organism colonizes the intestines to perhaps 99% of the total microflora (Gyllenberg and Roine, 1957; Haenel, 1970). The most obvious source of this bacteria would seem to be the human vagina, but examination of vaginal smears, while showing some differences in microflora, in no case disclose *L. bifidus* in sizable numbers until immediately prior to delivery. The bacterium then colonizes both colostrum milk and the skin of the lactating breast (see Sandine *et al.*, 1972). It shows up in infant feces within 24 hours after birth; it has gained control of intestinal microflora in 3–4 days. Breast-feeding alone stimulates its growth and development. For a general review of this topic see Sandine *et al.*, 1972; Speck, 1975; Mendez and Olano, 1979; and Sandine, 1979.

A variety of bacteria can and may colonize the intestinal tract of newborn infants. These include *E. coli, Clostridium perfringens,* group D Streptococcus, bacteroides, and lactobacilli. Hospitalized infants often show presence also of such organisms as *Klebsiella, Pseudomonas aeruginosa,* shigella, salmonella, and *Proteus* spp. But for as long as breast feeding continues, at least up to 1 year, *L. bifidus* remains a predominant species, and is thought active in subduing gram-negative pathogens. Although, obviously, other immune factors also play a role, incidence of infant infections and diarrhea is generally lower in breast-fed than bottle-fed infants.

Colonization of the intestinal tract with lactic acid bacteria apparently is accomplished in a manner different from that of disease producers. In this case, lipoteichoic acid may be the agent responsible. This acid, lipid in nature, accumulates near the surface membrane of the bacteria, close enough to react with antibodies, close enough to allow phage to absorb to the surface, close enough (according to some researchers) to provide an attachment mechanism to cells of the intestinal wall (see Reiter, 1978).

Eventually, certain other lactobacilli can and do replace *L. bifidus*. In weaned infants, the organism occurs much less frequently. Yet lactobacilli continue to make up a major portion of the flora inhabiting healthy individuals through adulthood, and their presence goes unaltered by the pattern of food choice and intake (Speck, 1976).

If *L. bifidus* shows up in breast milk, two reasons suggest themselves. Either breast milk contains a constituent that encourages and supports growth of the bacterium, or some other factor(s) in the milk suppresses growth of competing organisms. Both conditions may, in fact, play a role. Learned speculations include both possibilities. One group of researchers has isolated and named as *bifidus factors* a group of related compounds technically referred to as *N*-substituted *D*-glucosamines. A patent has been issued for the addition to infant formula of *N*-octanyl-*D*-glucosamine, *N*-benzoyl-d-glucosamine, or *N*-carboethoxy-*D*-glucosamine. The compounds do stimulate growth of *L. bifidus*. One unique characteristic of human milk is its high content of nonprotein nitrogen (NPN)—up to 25% of total nitrogen. Compounds making up this ready source of organic nitrogen (like those just mentioned) might be expected to play some special role in the infant's development. By comparison, cow's milk contains only about 5% NPN.

Still other factors may stimulate growth of *L. bifidus*. A compound found in carrot juice has been suggested. Pantetheine phosphate, a coenzyme A precursor, has also been identified as a possible factor (Kanao *et al.*, 1965). And another compound, this a derivative of lactose, has been conclusively shown to encourage growth of *L. bifidus* (see Mendez and Olano, 1979). Fortuitously enough, this latter compound, a ketose of lactose called lactulose, is generated when milk is heated to sufficiently high temperatures. For this reason it shows up in significant quantities in sterile liquid infant formula, but to low or negligible amounts in powdered formulas. Thus, its presence in some formula preparations has been inherent over the years, though its special value has perhaps gone unrecognized, generally, until quite recently.

Although not found in raw (unheated) milk, lactulose likely serves the bifidus organism in much the same way as certain other saccharides, some of which are present in raw milk. That is, it passes unabsorbed from the upper to the lower intestine, there to provide a source of nourishment for those bacteria with the enzyme system(s) necessary for its utilization. *L. bifidus* type IV, the organism that predominates in breast-fed infants, seems especially well adapted to this purpose, carrying both lactulase and α galactosidase activity. It appears better adapted even than *L. bifidus* type II (the strain associated with bottle-fed infants), despite the fact that lactulose is not a constituent of breast milk (see Mendez and Olano, 1979). Presence of either organism results in lower pH, high oxidation reduction potential, and low ammonium level, all of which tend to inhibit growth of gram-negative putrefactive bacteria.

Lactulose has been conclusively shown to be a factor promoting presence of bifidus bacteria in bottle-fed infants (see Mendez and Olano, 1979). At the same time, lactulose presence does not appear to greatly enhance implantation of *L. bifidus* in either healthy children or those suffering enteric disease. That is, a freeze-dried culture of the organism was found to successfully colonize the intestinal tract without lactulose, and in a large percentage of cases. However, a greater reduction in pathogenic *E. coli* occurred in those instances in which lactulose was fed along with the bacterial culture (see Mendez and Olano, 1979).

Although its origin yet remains shrouded in mystery, *L. bifidus* appears to serve a health-giving role in most infants. Not all authorities feel the role to be particularly important, at least not in relation to other immune factors of human milk. Yet pH remains one of the surest methods of control of food spoilage organisms generally, and cannot be discounted as a significant control mechanism in the human intestines, and to any disease organism unable to survive a low pH. This would include most of the enteropathogenic organisms common to the intestinal tract of infants.

To the extent pH (and perhaps certain other factors) is a significant deterrent to intestinal diseases, organisms other then *L. bifidus* can provide helpful, if not important, service in this regard. In fact, some such organisms ultimately show up and take over the role of *L. bifidus* simply as a matter of course. Most frequently, a variety of strains of *Lactobacillus acidophilus* are found. Thus, *L. acidophilus*, as well as *L. bifidus*, can serve an infant's—and an adult's—needs, similarly, if not identically. *L. acidophilus* has been used, in capsule form, as an aid in intestinal bacterial adjustment of premature infants (Vicek and Kneifl, 1964). It has served much the same purpose in treatment of certain adult diseases, but more often in establishing a healthy intestinal microflora following antibiotic therapy (Rafsky and Rafsky, 1955; Winkelstein, 1956; Gordon *et al.*, 1957). A sweet acidophilus milk has also been marketed widely in the United States and can maintain an appropriate level of the organisms in the intestinal tract. Intake of about 1 billion cells daily appears to be a valid dietary level (Speck, 1976).

It is apparent, therefore, that the presence of *L. acidophilus* could serve a useful purpose in infant formula. Not only could the organism provide the routine function of *L. bifidus*, especially for infants whose intestinal microflora is found lacking, but it could perhaps prove beneficial to infants plagued by diarrhea and other intestinal disorders. In Third World countries, where disease takes its heaviest toll in infant mortality, a formula supplemented with *L. acidophilus* might be nearly as useful as a more nutritious diet. A daily supplement of the organism would also be good preventive medicine during stress of weaning.

Stress alone is known to cause a change in intestinal microflora of both infants and adults. During periods of stress, lactobacilli are apt to be crowded out by a variety of organisms whose mode of action is the cause of diarrhea and other intestinal upsets. So significant is this problem that it was a major risk consideration in long-term flights of spacemen. Russian cosmonauts on a 120-day flight developed some rather severe gastrointestinal disturbances (see Sandine *et al.*, 1972). Type and balance of intestinal microflora changed significantly. Thus, a hazard to health arises, one that could be ameliorated by daily intake of *L acidophilus*. Weanling pigs are often treated with cultures of *L. acidophilus* to prevent diarrhea. Similar treatment may be rendered as therapy for scouring. Better weight gain and reduced enteritis (intestinal disease) have been noted in piglets fed *L. acidophilus* as a regular dietary supplement (see Sandine *et al.*, 1972). Special note should be taken of the fact that intestinal diseases of pigs and humans follow a remarkably similar pattern. The evidence therefore is mounting that lactic acid-producing bacteria have a possibly unique and important role in human health. This is especially true for infants, with intestinal disorders and during weaning. Weaning itself is stressful. The emotional trauma combined with the dramatic change in feeding may alter unfavorably a delicate microbial balance. In such cases, lactobacilli may be shut out, and coliform and other putrefactive and/or disease-causing bacteria may gain the advantage. Feeding *L. acidophilus* to formula-fed infants (and even as supplement to breast-fed infants) appears to be a significant step in public health maintenance.

Five different antibiotic compounds have been identified in cultures of *L. acidophilus*. These include acidophilin, lactocidin, lactobacillin, acidolin, and lactolin (Shahani and Chandan, 1979; Sandine, 1979). Different strains of *L. acidophilus* apparently differ markedly in the output of antibiotics. Quite possibly strains isolated from the human intestinal tract best serve the intestinal needs of humans. These organisms not only produce antibiotics but a variety of acids (lactic, acetic, and benzoic), which themselves are inhibitory to numerous spoilage and/or disease germs. Production of hydrogen peroxide, another feature of their growth, serves the lactoperoxidase system. Taken together, antibiotics, acids, and other possible inhibitors create an environment highly poisonous to many disease bacteria that may, or do, inhabit the intestinal tract. Specific evidence has been found of inhibitory action against a number of food-poisoning bacteria and coliform. Other lactic bacteria likewise are known to produce antibiotics and/or other inhibitory substances; thus, lactobacilli are not unique. However, lactobacilli do naturally inhabit the intestinal tract, and inference certainly suggests some possible function(s) there. They do appear to "crowd" out less desirable or disease organisms. They are active in reducing the coliform strains known to cause diarrhea, and they have been successfully used in treatment of infantile diarrhea. Following antibiotic treatment, they serve to restore "natural" intestinal flora. There is even evidence that their presence in the intestines causes an increase in blood urea nitrogen, hemoglobin, and iron. They may therefore serve to enhance a variety of nutritional needs particularly essential to infant health. Although research must yet be done to establish mode of action and possible value more conclusively, there is little reason to delay preparation for their more widespread use in infant formulas or weaning foods.

OTHER IMMUNE FACTORS

The immune factors and processes discussed to this point are by far the best researched and the best understood of all those that in some way defend against disease of the gastrointestinal tract. Of the nonmicrobial agents, all so far have been protein in nature. To these should perhaps be added properdin and conglutinin; both have been determined to be present in milk, the latter only in colostrum (see Reiter, 1978). Certain proteins also found in milk bind vitamin B_{12} and folic acid withholding the nutrients from bacterial uptake. Lacking these vitamins some bacteria compete less effectively for a place in the human intestine. An entire ecology is thereby altered, and favorably so for the infant.

As immune factors, proteins obviously perform well. Problems arise mainly in processing them for addition to infant formula. Thus, it is significant in more than one respect that an unsaturated fatty acid (C 18:2) has been shown to be lethal to certain staphylococci (Reiter, 1978; Kabara, 1980). These latter organisms have been scarcely mentioned thus far. They remain a major disease of cow's udders, through which formula ingredients are derived, and of the human breast, where they may both produce toxin harmful to infants or provide contaminating seed that enters the infants during suckling. Staphylococci are perhaps far more troublesome than many scientists suspect. They are a major foodborne disease as well as an infectious agent of the breast. The presence in human milk of a heat-stable, staphylococcal-killing fatty acid is good news. Certain fatty acids and monoglycerides are thought also to provide some protection against viral disease. Of the latter, monolaurin has been recommended for use in infant formula, along with polyunsaturated monoglycerides as a source of essential fatty acids.

Interferons

So great is interfon's potential that this substance could become the most prized medical discovery of the twentieth century. Time will tell. For now, only a few concrete statements can be made about it. First, interferon(s) is protein in nature. The amino acid sequence has yet to be worked out. More than one kind of interferon appears to be produced by the body. One originates in leucocytes. Another comes from fibroblasts. Still a third—immune interferon—is a product of T-lymphocytes. All are species specific. This last statement is important, for it says that only interferon produced by humans has the power to combat the diseases of humans. Thus, human milk can serve as a natural source, while cow's milk or milk of other animals cannot.

Interferons appear to function mainly against viruses and possibly against cancer cells. If, as some researchers suspect, both viral and nonviral forms of cancer exist, then interferon(s) show potential to inhibit both types. Immune interferon seems to be the most potent of the lot.

Interferon production is triggered by virus, viral nucleic acid, specific antigens, and nonspecific mitogens (see Archer, 1978). Thus mobilized, the agent acts as a kind of early warning system. It sounds the alarm that an invader is present. Those cells and immune defenses that can, produce more interferon. But the entire immune network seems to come to the ready. After infecting the first few cells, viruses now confront interferon and other defense forces almost at the doorstep of new cells slated for attack. Deterred there, unable to duplicate themselves, the attackers lose their foothold; the battle is over almost before it starts.

Either as an agent formed by the body or as a component of human milk, antiviral interferon carries out its surveillance and preventive actions along the stomach wall (see Archer, 1978). Though present in human milk in exquisitely small amounts, it nonetheless provides some level of defense for the infant. It is possible that the quantity of interferon in mother's milk varies upward to the extent of exposure of the mother to the same or possibly even other viruses. In any event, interferon shows potency against a broad spectrum of viral diseases.

Human interferon may one day become an ingredient in infant formula, but that prospect awaits development of methods of producing the substance in quantity. Until recently, there was little more than vain hope of such possibility. Now, however, human interferon, found nowhere else except in humans, and there only in infinitesimally small amounts, seems destined for tailor-made reproduction by bacteria. This would be done through recombinant genetics, that is, through the splicing of human and bacterial DNA in bacterial cells.

A comparison of the relative level of various immune factors in human and cow's milk is shown in Table 15.

NUTRITIONAL STATUS AND IMMUNE RESPONSE

Malnutrition (undernutrition) is a kind of two-headed vampire. The body is drained of vital building blocks needed to produce growth, to build healthy organs, and to energize and maintain itself; at the same time it is compromised in its ability to defend against disease. Infants, already handicapped with undeveloped life processes, are doubly jeopardized. Malnutrition may weaken the mother physically, and it may increase her susceptibility to disease. The child of this woman is similarly affected on both counts. In addition, malnutrition lowers milk yield. The infant's food supply is depleted, and it may be lost entirely. Lastly, the milk, whatever amount there may be, loses nutritional potency; it also loses immune potency. Either one of the latter two factors may result in the death of the child. Together, they form a bestial, unholy alliance.

It is misleading, perhaps, to generalize. Exceptions are occasionally the rule. At least it is known that populations differ; direct comparisons of cause, treatment, and effect of malnutrition are difficult to make. Malnutrition itself is many-sided. Both over- and under-nutrition pose problems. Both vary as to cause. For the undernourished, about which concern here will focus, mild versus severe lack of food (nutrients) are distinctly different situations. (For a general review, see Watson and McMurray, 1979.) Marginal malnutrition

TABLE 15

Comparative Level of Various Immune Factors in Human and Cow's Milk[a]

Immune factor	Human milk	Cow's milk
Lysozyme	++++	+
Lactoperoxidase	+	++++
Secretary IgA	++++	+
IgG	+	++++
IgM	+	+
Lactoferrin	++++	++++
Macrophages	++++	++++
B-lymphocytes	++	N.A.[b]
T-lymphocytes	++	N.A.[b]
B_{12} or folic acid binding factors	++++	++++

[a]Adapted from Goldman (1976).
[b]Not available.

may in fact shore up immune defense systems. Severe malnutrition almost always weakens them. Different defense systems respond differently to differing kinds of malnutrition. Even with a great paucity of data, that last statement appears uncontrovertible. For that reason, some attempt must be made to classify various forms of malnutrition. In this regard, three major forms of nutritional disease states are recognized: (1) kwashiorkor, (2) marasmus, and (3) protein/calorie malnutrition. The first reflects a deficiency of protein but an adequate calorie intake. The second, conversely, results from adequate protein but insufficient calorie intake. The third, obviously, is a lack of both protein and calories in the diet.

Out of the varied kinds of malnutrition often emerges a group of subtle, though important, alterations in the body's defense system. Malnourished children may show normal or even high amounts of circulating antibodies; the titer is right. The antibodies, however, may have lost their ability to neutralize disease. The child may be vaccinated against some crippling disease only to find that the vaccine doesn't "take" as well. It even fails at times. Severe malnutrition will cause this to happen. If the child is unable to develop a fully functioning thymus, because of a lack of food, its body will lack the activator of its T-cell immune defense. Lack of iron and zinc may likewise inhibit this response. Even in a state of moderate malnutrition a child's disease resistance is lowered. If the child is suffering both severe malnutrition (kwashiorkor, protein/calorie malnutrition) *and* infection, treatment may have to center first on the disease, especially diarrheal forms, then nutrient intake. A mother, herself a victim of malnutrition, likewise suffers weakened cell-mediated defenses. She herself is more prone to disease. Whether her milk (colostrum) shows lowered titers of lymphocytes and associated defense agents is not known. It is certainly possible. It is also possible that her weakened body might produce impotent cells. It is known, for example, that macrophages produced under a siege of malnutrition lack full power to synthesize complement proteins. The milk of undernourished test animals (rats) also shows lowered hemolytic complement values. The total white cell count of children appears uninfluenced by nutritional status, but the cells lack some degree of lysozyme activity. Secretory antibodies drop in number under the stress of protein/calorie malnutrition. Lysozyme activity decreases in body secretions, tears, saliva, and the mucosal secretions of the intestinal tract. Another secretion, mother's milk, would also be expected to show a loss in immune activity.

Although much remains to be learned, reason suggests that malnutrition of the mother produces, for the infant who must survive on it, a food enfeebled in immune competency. Moreover, it has been proven beyond doubt that malnutrition increases susceptibility to breast infection. This carries with it its own peculiar set of risks, both to mother and child. (See Chapter 5).

THE PROBLEM OF ALLERGIES

What might a mosquito bite and infant allergy to food have in common? Ill-effects of both conditions may come about, or be mediated, by the presence of IgE (Hamburger, 1976). Here is a situation, then, where the immune system itself becomes part of the problem. It occurs in one of two types of food allergy. An allergic response (hives, asthma, heartburn, headache, cramps, gas pains, or diarrhea) may develop quickly (within 1 minute to 2 hours) or slowly (perhaps 5 days after exposure to the offending allergen or antigen). The former kind of allergy may be called immediate (or obvious), the latter delayed (or occult). Some basic differences exist between them; the quick-response type involves IgE (Breneman, 1978). In this form of allergy, skin tests help in diagnosis (just as a red, itchy spot on the skin gives evidence of a mosquito bite). In this type, too, antihistamines usually provide relief precisely because of the reaction between IgE and certain components of body tissue (mast cells) and blood (basophils). The process could be described as follows.

Suppose, first of all, that the infant has inherited from its mother or father or both a tendency to allergy. This is an important consideration. Allergy is often an inherited ailment. Knowing such conditions exist in the family tree, a mother has one important reason for breast feeding, if at all possible. An allergy may indeed by avoided by so doing. For the moment, however, assume only that an infant is vulnerable. There must then be exposure to an allergen, perhaps a protein of food other than mother's milk, for example. About the only barrier to an allergen in the intestinal tract is sIgA. The infant, of course, lacks this antibody unless it is provided through milk of the mother. Assume that it is not. A protein, or an antigenic fragment of protein, will simply be absorbed whole. The body reacts to the offending agent by producing IgE. The IgE is one specially designed to recognize and bind to this specific antigen. There are, however, two ends to an antibody: the Fc, or base of the Y-shaped antibody, and the Fab, the two protruding fingers of the Y. The fingers are designed to bind to the antigen. The base, the Fc segment, binds in this instance to mast cells or basophils (Hamburger, 1976).

An infant has been exposed to an allergen. IgE has been produced. It has attached itself to mast cells of body tissue. Once again allergen, the same one, is introduced. IgE binds to it and, at the same time, issues a chemical command to the mast cell. In essence, the command calls for release of histamines from numerous small granules that reside in the cell. The order is given, and like soldiers reacting to a commander, the granules release histamines, which, in turn, cause the various disorders that accompany an allergic reaction.

Obviously the preceding has been an oversimplification. The process is terribly complex, and each individual differs. The number of mast cells varies greatly. The number of IgE binding sites per mast cell (or basophil) varies greatly. Even the amount of histamine in the cell and the amount that will be released upon command by IgE vary (Hamburger, 1976). These factors notwithstanding, some kind of allergic response becomes manifest. A mother, especially one aware of family history of allergy, best prevents a problem by breast feeding, that is, by providing nonallergenic food and, at the same time, ample doses of allergy-fighting sIgA (Breneman, 1979).

The newborn is particularly vulnerable. For some few days the stomach is porous, even to whole proteins. The milk of any nonhuman species is more likely to induce an allergy in sensitive infants than mother's milk. Certainly this is true of cow's milk. Similarities between cow's and goat's milk make it likely true for the latter. Soy formulas and infant formulas based on cow's milk, even "humanized" formulas, cannot be considered exempt. A protein carries not one but many potentially antigenic (allergy-causing) sites. Any one alone may incite an allergy. Various studies (Goldman *et al.*, 1963; Lebenthal, 1975; Taylor, 1980) show infants to have reacted to casein, the major milk protein, and to β-lactoglobulin and α-lactalbumin, both whey proteins and common ingredients of milk-based formulas. Some infants also react adversely to lactose, milk sugar. Although the scientific literature reveals fewer allergies to soy formula, the reason may lie partly in less overall use of these products, and therefore, in less exposure to the allergens therein. Also, infants will not react at all similarly. Allergies can be highly specific. Omission even of one ingredient of formula, assuming it is the appropriate one, can cure a food allergy. Ingredient substitutions, therefore, offer one means of treatment. A number of other processing considerations may also be introduced in formulation of special "nonallergenic" infant formulas.

More often than not, soy-based infant formulas become the first step in the treatment of cow's milk allergies. Substitution of soy for milk protein alone may suffice in this regard. Soy formulas are also formulated without lactose, and the absence of this ingredient can obviously make a difference. Thus, one alternative to cow's milk products stands readily available. Goat's milk, too, is another oft-considered substitute. Although success in this approach cannot be entirely discounted, the scientific literature gives little reason for high hopes. Both cow's and goat's milk contain lactose to similar levels. In addition, major protein components of cow's milk are likewise found in goat's milk. These include both β-lactoglobulin and α-lactalbumin. Admittedly, some structural difference exists between the β-lactoglobulin of cow's and goat's milk. The α-lactalbumin of goat's milk is apparently devoid of the amino acid methionine. This could be a significant difference, as could the absence from goat's milk of one fraction of casein. Goat's milk contains κ-casein, β-casein, and α_{s2}-casein; they are in close, though not necessarily identical, semblance of those same components of cow's milk. Goat's milk is devoid, however, of α_{s1}-casein (Jenness, 1980). If this lack offers hope, research yet remains to be done to prove it valid. In immunological tests considerable cross-reaction is found between goat's and cow's milk protein. This fact would suggest little benefit in feeding goat's milk to most infant victims of cow's milk allergy.

Of all proteins of milk, β-lactoglobulin is often the one most suspect in cases of infant allergy. This arises in part from knowledge that mother's milk is essentially devoid of this protein. Scientific findings also suggest a high frequency of involvement (Goldman et al., 1963a, b; Bleumink and Young, 1968; Lebenthal, 1975). It is possible, too, that it is not β-lactoglobulin per se but a reaction product between lactose and the protein that constitutes an antigen. This product would form when milk or lactose-containing formula is heated to a high temperature and undergoes discoloration, or browning. In addition, researchers have found allergenic properties in both native, whole protein and in fragments thereof—as, for example, in the breakdown products of β-lactoglobulin under the influence of pepsin, the digestive enzyme. Here, though, one must distinguish between problems of the newborn and the infant of even 2 to 3 months of age. The former, with its feeble digestive system and porous stomach, is more vulnerable to whole proteins and must deal, at the very least, with whole proteins as antigens. In the older infant, the digestion of protein is more complete. At that point, and with the stomach a more tightly-knit screen, the infant must cope with the protein digest. At least United States Department of Agriculture (USDA) researchers see it that way. Allergy-causing fragments of protein, according to this source, may originate in β-lactoglobulin, α-lactalbumin, serum albumin, and casein. If differences in the fractional component of casein are in fact meaningful and if, in fact, the absence of α_{s1}-casein in goats milk is significant, this might well be the circumstance.

It is important to note, however, that the diagnosis of food allergy is not easy to make (Taylor, 1980). Symptoms are similar for a number of disease states. Few precise diagnostic tools exist. Perhaps the best method of pinpointing food allergy is to introduce new foods or new ingredients of foods one at a time at 3–5 day intervals. If an allergic response is noted, the food may be removed and a retest made some time later. When one formula is exchanged for another, care should be taken to note carefully the specific ingredient in each so as to distinguish rather precisely the differences between them.

Luckily, allergy to milk often wanes or vanishes entirely with time. In anywhere from 17 to 85% of the cases, this happens by the end of the first year (Bahna, 1978). Those percentages go up at 2 years of age. Incidence of true milk allergy, as founded on rigorous scientific diagnosis, appears to run somewhere between 0.3 and 7.5% (Bahna, 1980). A problem exists, but it is not all-inclusive. Nonetheless, any mother with a known family history of allergy would do well to consider breast-feeding solely for 3–4 months. A problem could very well be avoided, or at least delayed, until such time as the infant is better able to cope.

It is important to note, however, that infants may exhibit an allergic response to breast milk. Kulangara (1980) has demonstrated the presence of wheat antigens in milk of lactating women consuming wheat as a regular part of the diet. Other food antigens (or fragments thereof), once ingested may also comprise a part of milk composition. Such antigens can produce typical allergic responses, including diarrhea, in breast-feeding infants. Kulangara (1980) warns of serious implications for sensitive infants, particularly Third World infants who, because of prenatal malnutrition—intrauterine malnutrition—are born "small-for-date."

ADDITIVES AND IMMUNITY

A disease bacteria produces illness by breaking down body defenses, that is, the immune system. Is it possible, then, that a food constituent might breach those same defenses? Is it possible that additives or naturally occurring food components might simply weaken the immune system at some point. If a leak is sprung, the body lies more prone to attack from other disease agents. These are possibilities, of course. Immune responses are fast becoming one of the most exquisitely sensitive measures of toxicity in matters of this kind. Thus, testing the nature of chemical compounds by this method is usually carried out *in vitro* (outside the body). Results do not necessarily apply to the situation *in vivo* (in the functioning human body). Evidence of an adverse response cannot be ignored. It should be viewed, however, with perspective and with understanding that this is a profoundly complex area of research.

At least one additive approved for the use in infant formulas has been found to suppress one immune body, the macrophage (Thompson *et al.*, 1976). Carrageenan, a stabilizer, in *in vitro* studies, gives evidence of tying up this immune agent. Carrageenan is not absorbed through the stomach wall, though. It could not, therefore, interfere with the activity of immune cells therein.

Other additives or their breakdown products have been found to block other immune processes. Gallic acid, a metabolite of the preservative propyl gallate, inhibits activity of T-lymphocytes under certain conditions (Archer *et al.*, 1977b). Tannic acid, native to tea, does much the same (see Archer, 1978). BHA, another preservative, has also been shown to sabotage the immune machinery (Archer *et al.*, 1977a). Neither propyl gallate nor BHA are recommended additives for infant formulas (see Appendix 6). They are evidence of a kind of risk, though, heretofore scarcely considered.

BUILDING IMMUNE FACTORS INTO INFANT FORMULA

A healthy mother generates a broad spectrum of immune factors directly into breast milk. Science now suggests that many of these same or similar components can be isolated from cow's milk and added to infant formula. Natural cheese whey, as one possible source, contains low levels of immunoglobulins, lysozyme, and lactoferrin. It has in it considerable amounts of lactoperoxidase. Interferon—of the type found in humans and now being readied for commercial production through bacteria treated by recombinant genetics (gene-splicing)—should one day be available in amounts and at a cost that make possible its use in formula. Other immune factors are available now.

You will recall that the main immunoglobulin of mother's milk is IgA. The cow produces far more IgG than IgA. The two are similar in action, however, and the latter could possibly serve nicely in lieu of IgA. Two forms of IgG exist: IgG_1 and IgG_2. Both are found in the colostrum of cows, but the former is at much higher levels. Thus, research has focused on this immunoglobulin as a replacer for IgA of mother's milk, and mainly in its potential to defend against various strains of disease-causing *E. coli*. (For a general review of this subject, see Nestlé, 1975.)

Bovine IgG_1 and native lactoferrin, also obtained from cow's milk, together achieve good inhibition of *E. coli*; they work together better than if either is used singly. The same is true for IgA and transferrin. For now, we will concentrate on the IgG system.

Obviously, it would be possible to concentrate natural IgG from colostrum of cows. However, that IgG, though having some potency against human disease, would not necessarily show the kind of specificity desired. In fact, it would be a comparatively weak agent. Thus, the major issue revolves around the production of IgG antibodies against specific intestinal diseases of infants.

The Problem

An infant formula is desired that contains immune agents similar to those found in mother's milk. It is preferable to start with those immune agents able to attack those bacteria most commonly the cause of infant diarrhea. The name given these organisms is *Escherichia coli*. Not all strains of *E. coli* cause intestinal disease, but they are all more or less inhabitants of the intestinal tract. Any time one or more disease-causing *E. coli* attaches itself on or along the intestinal wall, a predisposing condition to diarrhea is being met. If these outlanders are grouped together, they may be called *enteropathogenic coliform*. Entero means intestinal, for that's where they reside; pathogenic is used because they cause disease. Colonization of the intestinal lining is apparently essential to onset of the disease state. To aid the process by which colonies form, *E. coli* have evolved a mat of hairlike appendages (fimbriae). As single cells of the organism move along the gut wall, these hairs wiggle, feel, and grasp for a hold; their action resembles a mountain climber feeling his way up a shear rock face. These hairy feelers would undoubtedly find a hold and latch on were it not for the presence of immune agents, that is, antibodies. It is in the nature of an antibody response that a kind of slippery covering is thrown over the fimbriae. It is as though the mountaineer's fingers had been coated with grease.

Obviously it would be a miraculous advance if infant formula could be "fortified" with those antibodies known to defend specifically against human disease strains of *E. coli*. A nursing mother provides just this sort of protection. Her antibodies not only survive the harsh environment of the stomach, they even alter the germs, making them more vulnerable to the search-and-destroy missions of phagocytes, the large cellular bodies that envelope and suck from the disease agents the very juice of life. The question is, how do we get the same kind of defense mechanism built into formula?

Nestlé's Solution

In attacking a problem of this kind, scientists start with the scientific literature. They do this to find out what has been done anywhere in the world that remotely suggests a possible route of experimentation for the problem. Typically, they discover a lot of people working on bits and pieces of various segments of the puzzle, though perhaps (even likely) with entirely different goals in mind. In this case, they would find a possible line of attack. The idea originated with a University of Minnesota scientist renowned for his research on the cow's udder and the complicated mechanism by which it makes milk. The literature is crowded with his name, but what concerns us here is that segment of his work dealing with immune concepts.

The scientist, William E. Petersen, claimed that cows could be made to produce antibodies specific to the diseases of humans. This could be done by stimulating the cow to defend against those very diseases or poisons, and in a way not at all unlike the way a person would be "immunized."

Nonetheless, Nestlé and other scientists took up Petersen's idea (see

Nestlé, 1975; Hilpert *et al.*, 1975). They began by immunizing the cow during pregnancy. They took 13 various disease-causing strains of *E. coli* and brewed them into a vaccine, which was then used to give the cows a "shot." Theory held that the cows would respond by producing antibodies specific to those 13 types (called serotypes because they are distinguishable only by immunological methods) of enteropathogenic *E. coli.*

Cows, like other mammals, produce antibodies specific to diseases of the calf. Like other mammals, they assemble this arsenal for a single massive defense during the first 5–6 days of life, when the calf is most vulnerable. The colostrum that is produced during this time is extra rich in antibodies. If a cow is induced to produce antibodies against human disease, the colostrum would hold the richest store.

Antibodies in milk are found in the serum, the waterlike liquid remaining after large suspended materials are removed. Fat can simply be separated off as cream. Most casein drops out when rennin (curd-clotting enzyme) and acid (in this case citric acid) are added to pH 4.6. A centrifuge spins the serum clean. However, other contaminants (lactose and mineral salts) remain. For the most part, these are removed by ultrafiltration and diafiltration, which further refine the protein antibodies. Following this, all that need be done is to remove bacteria and other spoilage or disease agents. High heat or other harsh treatments cannot be considered because the antibodies themselves would be denatured (destroyed). Sterilization must be achieved by filtration. The microorganisms are filtered by running the antibody-containing liquid through what amounts to an extra fine sieve. A clear liquid suspension of antibodies percolates from the filter. To concentrate and preserve it, the material is freeze-dried under sterile conditions. The resulting powder, a somewhat refined fraction of colostrum milk, is the final product. It contains from 40% to 45% immunoglobulins. These must be proven to be active against those same 13 serotypes of disease-producing *E. coli.* This proof will require technical assistance from some specialists in immunology and pediatrics.

In Nestlé's experiment four specialists were added to a team of four Nestlé scientists (see Hilpert *et al.*, 1975). Two members came from Autonomous University School of Medicine, Children's Hospital of the Seguridad Social, Barcelona, Spain; a third from Children's Hospital, Cité Hospitaliére, Lille, France; and a fourth from the Department of Pediatrics, University of Geneva, Switzerland.

Three routes of attack can be used to test immune specificity of antibodies. "Test-tube" (*in vitro*) experiments are one approach. But such tests do not always reflect what happens inside the body (*in vivo*). Therefore, mice or other animals can be brought into the picture. Test animals like these can be exposed first to the disease agents, then to the antibody mixture. Controls will indicate whether or not the antibodies are effective. Nonetheless, although the physiology of humans and mice may be closely related, it is not one and the same. The mixture of antibodies will eventually have to be tested in clinical trials on human infants.

In the first step of the Nestlé experiment, antibody activity was checked against presensitized red blood cells of sheep. The results gave some evidence of the relative strength of the antibody titer. Next, the antibodies were mixed with cultures of the *E. coli* organisms that they were supposed to inactivate. This was done in a liquid medium containing minimum nutrients (along with 1% glucose) for *E. coli* growth. Various amounts of antibody powder were added to a known number of organisms, and the mixture was incubated at a temperature favorable for growth of *E. coli*. Samples were taken each hour, and the numbers of coliform were determined by standard culture plate methods. If the antibodies had no effect, the growth of *E. coli* would be uninhibited. All mixtures, irrespective of amount of "antibody" powder present, would show equivalent growth, or numbers, of *E. coli*. But this is not what happened. The numbers of *E. coli* were reduced in more or less direct proportion to the amount of antibodies added. Step number one was a success.

In the experiment done on mice, one test organism of *E. coli* was selected to serve as a lethal challenge to the animals. Culture 0111:k58(B4), as it was known, was diluted in 5% sterile hog mucin, and various dose-strengths, four in all, were made up. The four doses (500; 5,000; 50,000; and 500,000 bacteria) were then injected directly into mice of similar size and age; five mice were injected at each dose-rate. To one such group of mice, plain saline was given to serve as control. Three other such groups were given 10, 25, and 100 μg of antibody material. Another three groups were given similar doses of normal cow (unimmunized) antibody powder obtained by the same extraction process as the test material.

This test was easy to read; after 48 hours a count was made of the number of dead mice. Given saline, all mice at all levels of challenge died. Protected with only 10 μg of antibody material, all but 2 mice, these 2 at the lowest rate of challenge with *E. coli*, died (i.e., there were 2 survivors of 20 mice). At 25 μg of protective substance, only 9 of 20 mice were found dead, and at 100 μg of antibodies, all mice at all doses of challenge survived.

The preceding evidence strongly suggested the presence of antibodies specific to the strain of *E. coli* used as test disease agent. The same experiment, using other coli strains, produced similar evidence. However, questions remained: Was the protection afforded the mice a product of the hyperimmunization treatment of cows, or was it rather a protective component normal to colostrum milk of cows? The 60 mice (5 at each injection dose of *E. coli* $= 20 \times 3$ levels of "protection" with "normal" (unimmunized) cow antibody fraction) would provide an answer. The evidence was unmistakable. Every single mouse died.

Opsonization Tests

Opsonization is the process by which germs are altered by antibodies, altered in such a way that they are made more vulnerable to attack and destruction by roving phagocytes. This is a highly focused process, and only antibodies specific to a given germ appear to have opsonizing ability. Thus, proof of opsonization further adds to proof a specificity of a given antibody. If antibodies induced into cow's milk were going to function as human antibodies, they would have to show this ability. In turn, this kind of activity would be an aid in clearing from the infant body the germ(s) that would otherwise cause diarrhea.

In short, *in vivo* tests using mice gave clear evidence of the specificity of the cow's milk antibodies to the opsonization process.

Antibody Survival in the Human Stomach

Thus far in the experiment, the antibodies produced by cows seemed to be working just as though a human had produced them. Still, human milk antibodies had another well-known advantage. Somehow they managed to survive and carry out their protective function in the infant's stomach where acid and enzymes attacked other proteins with impunity. Would the cow's milk antibodies be able to do likewise?

Putting this question to test, the scientists first induced cows to produce antibodies against tetanus infection. (Antitetanus activity is easy to detect and is a more or less foolproof measure.) These antibodies, obtained in exactly the same way as the others, were first submitted to testtube conditions similar to those encountered in the stomach. Acid (or alkali) was added to appropriate pH levels. Trypsin was then given a chance to break down the antibody over 2 hours of exposure. Then pepsin (at a pH conducive to its activity) was given a like opportunity. After this combined treatment, the level of activity of the antitetanus antibody was checked by a standard hemagglutination test. The results showed that "considerable" antitetanus activity yet remained. Although that was promising, the true test had to be done on infants. Test tubes and test-tube conditions are simply not the same as those present in a living human. Therefore, clinical trials were set up.

Clinical Trials

The first clinical studies on human infants were done at Children's Hospital in Geneva, Switzerland, and were designed only to determine whether or not "human" *E. coli* antibodies produced in cow's milk could survive the digestive process of the human stomach and intestines (Hilpert *et al.*, 1975). In all, 11 infants became test subjects. All were patients of the hospital, and all were admitted for reason(s) other than the presence of gastrointestinal distress. Their ages ranged from 2 weeks to 13 months.

In these trials the infants were fed 2 g antibody substance/kg body weight; this was divided between the meals taken over a 1-day period. Both the first and last feedings were tagged with a harmless red dye. Stool samples were taken both 12 hours before and up to 48–60 hours after the last feeding of antibodies. These specimens were then checked for any remaining cow's milk anticoliform antibodies or fragments thereof. The antibodies themselves or the pieces that remained were identified by an analytical procedure called immunoelectrophoresis. Lastly, any intact or even fragmented antibodies were repurified and tested for activity in mice, just as earlier tests had done.

Again, results were positive and clear-cut. Both intact and fragmented antibodies were found in the stool samples. One such fragment, thought to occur under normal stomach conditions but yet possessing antibody activity, was even tested for opsonization potency. Activity was found to be nearly as great as in the native antibody. When the purified stool antibodies were tested in mice, they fought off *E. coli* with a fierceness that equaled their "undigested" counterparts.

Final Proof

In the end, the only truly valid test of immune potency of cow's milk antibodies must come in feeding trials of infants. Even then, two avenues of research might be undertaken. One would be use of cow-produced antibodies as preventive medicine, so to speak. The other would be their use in treating a disease state. The scientists in this instance chose the latter, and Children's Hospitals in Lille, France, and Barcelona, Spain, became the focuses for experimentation.

In total, the French hospital treated 61 cases of infant diarrhea, the Spanish hospital 95. Treatment consisted solely of feeding cow's milk antibodies at the rate of 1 g/kg body weight, along with an otherwise normal diet. No drugs were given. All infants were under 7 months of age. Treatment carried through 10 days when conditions seemed to warrant it. Stool specimens were examined at regular intervals for numbers of *E. coli*. In addition, other symptoms were evaluated as under routine medical practice. Finally, 43 cases of infant gastroenteritis served as controls. These infants were fed only cow's milk antibodies from nontreated (nonimmunized) cows.

Table 16 summarizes the test results. Note that the results were grouped according to four clinical possibilities: (1) disappearance of both *E. coli* in stools and of symptoms of disease, (2) disappearance of *E. coli* but

TABLE 16

Success Rate of Treatment of Infant _E. coli_ Gastroenteritis with Cow-Induced Immunoglobulins of Milk[a]

Code No[b]	Barcelona, Spain 95 cases	%	Lille, France 61 cases	%	Total 156 cases	%	Controls 43 cases	%
1	42	44.2	34	55.7	76	48.7	14	27.7
2	14	14.7	—	—	14	9.0	—	—
3	18	18.9	12	19.7	30	19.2	—	—
4	21	22.1	15	24.6	36	23.1	29	67.4

[a] Adapted from Hilpert, _et al._ (1975). Courtesy of the editor of the XIII Symposium and of the Swedish Nutrition Foundation, Goleborg, Sweden.

[b] Code 1: Disappearance of _E. coli_ from fecal cultures and also definite clinical improvement of the infant. Code 2: Disappearance of _E. coli_ from fecal cultures, but clinical symptoms remain. Code 3: Clinical success, but _E. coli_ still detected in fecal cultures. Code 4: Within 10 days of observation, symptoms of disease remaind, as did presence of _E. coli_ in fecal samples.

symptoms unchanged, (3) disappearance of symptoms but _E. coli_ still remaining in stool samples, and (4) presence both of _E. coli_ and symptoms of disease. Data in this table are taken from only the first 10 days of experimentation. In those cases where further treatment was considered desirable, the antibody feeding continued over an additional 10 days. In several such cases, _E. coli_ were found eventually to disappear.

A glance at Table 16 gives good evidence of the effectiveness of feeding cow's milk antibodies. Nearly half the infections cleared up within 10 days; that is, the _E. coli_ were eliminated, and the symptoms of ailment vanished. In contrast, using the same standard, the success rate among the control group ran only about 28%. Total failure in the control group hit 67.4%. Among infants given active _E. coli_ antibodies, failure rate ran less than 25%. Another 28.2% either improved in bacteriological or clinical symptoms. Overall, then, some improvement in the status of the disease state took place in over ¾ of the "treated" infants.

A few other important facts should be noted. First, in those cases where fecal cultures came up negative for coliform, stool consistency improved faster on lactose-free formula. Second, in general, best results were obtained using high doses of immune agent over a short period. Third, since this work was done, additional benefit has been shown to occur through addition of serum antibodies of vaccinated cows and horses. In addition, further clinical trials on premature infants have also proven successful; moreover, the results have been rated as highly statistically significant. It should be remembered that, although immunoglobulins serve best in combination with other immune factors, IgG alone was tested in these trials. IgG potency could be greatly enhanced with the addition of lysozyme, lactoferrin, and lactoperoxidase. Further help could come from D-mannose and α-methyl-mannoside, both of which inhibit adhesion of bacterial cells to the intestinal wall at concentrations as low as 0.003 mg/ml. The bifidus factor or *L. acidophilis* could supplement the entire mix.

All clinical trials thus far performed have all been made to test the cure rate of diseases already established. The use of "immune" formulas as preventive of disease opens a whole new world of possibilities.

5

Mammary Infections, Drugs, and Environmental Pollutants

MAMMARY INFECTIONS

Mastitis, a disease state of the mammary gland, is the most common ailment of milking animals. Infections of the udder occur almost universally among the cow population, but they are not always serious. More often than not they go unnoticed. Nonetheless, they occur at a high rate of incidence. Where sanitation practices are good, the rate of infection runs nearly 50%. Although less than 2% will show clinical signs, that is, redness (inflammation) and swelling, a disease state exists in all cases. In some few ways the milk supply will reflect that fact.

Serious infections cause changes in milk composition and, worse, loss of yield. Under seige, milk-making functions are befouled; the debris of defense battlements, immune bodies, litter the food. Upon healing, scar tissue replaces milk-making tissue. Some or much of the ability to produce milk is lost. Rarely does mastitis cause extreme damage, except when medical aid and drugs are lacking. Mild infections create little permanent harm, but compositional changes in milk take place anyway. The difference is one mainly of degree.

A disease of the mammary gland obviously adds immune bodies to milk. These may persist for some time after the infection has cleared. In milk of cows, fat content usually drops. Casein commonly remains relatively constant or decreases slightly. Other proteins, such as globulins and albumins, increase. Because the inner flesh of the mammary gland is being eaten away, certain blood components flow into the milk more or less unimpeded. Thus, chlorides and sodium content go up. To compensate (osmotically) for the increase in chlorides, a corresponding decrease occurs in lactose content. The pH rises because alkaline compounds are released into the milk from the blood. In addition, there is a slight decrease in calcium level, but magnesium, iron, copper, and zinc all increase to some small extent. Quite likely the increases in mineral content (with the exception of calcium, which is associated partly with the casein, and therefore influenced differently) are due to a general lowering of milk yield. All factors considered, milk of mastitic cows is a poor source of food for infants.

Data on changes in human milk composition during breast infections are sketchy indeed. In relatively mild cases, the protein and ascorbic acid levels decline. In more severe cases, the fat and lactose content drops, and the levels of zinc, aluminum and silicon fall. Both copper and manganese content tend to rise (Grebennikov and Luzhkovaya, 1977). In one comparison of mastitic versus healthy lactating women, protein content averaged 1.4% in milk of the former and 1.6% in the latter. The pH of human milk is naturally higher than in cow's milk, and may range from 6.7 to 7.4 in colostrum (Ansell *et al.*, 1977). Evidence of changes due to infections is lacking. The cell count of the milk does increase, obviously, and in serious infections reaches 4.5 million/ml (Chumak and Kozyrev, 1973). Normally, the cell count in human milk averages near 600,000 at childbirth.

Comparing milk of an infected breast with milk of an uninfected breast of the same woman, researchers in the United States found higher levels of sodium and chloride in the former, as would be expected. The magnitude of this difference is perhaps more surprising. The average sodium content was 108 mEq/liter, chloride 88.0 mEq/liter. Milk of the healthy breast averaged 3.0 and 7.0 mEq/liter, respectively (Conner, 1979). Such findings are, of course, of practical significance. High levels of sodium and chloride impart to milk a salty flavor, and infants are known to reject such milk. Chronic infections of the breast, then, must be seen as at least one cause of poor feeding habits of breast-fed infants. If the flavor of the milk is not alone to blame, the difficulty in extracting milk—that is, in suckling—may add another factor.

Aside from the preceding potential causes of infection, is it possible that infant food itself can promote disease? For infant formula the answer is yes. Any of a number of disease germs might find their way into the food and cause illness. Although the function of food processing is to prevent that, it can happen. Less apparently, mother's milk may also be a carrier of disease by a process not unlike that which poisons an infant formula.

A rather large number of infecting germs can cause mastitis. This is true of both animals and humans. For the cow population at least, the evidence is strong that introduction and extended use of antibiotics have done little or nothing to reduce the rate of infection. Instead, these drugs have only altered the ratio of various infecting germs to each other. At one time streptococcal bacteria accounted for over 50% of mastitis infections. This group now accounts for less than 40%. Another group of bacteria, staphylococci, once far less significant, now tops the list at nearly 60%. Treatment with antibiotics only paved the way by killing off the more sensitive (to antibiotics) competition. Udder infections of dairy cows still run high.

The data on the extent of mastitis among humans are so scarce as to be practically nonexistent. One can only assume that it ranges much higher than is apparent on the surface. As mentioned, most such infections create no visible signs of ill health in the nursing mother. Only a few medical researchers, confronted by infant illness, take the laborious steps necessary to track the illness to its source. Few surveys are taken among lactating women generally. It is not surprising that far more is known of mastitis of cows than of the human family. Nonetheless, the meager evidence gleaned thus far deserves mention. First, the rate of mastitis infections seems to run higher among women who deliver their children outside of hospitals or professional clinics (Mares *et al.*, 1975). This would not appear unusual in that sanitation practices obviously play a major role in the contraction of breast infections. Some observers state that the infection rate in hospitals, under ideal conditions, can be held to less than 1% (Kohler and Amon, 1974). However, this may be true only of serious infections. Acute mastitis has been diagnosed in 2.5% of breast-feeding mothers in one study in the United States. Importantly, *Staphylococcus aureus* was the offending organism in 23 of 48 samples of infected milk brought under scrutiny (Marshall *el al.*, 1975). But again, these were cases of severe mastitis. In a Polish investigation (Nowakowski, *et al.*, 1976), which is very likely quite repeatable elsewhere, milk samples from 100 women, selected at random and showing no overt signs of infection, were found to contain staphylococci in many cases. *Staphylococcus epidermis* and *S. aureus* were detected in 63 of the 100 samples. Over 82% of 60 strains of *S. aureus* were found to produce toxins. Though *S. epidermis* is a generally less virulent microbe than *S. aureus*, it has been shown to cause alterations in the mammary gland of mice, and some strains are know to produce toxin.

Most common among infectious agents of the human breast are staphylococcus. Other infecting organisms include *Proteus*, coliform, *Streptococcus, Pseudomonas, Klebsiella,* and *Candida*, and possibly descending in incidence in the order of presentation. Again, data are most scarce. However, taking lessons from the scientific literature on both cows and humans, some pertinent assumptions can perhaps be made:

1. The rate of infections of the human breast likely runs far above visible or palpable evidence of their presence.
2. The infection rate may run relatively high even in clean, sanitary surroundings, and under hygienic practices of infant feeding.
3. The rate of infection and specific types of pathogens involved may vary widely within a community and over the world.
4. Unsanitary conditions and practices can only be expected to increase the rate of infection and add to the disease burden of the breast-fed child.

Of the many disease germs that may infect the human breast, staphylococci perhaps pose the most serious threat to the feeding infant. They are everywhere. They are in soil. They inhabit the human body. The nose, hands, and skin can be carriers. A nursing infant may spread staphylococci to the mother by the very act of feeding itself. The mouth is a potential reservoir; boils, pimples, and other skin eruptions are additional sources. Soiled diapers harbor the organisms. They invade and reside in the human intestinal tract. A nursing mother may bathe in polluted water; if fresh water or the fuel to boil water is lacking, that same water may serve to liquefy dry infant formula. Both the mother and the formula will carry disease. A mother might also use a dirty wash rag for sponging off the breasts. The transfer of disease is a mindless matter. It is made better or worse only by the environment in which humanity must live.

Polish scientists have found disease-causing strains of staphylococci to occur "very often" in human milk. The literature substantiates that fact (Knorr, 1957; Montgomery *et al.*, 1959; Rantasalo and Kauppinen, 1959; Foster and Harris, 1960; Burbianka *et al.*, 1973). The unresolved question is, To what extent do such infections cause infant illness? The toxin(s) in this case must be produced as the bacteria grow and multiply in the breast of the nursing mother. It must then be present in sufficient amounts or be sufficiently toxic to produce, upon feeding, symptoms of disease. Evidence suggests that it happens possibly far more frequently than one might suspect. Because it can happen during low-grade (subclinical) infections, and because no pain or no visible signs of infection may be present, it may escape detection. However, characteristically, the infant becomes ill shortly after feeding.

Just how significant is the problem? Some scientific findings may help provide perspective. First, pathogenic staphylococci are the major cause of acute and chronic disease of the mammary gland of both cows and humans

(Niskanen *et al.*, 1978). Major toxins produced in both species appear to be α and β hemolysins. Toxin has been found in milk of cows with as low as 100–1000 organisms/ml (Niskanen, *et al.*, 1978). Injection of as little as 1.0 μg toxin (in a milk suspension) into an udder causes a reaction (irritation). Toxin has also been found in human milk with counts of staphylococci as low as 100/ml. Counts as high as 30,000/ml have been noted. The level of toxin intake by infants can approximate 1–2 μg per feeding. In the study from which the latter facts were established, Polish scientists (Burbianka *et al.*, 1973) determined the relative prevalence of this disease state; infant illness was used as a reason for evaluating the milk. Two sources of milk were analyzed. One came from women who were providing milk to a "lactarium," where their milk was being used as infant food. The other source came from medical doctors who took samples from nursing mothers whose infants were showing signs of intestinal disorders. Of 214 samples from the former source, 43 showed positive for presence of pathogenic staphylococci. Of the latter, 90 of 215 samples were positive. Certainly these are relatively high percentages of staphylococcal infection. Not all may have produced disease symptoms in the infant, but the potential was there. Moreover, these results were found in a nation that takes above-average steps to nurture its infants and children properly. The scientists in this case concluded that the amount of toxin(s), though small, was sufficient to provoke illness. Sensitive infants might respond to levels as low as 1 μg. Finnish scientists (Niskanen *et al.*, 1978) came to a similar opinion. They reported that enterotoxins produced by *Staphylococcus aureus* in the milk of nursing mothers may represent a danger to the health of the infant.

Further evidence comes from another Polish study (Dluzniewska, 1966), one which no doubt prompted the work cited earlier. The subjects were breast-fed infants showing symptoms of stomach trouble. Milk from the mothers was analyzed, and a large number of these samples were found to be harboring staphylococci. This was often the case even when visible signs of infection were missing. Infants, though, evidenced all the classical symptoms of staphylococcal food poisoning: stomach cramps and vomiting soon after feeding, diarrhea shortly thereafter, and eventual loss of body weight. Continued feeding led to more generalized illness. Upon switching to infant formula, disease gave way to "quick improvement" in health.

These findings should not be taken to mean that all infant formula is free of toxin(s) from this source. What they mean is that cow's milk formula, under sanitary conditions of production and processing, may very well represent less overall hazard than breast milk of *some* nursing mothers. Where sanitation and other conditions are generally bad—as reflected in the masses of unschooled, poverty-stricken persons of the world—the infant is literally placed in double jeopardy. Any survey of the cause of infant death that fails to distinguish these two vectors of disease misrepresents the facts. The true villain can never be the appropriate use of high-quality formula for feeding infants. Rather, ignorance and poverty make of its use a travesty and a sham.

A report presented at the 1981 meeting of the American Society for Microbiology also implicated *S. aureus* in the disease that is termed *toxic shock syndrome*. At first the disease was thought to be restricted to women who used tampons. Now reports of health authorities confirm cases in a small number of women who do not use tampons and in males. The disease has been observed to occur following surgery or, in some women, following birth of a child. Irrespective of the cause, however, the toxin associated with the syndrome has been found in breast-milk of afflicted women. Thus far it is known only that toxin reaches the milk. Whether or not the disease itself can be transmitted through the milk supply is not known.

As for the common kinds of breast infections, the mother herself is obviously the best safeguard against them. Diagnosed at an early stage, such infections are more readily treated, and often without resort to drugs. A concerned mother will therefore keep watch for cracked nipples or unusual redness or swelling of the breast(s). Treatment of cracked, sore nipples may call for little more than use of lanolin, or exposure of the breast(s) to air or to heat of a 75-watt light bulb. Breast infections per se, often respond to continued milking—by hand expression if necessary—plus applications of heat in the form of hot washcloths, a plastic overlay, and low heat from a heating pad. As a general rule, nursing women should avoid use ot tight-fitting bras that may cut off blood circulation. For severe infection, antibiotic or other drug treatment may be indicated. In this event, only those antibiotics or those drugs generally considered both effective and *safe* for the breast-feeding infant (if breast feeding is continued) should be used. Consult a medical counselor for advice in this respect. It is also well to know that antibiotics are more quickly shed from the milk supply by frequent, complete expression of milk from the affected breast(s). Not only is the level of the antibiotic more quickly reduced, stasis—stoppage of the flow of blood and healing fluids—is prevented. The need for the continuous expression of milk for either reason cannot be overemphasized, at least in most cases.

If the above treatment serves the nursing mother, it is equally important for the same reason in handling infected or drug-treated cows. At issue are the composition and nutritive quality of the milk as food (or ingredient in infant formula) for infants, and also the residues of the antibiotic in the milk. The amount of antibiotics used on diseased cows is literally measurable in tons per year. The level of residue is strictly monitored and is especially important for milk to be used in infant formula. By regulation in the United States, milk from antibiotic-treated cows must be withheld from markets, usually for 72 hours. Normally, with continued milking of treated animals, antibiotics will have cleared the milk within this period of time. Any residual will—or should be—below the level of detectability of methods currently applied in determining presence of antibiotics in milk. On individual farm supplies, this implies an amount of 0.05 units or less of penicillin per milliliter. For pooled, stored supplies of milk ready for processing, the level drops to nearly 0.005 units/ml, or to some level preset by the regulatory authority. In any event, the final level of residual can only be as low as the sensitivity of a given method of measuring antibiotic residues. Procedures have improved greatly over recent years, and, along with them, the level of detectability of antibiotics in milk has become more sensitive.

There are reasons for emphasizing the preceding facts. One has to do with the possibility of an infant reacting adversely to intake of antibiotics. Some very few infants may be most sensitive indeed. Either mother's milk or cow's milk (or milk-based formula) could be a source. There is also growing evidence of the evolution of antibiotic-resistant strains of disease bacteria. The more widespread the use of antibiotics, and, therefore, exposure of germs to them, the higher the probability that mutant or otherwise resistant strains will emerge. This is a growing problem. Antibiotic treatment, some-times sorely needed, becomes that much less effective. There is also a small body of evidence that antibiotics, though serving to destroy a disease agent, may in some meaningful way, in infants particularly, curtail one or the other of the infant's own emerging immune systems. In such case, one is struck by the obvious advantage of the use of "immune" formula and of antibodies more or less native to the human body. However, these remedies are still largely in the future. For the present, one should keep in mind the problem of antibiotic residues in milk and remember that a treated, unknowing mother can feed to her infant a massive dose through breast milk as compared to any well-monitored residual of cow's milk or milk-based formula.

Antibiotics constitute only one group of an almost limitless number of other drugs that may enter the milk of a nursing mother. In today's society, this fact is of particular importance.

DRUGS AND THE NURSING MOTHER

Consider the young mother of a first-born; she may be tense, and anxious, and have access to a supply of diazepam (Valium). Possibly there remains in the medicine cabinet a stock of barbituates that might also provide relief. A constipated mother may resort to use of a laxative. A mother may take reserpine, for hypertension, or lithium as an anti-depressant, or pheno-barbital as an anti-convulsant. Finally, consider a heroin addict, whose infant became an addict in the womb or an addicted mother who now seeks control over her addiction through regular use of methadone.

Pills and drugs are a way of life for many. One of the most serious risks to breast-feeding infants is the drug needs—or habits—of the mother. Whether she sniffs it, eats it, inserts is as an anal or vaginal suppository, or injects it, more or less of the drug courses the tissues and blood and finally enters the breast milk. The difference in method of administration determines the amount of drug that finally enters the blood and the speed with which it reaches the capillaries of the breast (O'Brien, 1974).

For some drugs, level attained in breast milk may be small, perhaps even miniscule. Some drugs are not considered particularly harmful; possibly, then, no great risk is posed. But, as in other hazards to health, the infant's size, immature kidneys, and relatively undeveloped enzyme system make it particularly vulnerable. Binding of chemicals to glucuronic acid, for example, is one of the major routes by which potentially harmful components are rendered "safe" to the body. Two other processes—acetylation and oxidation—are likewise useful detoxification mechanisms. Yet neither these nor the former become fully functioning systems for 2 or more weeks after birth (see O'Brien, 1974). An infant's age and relative size are therefore significant factors. Although an infant may ingest only a miniscule amount of a drug during any one feeding, an infant feeds several times a day. The drug may accumulate to an amount that can even be considered therapeutic. That in itself may not be greatly harmful, depending upon the specific drug involved. But it can be. Mothers should be forewarned that many pertinent considerations remain unclear and untested, and that research, often done on animals, may not apply to the human body.

The mother's health also may play a role in amount of drug reaching her milk supply. If the kidneys are weak or diseased, more of every dose of drug she takes is carried to the milk. The same is generally true for smaller women. A smaller person may find withdrawal time—the time necessary for any given amount of drug to clear the body—lengthened. Even the kind of food consumed before, with, or after a drug is taken may effect overall amount reaching the blood and, therefore, the milk.

Several other factors determine the degree to which a drug contaminates the milk. These include (1) various aspects of milk composition, (2) degree of ionization of the drug (pK), (3) solubility of the drug in fat, (4) protein-binding capacity, and (5) presence of active transport mechanisms. In terms of milk composition, milk undergoes three major changes during lactation. Colostrum, milk secreted during the first 4 or 5 days, is very high in protein content, but lower in both carbohydrate and fat than milk produced at later stages; pH is generally higher, in fact, alkaline. Transitional milk lasts through the second and perhaps into the third week of lactation. The composition of this milk reflects a transition between colostrum and the more stable, long-lived composition of later stages of lactation. *Mature* milk comes into being about the third week and remains, with much slower changes in overall composition, for the duration of lactation. This milk contains less protein, more fat and carbohydrate; it is also more neutral or slightly acidic in pH. Lowered protein levels may mean there is less potential to bind and thereby carry drugs into the milk. However, milk with fat can contain more fat-soluble drugs. Fat content not only changes throughout lactation, but it also varies throughout a day, and even during a single feeding. Thus, the amount of fat-soluble drugs in mother's milk also can fluctuate a great deal.

A drug enters the milk by passing first from blood plasma through the endothelium of capillaries supplying the mammary gland. Once across this barrier, the drug, now located in alveolar (milk-producing) cells, must then be transferred into the lumen. The entire process occurs mainly through diffusion, the rate and extent of transfer dependent upon the concentration gradient existing across cell (membrane) walls. In turn, the difference in concentration varies with pH and the dissociation constant (pK) of the drug in question. Those drugs that react as weak bases ionize (dissociate) to a greater extent in acidic medium, and vice versa. Because mature human milk is slightly acidic (pH 6.8) in comparison to blood plasma (pH 7.4), it tends to attract and, in a sense, to trap drugs that react as weak bases. For this and other reasons it is quite possible for level of contamination of milk to equal or exceed levels in the blood. Colostrum, an alkaline medium, may produce a much different milk/plasma drug relationship than milk of later lactation. Both the nature of the drug, therefore, and the varying compositional nature of milk influence kind and overall level of drug(s) in milk.

In addition to natural laws of diffusion, a number of active transport systems operate. These systems are special biological or chemical mechanisms by which drugs are transferred across membrane walls. Protein binding and solubility in fat are but two factors, albeit important ones. In addition, some antibiotics act as ionophores, substances that form fat-soluble complexes capable of serving as highly selective carriers of a variety of ions. A smaller number of antibiotics are able to complex and transfer to milk certain amines (see Cowie and Swinburne, 1977). In sum, therefore, the forces acting upon drug transfer to milk are many, the interactions complex.

Moreover, some drugs, like aspirin, considered safe at normal level of use, and mainly because concentration in milk is low, have not been evaluated at high use-rate. The same may be said for various tranquilizers, for streptomycin, the antibiotic, and quinidine (Yaffe and Waletzky, 1976). These specific drugs are mentioned because of the need, at times, to prescribe heavy or prolonged dosages. O'Brien (1974) considers risk of streptomycin to outweigh benefits of breast-feeding. This same authority would suggest the need to monitor a breast-feeding infant whose mother consumes aspirin in "moderate" amounts (O'Brien, 1974).

It is possible that some drugs, at normal rate of intake, simply never reach the milk supply. Warfarin sodium, an anti-coagulant that binds tightly to protein, may represent one example (Orme et al., 1977). Possibly Heparin is another (see Yaffe and Waletzky, 1976). Some drugs taken at normal dosage that do reach the milk supply are considered to be relatively harmless. Bishydroxycoumarin and aspirin would appear to belong in this category, also propoxyphene, morphine, demerol, and codeine (see Yaffe and Waletzky, 1976). Certain antihistamines also appear to be relatively safe, though their level in milk may exceed the level in blood plasma. The heart medication, digozin, reaches only very low concentrations in milk and, again, is thought relatively harmless to the feeding infant (Yaffe and Waletzky, 1976). Several antibiotics and a number of drugs that act on the central nervous system are likewise considered safe at normal rate of use (see O'Brien, 1974).

Table 17 shows a number of drugs thought to be potentially harmful to the breast-feeding infant whose mother uses them. Several are sedatives or products used to relieve tension. Often the symptoms of drug intake in the infant correspond to those of the mother. Drowsiness is common in an infant feeding off mother's milk contaminated with sedatives. Lithium and reserpine produce a bluish tint to the skin, along with other disorders. Heroin or the painkiller Darvon can lead to infant addiction. A mother's addiction to heroin is especially problematic, because the treatment of addiction with methadone has been documented as a cause of one infant death (Smialek et al., 1977).

Note in Table 17 that two drugs taken by the mother to prevent blood clotting may cause bleeding problems in nursing infants. Two such anti-coagulants are listed. There are several drugs to prevent convulsions or epileptic seizures (Table 17 lists a few). In some cases effects on breast-feeding infants are known, but often long-term effects cannot or have not been adequately assessed. Phenytoin, administered regularly to the mother, reaches levels of 1–5 μg/ml milk. Carbamezine will be found in human milk at about 60% of the concentration present in blood serum (see Cowie and Swinburne, 1977).

Japanese scientists (Kaneko et al., 1979) evaluated five anti-convulsants: diphenylhydantion, phenobarbitol, primidone, carbamazepin, and ethosuximide. The amount of these reaching human milk, as percent of that present in blood serum, ranged all the way from 18% to 81%. Concentration in serum averaged 4.5, 19.3, 2.8, 4.3, and 29.3 μg/ml, respectively. Percentages of these levels found in mother's milk were, respectively, 18, 46, 81, 39 and 79. In one case, an infant received 16.5 mg phenobarbitol daily

TABLE 17
Some Maternal Drugs Known to Pose Potential Health Problems for the Breast-Feeding Infant[a]

Drug	Possible symptoms or effects on infant
Anticoagulant	
Ethyl biscoumacetate	Bleeding problems
Phenindione	Bleeding problems
Anticonvulsant	
Mysoline	Drowsiness
Phenobarbital	Hypnotic effect
Phenytoin (diphenylhydantoin)	Methemoglobinemia
Carbamezine	Long-term effect unknown
Antidepressant	
Lithium	Loss of muscle tone, lowered body temperature, bluish skin
Antihypertension	
Reserpine	Nasal congestion, weight loss, bluish skin
Antimetabolite	
Cyclophosphamide	Bone marrow depression
Methotrexate	Bone marrow depression
Antimicrobial	
Chloramphenicol (chloromycetin)	Refusal to nurse, sleepiness, vomiting
Metrondiazole (flagyl)	Causes cancer in test animals
Nalidixic acid	Hemolytic anemia
Nitrofurantoin[b]	See footnote
Sulfonamides[b]	Hemolytic anemia
Antithyroid	
Iodide	Altered thyroid synthesis and release
Thiouracil	Altered throid synthesis and release
Radioactive iodine	Cancer, loss of thyroid activity
Autonomic drugs	
Atropine	Constipation
Laxative	
Anthraquinone derivatives: (Dantron, Dialose Plus, Dorbane Dorbantyl, Doxiden, Pericolace)	Bowel problems
Aloe	Bowel problems
Calomel	Bowel problems
Cascara	Bowel problems
Danthron	Bowel problems
Narcotic	
Heroin	Addiction
Methadone	One death recorded
Oral contraceptives	Gynecomastia, long-term effects unknown
Pain-killer	
Propoxyphene (Darvon)	Addiction

TABLE 17 *(continued)*

Drug	Possible symptoms or effects on infant
Sedative	
Barbituates	Drowsiness
Bromides	Drowsiness
Chloral hydrate	Drowsiness
Diazepam (Valium)	Lethargy, jaundice, weight loss
Steroid	
Prednisone	Poor growth
Prednisolone	Poor growth
Miscellaneous	
Dihydrotachysterol	Renal calcification
Ergot alkaloids	Ergotism
Gold thioglucose	Rash, hepatitis, hematogocic alteration

[a]Adapted from Yaffe and Waletzky (1976) and Hecht (1979).
[b]This drug causes problems mainly in infants suffering the inherited enzyme deficiency glucose-6-phosphate dehydrogenase.

from 500 ml of mother's milk. For this infant, bottle feeding was recommended. Beyond this one problem, though, the above figures point out the relative disparity in the level of transfer to milk of various drugs—even drugs within the same class of medical aids. This fact should perhaps be apparent for the reasons cited above, but it seems worthy of emphasis in certain specifics.

Many drugs perform their function through action on the central nervous system. Cowie and Swinburne (1977) list a large number. What is important to recognize, perhaps, is that such drugs may be prescribed for widely diverse illnesses: codeine or alcohol (ethanol) as ingredients in medicines for the common cold, valium for tension, aspirin for a headache. Valium residuals in mother's milk induce lethargy in the breast-fed child (see Yaffe and Waletzky, 1976). Their presence could lead to hyperventilation. Both valium and its dimethylated metabolite find their way into breast milk. And evidence indicates that the infant is able to process valium from breast milk into the metabolic breakdown product. The efficiency with which it is able to do so increases with age. Where drugs are concerned, nothing is static. Their presence in the mother's body and in her milk, their presence in the infant body, is in a state of constant, dynamic change.

Lithium carbonate, another drug that acts on the central nervous system, may be prescribed for relief of manic depression. Symptoms of intake in infants nursing on breast milk of treated mothers include lowered body temperature, loss of muscle tone, and bluish skin. About one-half of the lithium reaching the bloodstream will find its way to the milk supply (see Cowie and Swinburne, 1977). Level of trichloroethanol, a breakdown product of dichloralphenazone, is secreted in milk in amounts somewhat less than that found in plasma. And Halothane, an inhalant anesthetic, has been reported as present in human milk of a single individual at a concentration of 2 μg/ml (see Cowie and Swinburne, 1977).

Reserpine is taken to relieve hypertension. Along with diuretics, it may be prescribed for victims of heart attacks. Ingested in breast milk, a nursing infant may show signs of nasal congestion or weight loss; the skin may take on a bluish tint. Other drugs used in treatment of heart disorders and also detected in human milk include deserpidine, dextrothyroxine, guanethidine, methychlothiazide, methyldopa, and benzothiadiazides (see O'Brien, 1974). Not all present problems for the breast-feeding infant.

Both cyclophosphamide, and methotrexate cause bone marrow depression when ingested by infants. Both enter the milk of treated mothers. The former has been found to contaminate the milk supply 6 hours after an intravenous injection of 500 mg. The former has been detected to a level of 2.6 ng/ml of milk after oral intake of 22.5 mg/day (see Cowie and Swinburne, 1977).

A variety of disorders follow intake by infants of breast milk contaminated with anti-microbial agents of one kind or the other. Other than those shown in Table 17, sulphanilimide and sulphapyridine have been detected in breast milk and are known to cause skin rashes in nursing infants (see O'Brien, 1974). Sulphanilimide also causes hemolytic anemia in infants suffering the inherited enzyme deficiency of glucose-6-phosphate dehydrogenase.

Penicillin, one of the most widely used antibiotics, is perhaps a most serious risk only after presensitization. Amounts ending up in breast milk are usually well under therapeutic doses for infants. However, a case is documented in which an allergic response occurred in a sensitive infant pretreated with 10 units of penicillin (by injection) and then exposed to penicillin in mother's milk (Catz and Giacoia, 1973). Complicating factors must always be considered, therefore, and drug use given due caution. To avoid problems to the extent possible, some drugs, at least, can be prescribed to be taken immediately following breast-feeding or at bedtime.

Aside from penicillin per se, other penicillin derivatives have also been detected in human milk. O'Brien (1974) makes note of the following: benzylpenicillin, benzathine penicillin, ampicillin and carbenicillin. One other, oxacillin, apparently has not as yet been found in milk of humans. Penicillin compounds are known to transfer readily to milk of cows and other mammalian species.

The scientific literature carries no evidence of presence of the antibiotics cephalothin or cephalexin in human milk, but streptomycin not only has been traced to human milk but persists there for extended periods of time (see Cowie and Swinburne, 1977). Other antibiotics that have been detected in human milk include kanamycin, chloramphenicol, novobiocin and erythromycin (see O'Brien, 1974). Chloramphenicol injested by infants may cause sleepiness or vomiting or refusal to suckle. Metronidazole, another anti-microbial agent, while untested in humans, is known to enter the milk supply of lactating women and to cause cancer in laboratory test animals. Like sulphanilamides, nitrofurantoin, has been found to produce hemolytic anemia in infants lacking glucose-6-phosphate dehydrogenase. Two of four women treated with 200 mg of this anti-microbial agent were found to yield milk with 0.3–0.5 μg/ml of the compound (see Cowie and Swinburne, 1977). Hexachlorophene has also been detected in milk of humans at levels of up to 9.0 ng/ml (see Cowie and Swinburne, 1977).

The final word on tetracycline antibiotics has yet to be written. These compounds have been detected in human milk (see O'Brien, 1974), and the levels may in fact exceed those in blood serum. But some authorities feel that tetracyclines are complexed by the milk and thereby withheld from uptake by the feeding infant. The issue is serious, for these antibiotics are known to combine with calcium of children's teeth. It becomes a part of the basic core (dentin) of teeth and causes a permanent (unremovable) yellow/gray stain. FDA advises against use of tetracyclines by pregnant women and all children under 8 years of age. Taken at any time between 3 months and 8 years, the drug may cause discoloration of the permanent teeth as they begin to show up. Infant drops of tetracycline were withdrawn from the market in the United States in 1978. The drug is still around, though, as medicine for adults, and prescriptions for its use by children continue to be written. A number of tetracycline compounds exist. These include oxytetracycline, chlortetracycline, demelocycline, doxycycline, methacycline, and minocycline. Their presence and use should, indeed, be questioned.

Radioactive elements may reach the milk of humans as environmental contaminants ingested with food, as medications against disease (radioactive iodine, for example), or as components of diagnostic tests. Gallium is an example of the latter and has been used in whole body scans to aid detection of tumors. The procedure does result in significant amounts of the unstable element appearing in milk of lactating women (see Cowie and Swinburne, 1977). Radioactive iodine, used in treatment of thyroid disorders, also transfers to the milk supply and might possibly lead to cancer in feeding infants (Hecht, 1979). Presence of the element does lead to loss of thyroid activity in the infant (see Yaffe and Waletzky, 1976). Another anti-thyroid compound, thiouracil, attains higher levels in milk than blood (O'Brien, 1974) and may cause goiter in nursing infants.

Although the emphasis here is on medications as source of contaminants, it is nonetheless important to note that a number of radioactive elements are known to transfer from feed to milk of lactating cows. The feed to milk transfer coefficient for radiobarium is 0.03–0.04%, for radiocesium 12–14%, for radiomanganese, polonium, and radium, 0.05%, 0.18%, and 0.02–0.07%, respectively (see Cowie and Swinburne, 1977). Transfer of radioactive strontium to milk, either of cows or humans depends to a great extent on level of intake of alkaline earth metals, chiefly calcium. The more calcium ingested the less the radioactive strontium passing to the milk supply. Technologies for removal of radioactive isotopes from milk do exist, but truly constitute a last-resort response to an already untenable hazard.

"Safe" laxatives include milk of magnesia, caster oil, mineral oil, Dulcolax, senna phenolphthalein (nonprescription Ex-lax) and fecal softners (Yaffe and Waletzky, 1976). Among other drugs used in gastrointestinal disorders and known to transfer to milk, O'Brien (1974) lists anthraquinone, aloes, cascara, emodin, rheum-rhubarb, and sagrada. Bowel problems may be symptoms in infants feeding on milk contaminated with such compounds.

It is also probably best not to consume alcohol during lactation. Evidence suggests little potential harm to breast-feeding infants if the mother's intake is moderate. Alcohol per se does reach the the milk supply and in concentrations similar to that present in the blood. A major metabolite, acetaldehyde, has not been detected in human milk, however (see Cowie and Swinburne, 1977). Excessive intake of alcohol by a nursing mother has been found to cause delayed growth in at least one breast-fed infant (Binkiewicz, *et al.*, 1978). In general, level of alcohol intake of the mother appears a far more serious problem to the unborn fetus than to the nursing infant. For the fetus, serious birth defects may arise when the mother consumes little more than two alcoholic drinks per day, or drinks excessively at about 3 weeks into pregnancy.

Scientific literature cites no specifics of the transfer of D-lysergic acid diethylamide (LSD) to milk. But compounds not far removed in chemical structure have been detected in human milk (see Cowie and Swinburne, 1977).

Smoking is another matter. Nicotine of cigarettes does enter the milk of humans and definitely can cause nicotine poisoning of the breast-feeding infant. Infants 3–4 days of age whose mother smoked 6–12 cigarettes were reported to refuse to suckle, become apathetic, vomit, and retain urine and feces (Majewski, 1979). In a chain-smoking mother, nicotine content of milk reached 75 μg/liter. Urine of the breast-feeding infant showed a nicotine level of 4 μg/liter (Perraudin and Sorin, 1978). Cigarette smoke also contains cancer-causing compounds, and one of these, benzopyrene, has been found to enter the milk supply of lactating mice when introduced to the animals through the trachea (see Cowie and Swinburne, 1977).

But if cigarettes pose a threat in this regard, marijuana is much worse, with 50% more carcinogens than tobacco smoke (Tashkin, 1980). To the marijuana smoker, dangers of lung cancer are real. To date, though, no work has been done to determine the amount of carcinogens that reach the milk supply of a pot-smoking, nursing mother. Beyond any doubt, however, contamination does occur. Moveover, scientific evidence leaves little doubt of the transfer of the active constituent of marijuana, tetrahydrocannabinol, to milk of various test animals. That the same potential exists in humans seems clear.

Because of the increasing number of teenage users (estimates put marijuana use at 4 million Americans between the ages of 12 and 17), this type of contamination of mother's milk may have serious consequences in the future.

Like alcohol, caffeine of coffee, cola drinks, and various medications may pose a more serious threat to the unborn fetus than the nursing infant. As yet there is no conclusive proof that caffeine has caused birth defects in humans, but evidence shows that it does in rats, and at levels of intake not much higher than women would normally consume (on an equivalent basis). Present in human milk, caffeine, a stimulant, could cause a response in infants similar to those noted in adults—wakefulness and irritability. Some small amount, however, seems to be without risk, at least at this time. Another stimulant, theophylline (found in the drug aminophylliné), likewise enters the milk of treated mothers (see Cowie and Swinburne, 1977).

At one time cyclamates were a common "artificial" sweetener in food products. It is now banned from use in the United States, but not necessarily all countries. Nevertheless, cyclamates have been shown to reach the milk supply as a food ingredient ingested by laboratory test animals. Vitamin D, an essential nutrient but one which can be toxic in overdose, appears in human milk, following intake in pharmacological amounts, as the active metabolic product, 25–hydroxycholecalciferol (see Cowie and Swinburne, 1977).

Hormones constitute a whole class of compounds in themselves, and are naturally present in human milk. Hormones are also prescribed for a number of reasons and their content in milk increased as a result. Two of them, prednisone and prednisolone, when ingested by breast-feeding infants, have been found to cause poor growth (see Yaffe and Waletzky, 1976). Those used as oral contraceptives may both alter the nutrient content of milk and also effect a nursing infant's health. With regard to the former, long-term use results in milk of reduced vitamin B_6 level (Roepke and Kirskey, 1979b). Though the amount of calcium, magnesium, zinc, copper and iron seem uninfluenced by previous use of the "pill," manganese concentration drops significantly (Kirskey et al., 1979). Thus, there are both long-term and short-term direct and possibly indirect effects of drug use. Some oral contraceptives are formulated with high levels of both estrogens and progestin. Their use may suppress lactation and lower milk yield. High doses may transfer to milk in levels so great as to provide pharmacological amounts to the breast-feeding infant (Atkinson, 1979). If it becomes necessary, therefore, to use contraceptives during lactation, it is preferable to use those that contain progestins only and then only at the lowest possible dose. Gynecomastia, the abnormal growth of breasts in male infants, has been attributed to presence of contraceptive steroids in human milk.

To know what level of hormone in milk may be considered safe, it is necessary to know the natural level that is present. Although research in this area is incomplete, evidence suggests higher levels of hormone in blood of women than of ruminants. One might expect milk levels to show corresponding differences, at least in some instances. Pregnanediols have been detected in human milk, but progesterone is apparently missing. A form of the former has been mentioned as a possible cause of infant jaundice (see Cowie and Swinburne, 1977). Both norethylnodrel and mestranol have been detected in milk of women following intake of the hormones. Thyroxine is naturally present in human milk and level appears to increase markedly over the first 3 weeks of lactation.

The foregoing gives unmistakable evidence of risk to breast-feeding infants, and a nursing mother will do well to heed advice on use of drugs; little may be presumed. Some authorities warn that drugs cannot be considered necessarily safe even in light of previous studies to the contrary (Stanway, 1978). The science(s) involved have not been without error. It is no simple matter to assess presence of drugs or their metabolites in the complex environment of milk.

A nursing mother or expectant mother must be willing to forego all but the most essential of drugs, and to take any one of them only when in absolute need. A nursing mother would likewise do well to avoid foods known to be sources of drugs, including a number of herbs, and plants that contain a variety of mind-altering or other toxic components. A nursing infant can be exposed to these components and receive a shock, possibly violent, to his or her mind or body. Lastly, when drug use is essential and when the drug is thought to pose a hazard to the nursing infant, be prepared to use infant formula or other infant food. Formula can serve, certainly, in the interim, even in longer periods made necessary by use of drugs that are slow to leave the body or by extended drug use needed to treat a more prolonged disease state.

Perhaps one of the best sources of information on drugs in relation to human milk and infant health is the family pharmacist. Also, always read the product label. Often precautionary statements are presented, and this may be true for drugs of most any vintage. Effective December 26, 1979, however, all manufacturers of drugs in the United States were required to provide relevant information on the label of new drugs developed and marketed after that date (Federal Register, 1980b). Whatever is known about excretion of the drug into milk, whatever is known of the effect or possible effect on the infant will be indicated on the label. If nothing is known, the label will state that fact. In such a case, and in all use of drugs, the prudent mother will exercise due caution.

ENVIRONMENTAL POLLUTANTS

As the result of a human error in Michigan, a large stock of meat, milk, poultry, and eggs become contaminated with polybrominated biphenyls (PBB's). After an industrial discharge violates an ocean-going river, a Japanese fishing bay absorbs a deadly dose of methylmercury. Twenty years after it is banned, DDT is detected in bread, in health food stores and supermarkets, at 4–5 parts per billion. A diseased animal gets a shot of antibiotics and, failing to respond, is trucked off to the stockyards. For a destitute, unemployed day-laborer, a batch of moldy peanuts becomes a meal. A weed killer sprayed from an airplane drifts slowly onto an alfalfa crop of a neighboring farm.

A woman sits at the very top of the food chain and consumes every pesticide residual, drug residual, heavy metal, and other industrial pollutant that finds its way into food. Although a thousand complexities enter in, some small amount of the total intake may ultimately come to reside in mother's milk.

Some 150 different herbicides now assist the farmer in killing weeds. As many or more insecticides help destroy the insects and parasites that feed on plant and animal. Drug use on meat-producing livestock in the United States alone measures in tons. Little doubt exists that some small amount of these agricultural aids must remain in the food one eats, and some must reach the human breast. However, it is not enough to advocate a food system free of chemical aids. That course may produce a food shortage or a food supply amply sprinkled with insect parts, parasite eggs, and the cancerous toxins of mold growth. Various contaminants also find their way into the ingredients of infant formulas, whether based on milk, soy bean, or other food source. Such contamination, though, is on a monitored basis and, in the case of cow's milk is screened to some extent by the animal's own body. In human milk, the kind and amount of environmental pollutants depend primarily on the eating habits of the mother and the level of contamination in foods common to her diet.

In order to avoid confusion to the extent possible, it seems worthwhile to categorize and treat separately the various contaminants of human milk. Although some overlap exists, I propose to consider briefly four subgroups: (1) pesticides, (2) mycotoxins, (3) heavy metals, and (4) organic industrial pollutants. Within each category are compounds known to enter the milk supply of nursing mothers and to cause some risk to breast-feeding infants.

Pesticides

The most famous—or infamous—member of this group of contaminants of human milk is the insecticide DDT. If anyone has any doubts of the widespread presence of DDT over the planet, he or she has only to look at the scientific literature on human milk. Even the most recent literature continues to give evidence of the dogged persistence that this chemical achieves, though banned in some nations of the world. In Switzerland, human milk still averages 3.0 mg/kg fat. Some samples reach to over 15 mg/kg fat. The acceptable daily intake is set at 0.005 mg/kg body weight. Calculations put the level of intake in excess of this amount in 78% of breast-feeding infants in Switzerland (Schupback and Egli, 1979). In Guatemala, where DDT is still used on cotton fields, the level in breast-fed infants breaches the acceptable daily intake by "many times" according to researchers in that nation (Olszyna-Marzys, 1978). A survey in Poland for the years 1975–1976 found the level of DDT in human milk to average from 3 to 7 mg/kg fat, depending upon the province from which samples originated. In cow's milk, at that same time, the level ranged from 0.11 to 0.18 mg/kg fat (Smoczynski, 1979). Thus, cow's milk reflected a considerably lower concentration of the insecticide than mother's milk. This is not unusual. A study in the German Federal Republic found a level of DDT of 0.19 mg/kg fat in 64 samples of human milk taken the first week after delivery. The level in reconstituted infant formula was given as 0.01 mg/kg fat. As the authors of the report pointed out, mother's milk would not comply in this regard with regulations in effect for cow's milk (Muller and Schroder, 1978). This was true not only for DDT but for hexachlorobenzene (HCB) and hexachlorocyclohexane (BHC) as well. Likewise, Czechoslovakian scientists found a "high" level of intake of DDT and lindane in breast-fed infants (Szokolay *et al.*, 1977).

All the preceding reports are from the late 1970s and early 1980s. Problems, therefore, are still widespread. Issues also reach beyond DDT and its breakdown products, DDD and DDE. Canadians have found mirex in samples of human milk of women residing in cities on Lake Ontario (Mes *et al.*, 1978). Dieldrin and heptachlor epoxide are still found in the human milk of Europeans (Gatti, 1975). In a recent survey, malathion appeared in the milk of Taiwanese women to a level of 0.0356 ppm (35.6 μg/kg) and lindane at 0.0842 ppm (84.2 μg/kg) (Yeh *et al.*, 1976).

What do such facts tell us? First, it still remains to be proven whether or not a significant long-term hazard exists from the routine intake of low levels of most pesticides. One would be less than candid to say otherwise. It is also true, however, that some of these compounds are known carcinogens. They have been banned in some instances for this very reason. Scarcely any comparison between the levels of pesticide in mother's milk and infant formula show anything but significantly lower levels in the latter. This would include a range of compounds from DDT through DDE, chlordane, hept- achlor, dieldrin, mirex, HCB, and BHC. As in the case of any toxic substance that enters the body in very small amounts, no apparent harm may evolve over a normal life span. That some obviously inflict harm at "high" levels of intake can only be noted through some tragic accident of excessive exposure. This was the case in Turkey a number of years ago when townspeople ate seed grain treated with HCB. Mercury-treated grains have triggered similar tragedies. Suffice it to say, perhaps, that a risk is associated with intake of any and all chemicals, both those inherent to and/or a contaminant of food. At present, most pesticides occur to higher levels in human milk than in cow's milk or infant formula, and the amount in human milk often exceeds the maximum allowable level set for cow's milk by the World Health Organization (WHO) (see Yaffe and Waletzky, 1976).

Mycotoxins

The contamination of mother's food or milk with pesticides is a serious problem. Nonetheless, even in the absence of pesticides, a second hazard exists. Here the problem is molds; this includes molds that spoil foods—

especially fruits, vegetables, and cereal grains—and molds that may also produce poisons during their growth on food. The most common of these molds belong to the genera *Aspergillus, Alternaria, Cladosporium, Fusarium,* and lastly *Penicillium,* the latter being the one from which the most famous of all antibiotics derives. Molds of all these genera cause food spoilage. One produces one of the most deadly poisons (carcinogens) known to humankind, aflatoxin B_1.

Only recently have scientists recognized the full significance of growth of *Aspergillus* on such major crops as corn and wheat, tree nuts, ground nuts (peanuts), and cottonseed. One species (*A. flavus*) produces aflatoxin B_1. The mold (or its toxin) may become a part of those foods (or products made from them) on which it grows. It is known to occur on foods like bread and cheese. If cows consume mold-infected feed, the milk supply may yield an amount of poison. Having been metabolized by the cow, aflatoxin B_1 is converted to a much less harmful cousin, aflatoxin M_1. If the cow is taken out of the chain, however, humans must deal directly with the more poisonous variant.

On corn crops, an insect, the corn borer, most often paves the way for infestation with *A. flavus.* It would be difficult to weigh the risk of applying an insecticide to stop the borer versus the risk of growth of the mold.

Aflatoxin produced by *A. flavus* must be considered a naturally occurring poison. It is not one that derives mainly from processing functions. For perspective, it seems well to point out that many different molds will grow on food. In all cases a form of spoilage results, but relatively few molds produce toxins. Even molds within the same genera vary in inherent ability to elaborate poisons. Thus, some are very harmful; others may in fact be used to produce the tangy sharp flavor of a blue-veined cheese. When toxins are indeed present, mother's milk is vulnerable to the toxin itself or some breakdown product.

In the home, molds will be found growing in foods held at refrigerator temperature. They grow best, however, on foods high in moisture content and in a warm atmosphere. Because they are especially vulnerable, some foods contain a small amount of additive designed to inhibit growth of mold. Use of additives of this kind is regulated. Again, a choice must be made, this time between a risk associated with an additive and that posed by growth of molds. In a world short of food, the choice must tilt in favor of preservatives.

The FDA has set guidelines in food for admissible levels of aflatoxin; these levels generally reflect the lowest levels of detectability, and range from 0.5 up to 20 parts per billion. Precise tolerances are still a matter of debate in some instances.

Heavy Metals and Arsenic

Industrial pollutants are a scourge unto themselves and heavy metals are the worst of the lot. All the major ones have been found in human milk. Three of them—mercury, cadmium, and lead— will be detailed here.

Mercury

Mercury has been a frequent offender as industrial pollutant of late. Accidental poisonings have occurred in scattered spots throughout the world. On two occasions, mercury-treated seed grain lay at fault. In Iraq in 1971–1972, bread prepared from treated grain caused a major poisoning. Human milk in this instance was found to contain as much as 100 ng/ml of mercury. Blood of the breast-feeding infant reached mercury levels of 1.0–1.5 μg/ml (see Cowie and Swinburne, 1977).

Other mercury poisonings have occurred; one in Minamata Bay, Japan, was a major disaster. In this instance industrially polluted seawater caused contamination of locally caught seafood. Twenty-seven unborn infants were poisoned. I have found no research on the mercury level of these mother's milk.

Even in relatively nonpolluted regions, it is difficult to escape mercury. You will find it in small but varying amounts in fruit, vegetables, grains, meats, and dairy products. Content tends to run distinctly higher in marine foods, especially tuna and swordfish. But it is found too in walleye or trout fished from the remotest of wilderness lakes and rivers.

To find mercury in human milk comes as no surprise. Level, of course, varies. Spot surveys in Japan (Fujita and Takabatake, 1977) and Poland (Juszkiewicz et al., 1975) detected averages of 3.6 and 6.0 μg/kg of milk, respectively. Range of mercury in milk of Polish women ranged from 1.1–15.8 μg/kg. These are levels similar to those found in other countries. In a breakdown by age, in one study at least, content of mercury in mother's milk was higher in women over 30 years of age (Juszkiewicz et al, 1975). Possibly this finding can be construed to reflect the longer exposure time of the older women. Like other heavy metals, mercury, once consumed, accumulates in the body. The body cannot readily rid itself of mercury, though some obviously escapes in mother's milk—but only to accumulate in the breast-feeding infant.

Cadmium

Cadmium, once solely a metallic by-product, now is found in just about every major industrial product, from tractors to hardware tools, from business machines to television sets and printer's ink. Taken in from the environment by plants, animals, and marine life, cadmium becomes a background contaminant of the foods we eat. Like mercury, it accumulates in the body. The symptoms of cadmium toxicity range from shortness of breath to bronchitis, kidney disease, and, in severe poisonings, death. Assuming low levels of prior exposure of nursing mothers, cadmium content of breast milk should be minimal, that is, undetectable. Fresh cow's milk may also be found missing detectable levels (Woidich and Pfannhauser, 1980). But regional differences are known to occur, and cadmium levels in cow's milk in the United States have been found to vary from 17 to 30 ng/ml. Market milk in Sweden and the United States (California) have shown levels of 0.2 to 6 ng/ml, respectively. Regional differences might very well be expected in cadmium level in human milk as well. In a limited United States study (14 women), cadmium content of human milk averaged 10.9 μg/kg of milk (Pinkerton et al., 1972). Cow's milk, evaluated at the same time, averaged 42 μg/kg. On a dry weight basis, Austrian scientists report a range of 0.02–0.31 mg/kg in dry milk produced in that country (Woidich and Pfannhauser, 1980). A World Health Organization study of milk of Swedish women reported a median level of cadmium of 0.1 μg/kg (Larsson et al., 1981). Obviously, milk-based infant formula (or, for that matter, other types of formula) can serve up some small amount to feeding infants. Infants are indeed more vulnerable to heavy metals of all kinds than are adults. Their small size alone greatly increases their sensitivity. Their diet, focused as it is on one (or very few) source of food, excludes variety, which might otherwise reduce exposure. In general, though, the problem of cadmium poisoning poses a less serious threat than the potential for lead poisoning, either from mother's milk or infant formula as source.

Lead

Several facts are most important where lead is concerned. First, lead ingested during pregnancy transfers in part to the fetus. In excessive amounts—development of fetus is impaired. Second, any amount of lead taken in during pregnancy carries over and causes an increase in lead content of milk following childbirth. Thus, the infant is placed in double jeopardy. Lastly, lead consumed by the lactating mother also enters the milk supply to some extent (Keller and Doherty, 1980). If any consolation exists, it lies in the fact that by some quirk of physiology infants are somewhat better able to expel lead (in relation to body weight), at least during early months, than older infants, children, or adults (Ryu et al., 1978). In no way, however, does this fact justify any but the most rigorous attention to all factors important to control of intake of lead either by the mother or the infant. Because dietary lead has no essential function in the body, any amount can be considered too much. As a practical matter, however, some lead must enter the body from environmental sources. Leaded gasoline guarantees that much. The presence of lead water pipes, particularly in poorer or older neighborhoods, ensures a given level in some water supplies. To infants and young children, lead-based paints remain a hazard. Food itself, specifically milk, constitutes a major source of lead to the infants who feed almost exclusively upon it. In the majority of cases, the lead intake of infants will likely be greater from foods other than mother's milk. This does not exempt human milk as an important source; it says only that the level of contamination of most milk (and milk-based formula) products runs higher than mother's milk. This appears to be true both in industrial and Third World nations. In the United States the heaviest burden falls upon the infants of the poor. Not only is the mother more likely to live in an environment concentrated with lead, but current social and economic problems necessitate more dependence on bottle feeding. Thus, the level of exposure in the food of infants is generally higher, no matter the source, and the burden from the environment is also that much greater.

A further complication turns on considerations of "safe" levels. As mentioned earlier, any amount of lead intake can perhaps be thought to be too much. Yet some amount is ingested, almost universally, and some amount appears therefore to be tolerable. Scientists fail to agree, however, on what should be considered the cutoff point, that is, the "daily permissible level." A specially constituted national committee in the United States suggests a daily intake not to exceed 300 μg of elemental lead per day (Walker, 1980). Other authorities propose a lower level, in one case, 93–133 μg/day (Baltrop and Killala, 1967); in a second, 87 μg/day for the newborn infants, 153 μg/day for infants 6 months of age (Chatranon et al., 1978). Part of the problem of setting standards rests on the difficulty in determining an injurious response. The level that manifests a clinical symptom(s) may be higher than that which induces a psychological disturbance of some kind. Data to this effect have already been reported, with classroom performance shown apparently to fall at levels of lead exposure lower than that in which physical ailments appear. Such findings would seem to justify recent trends to consider as threshold of risk even lower concentrations of lead in blood. Of late, this amount has been decreased from 40 μg to 30 μg of lead/ml of whole blood during early infancy (Walker, 1980). Efforts in the last few years to reduce lead content of infants foods seems well advised.

Studies on levels of lead in human milk and cow's milk products lend a necessary perspective. One limited United States investigation (using 14 women) found human milk to average 1.1 μg/100 ml (Pinkerton et al., 1972). Taken at the same time, data on fresh cow's milk showed an average of 2.6 μg/100 ml. Studies in Great Britain, Sweden, and California produced average levels of lead in cow's milk of about 2.0, 0.2, and 8.8 μg/100 ml of milk (see Cowie and Swinburne, 1977). The highest level found thus far, and this in a cow suffering from lead poisoning, was 22.6 μg/100 ml of milk (see Cowie and Swinburne, 1977).

At least one researcher suggests that there has been no substantial increase in lead content of human milk of American mothers during the 40 years preceeding the early 1970s. Data from this study showed an average of lead content in human milk of 2.1 μg/100 ml. The range went from 0.6 to 5.8 μg/100 ml. Number of samples was only 29, however (see Cowie and Swinburne, 1977).

In a fairly extensive Washington, D.C. survey (Walker, 1980), lead content of human milk ranged from none up to 5 μg/100 ml. The average was 2 μg/100 ml. Samples of homogenized-pasteurized cow's milk averaged 1 μg/100 ml, half the level of human milk. The highest level noted for this product was 2 μg/100 ml. Evaporated milk, as is often the case, yielded quite different results. The average was 30 μg/100 ml, with a range of 29–36 μg/100 ml.

As for infant formula, most studies seem to indicate level of lead to have reached an all-time low in the United States. This should not be construed to imply a satisfactory content of this heavy metal in all instances. It does, however, reflect an earnest control effort on the part of industry and regulatory agencies. In the Washington, D.C. survey cited, eleven brands of infant formula averaged from 5–50 μg of lead/100 ml. The grand average was 13.5 μg/100 ml. And all but two products contained less than 10 μg/100 ml. Considering total range of lead concentration, however, one sample was found to carry 90 μg of lead/100 ml. The average for this brand was 7.0 μg/100 ml. To convert these values to level of intake of infants, consider average intake to run from 168 to 178 ml of formula per kg of body weight per day. These were averages found in two independent studies. Given an intake of 550 ml during early infancy, lead consumption from the "average" formula would come to 74.3 μg of lead daily. The same level of intake of human milk at 2 μg of lead per 100 ml produces a daily infant intake of 11 μg. The difference is very clear. It is likewise confirmed in separate studies that much larger doses of lead will be consumed in either concentrated infant formula or evaporated milk than in dry milk (if reconstituted with water of low lead content), fresh fluid milk, or human milk.

By way of comparison, a quite extensive survey in Thailand produced the following data. Mother's milk averaged 8.5 μg lead/100 ml, infant formulas averaged 15.9 μg/100 ml (Chatranon et al., 1978). Though higher than comparable data of American studies, infant formulas contained twice the amount of lead as human milk.

One other emerging fact seems worthy of note. Animal studies produce evidence that lactose enhances lead absorption in the intestines. Other milk components, notably calcium, phosphorus, zinc and protein, impede uptake of lead. Net balance, in presence of both lactose and other milk constituents, leans decidedly to reduced uptake. But to realize the full potential to protect against absorption of lead, the milk product must itself be free of lead.

Arsenic

Arsenic is another poisonous element that ultimately may come to reside in mammalian milk. In milk of Austrian women, level of arsenic was found, in a relatively small sampling, to average 3.74 μg/kg of milk. Level in cow's milk in the same area hovered near the same value (Woidich and Pfannhauser, 1980). Other researchers find level in cow's milk to range from 3.0 to 6.0 μg/100 ml, and to pass to milk only as concentration reaches levels high enough to show evidence of poisoning, in which case the amount in milk may reach 45 μg/100 ml (see Cowie and Swinburne, 1977).

Organic Industrial Pollutants

I will draw attention here to only four industrial pollutants. Nonetheless, the story they tell is the story of pollution generally.

Polybrominated biphenyls

A single human error and contamination with polybrominated biphenyls (PBB's) ultimately resulted in the need to destroy 23,000 head of dairy and beef animals, 36,000 hogs, 500 sheep, and 1¼ million chickens. The same catastrophe put to ruin 2,600 pounds of butter, 34,000 pounds of dry milk products, 1,500 cases of evaporated milk, 18,000 pounds of cheese, 5 *million* eggs, and 865 tons of feed. The fallout ultimately led to contamination of 96% of breast milk samples of the female population of the largest part of an entire state.

The story behind this devastation is as follows: A chemical company produced a feed supplement for cattle called Nutrimaster. It is a white, granula chemical, magnesium oxide. The same company also produced a fire retardant called Firemaster made up of PBB's. Usually Firemaster is a coarse *brown* substance. During some experimental work, several batches of Firemaster are ground into a fine *white* powder.

Usually the compounds—PBB and magnesium oxide—were packaged in bags of distinctively different color combinations. At this time, however, a paper shortage caused the company to package both products in identical brown paper bags.

In error, the PBB's were shipped to a feed mill. Taken for a feed nutrient, the white power was mixed into a number of animal and poultry feeds and sold to Michigan farmers. This probably happened sometime in early 1973.

The story now jumps ahead to about March of 1974. A dairy farmer puzzled over the poor health and poor production levels of his cows was determined to find out what was wrong. After one or two false starts, he sent feed samples to the National Animal Disease Center in Ames, Iowa, for analysis. There a technician placed samples in a testing device, went to lunch, and left the equipment running. Upon his return, the technician spotted a strange new peak automatically traced onto the graph paper during his absence. It turned out to be PBB.

In the animal and human body, PBB tends to collect in the fat. There it is shed very, very slowly. Some experts say that the chemical may never be entirely eliminated from the exposed Michigan herds.

The question of how much risk such exposure of PBBs poses is not clear. If one looks at the LD_{50} of PBB, it appears relatively benign. LD_{50} is the amount of any substance that causes death of 50% of the test animals to which it is fed. The tabulation here provides a kind of bench mark of toxicity:

Compound	LD_{50}
	(mg/kg)
Caffeine	200
DDT (insecticide)	285
2,4-D (weed killer)	500
Malathion (insecticide)	1,156
Table salt	3,000
PBB	21,500

The lower the LD_{50}, the more toxic the compound. Any value less than 5 is extremely toxic: 5–49 very toxic; 50–499, moderately toxic; 500–15,000, almost nontoxic. The level of PBB is 21,500, which is almost nontoxic and far safer than salt or caffeine of coffee.

Nonetheless, LD_{50} is not the only measure of injurious response. As mentioned earlier, certain additives of infant formula have been shown to possibly interfere with the immune response. Such measures are exquisitely sensitive, very new, and very much open to various interpretations. These facts notwithstanding, researchers of the Mount Sinai Medical Center in New York (Selikoff, 1979), conducted a health survey of 1000 Michigan farm residents, found certain defects in cellular immune components. Theory says such persons might well be somewhat more prone to infections, allergies, and possibly even cancer. Indeed, the Mount Sinai study revealed what appeared to be a correlation between PBB contamination and ear infections, sore throats, and colds in adults. The researchers, however, could not exclude the possibility of chance effect because similar relationships could not be drawn for children who were also exposed. University of Michigan scientists even report of "reassuringly negative feelings" for a number of potential human disorders that could result from PBB intake. But the final word remains qualified. Uncertainty of the health effects will persist "for some years" say these scientists (see Food Chemical News, 1979). Such uncertainty now includes the possibility that PBB may cause cancer. These are the latest findings of a 2-year study by the National Institute of Environmental Health Sciences (see Minneapolis Tribune, 1981). Tests were conducted solely on rats and mice, and may not apply to humans. Yet in the rodent species the chemical was found to be carcinogenic. Tests on rodents are most widely used in evaluating the potential of any chemical compounds to cause an injurious response in the human body. Although findings may not be conclusive and may not be directly transposable to human life, at the same time evidence of this kind cannot be discounted.

At this point, perhaps only two facts appear unequivocal: PBB's resist breakdown by the body. They are excreted only through breast-milk. At an equivalent rate of contamination, nursing mothers would, therefore, show lower body levels of PBB's than other persons.

Polychlorinated biphenyls

Polychlorinated biphenyls (PCB's) are close cousins to PBB's. But close in chemical terms can mean a world of difference. For example, PBB's may be five times as toxic as PCB's, though the latter has been found to cause reproductive failures, stomach disorders, birth defects, and tumors in laboratory test animals. Accidental human exposure has resulted in digestive distress, skin rash, throat and respiratory irritations, and severe headaches. Fetuses exposed in the womb come forth into the world with a yellow/brown discoloration of the skin. Nine such infants were later found to lack endurance, to be apathetic and sullen, and to have dull, expressionless faces (Miller, 1977).

PCB's are now recognized as a serious pollutant. Literally thousands of contaminated environmental samples from all over the world give stark evidence of the extent of PCB contamination. Industrial application of PCB's goes back to 1929. It took at least nine separate and unrelated incidents of food contamination over an entire decade (1971–1979) to awaken us to its hazards (Federal Register, 1980c):

1965 Reproductive problems were noted in commercial mink. Several years later, after appropriate testing tools had been devised, PCB's were found to blame.

1967 A PCB-containing sealant, used on the inside wall of a silo, eroded into the silage, was fed to dairy cows, and led to contamination of milk.

1968 A heat exchanger was being used to process rice oil in a plant in Yusho, Japan. Heat exchangers are a common piece of equipment in food-processing plants. PCB's are often used as a fluid medium in the transfer of heat. This heat exchanger sprung a leak, and rice oil was contaminated. One thousand rice-oil consumers accumulated an average of 1 g of PCB's per person. Among other symptoms of trouble, infants were born with a strangely discolored skin.

1969 Spent PCB transformer fluid was used as a carrier for an herbicide, which was sprayed along a power-line right-of-way. Milk from several West Virginia dairy farms was found contaminated as a result of dairy cows feeding near the right-of-way.

1971 Another heat exchanger leaked PCB's into fish meal processed by a firm in North Carolina. Over 16,000 tons of meal were contaminated and ultimately used as an ingredient in the feed of meat animals, poultry, and fish.

1976 A Bloomington, Indiana, electric firm discharged PCB-containing waste into the local municipal sewage disposal system. Residents of the city used the sewage sludge as fertilizer for home garden plots. Sludge samples showed 479 ppm PCB's, and soil samples of contaminated gardens contained 17 ppm.

1977 A fire broke out in a Puerto Rican warehouse in which fish meal was stored. Electrical transformers housed in the same facility were damaged. PCB's leaked from the transformers to the fish meal, which was later used as chicken feed. In total, 400,000 chickens and 15,000 dozen eggs had to be destroyed.

1979 A farmer who had purchased nine barrels of waste transformer oil 7 years earlier, mixed it with insecticide (as carrier) and applied it directly to the skin of cattle. Upon analysis, the oil was found to contain 500,000 ppm (50%) PCB's. Even at concentrations 100,000 times lower than that, contamination of the animals would have neared the FDA's action level of 3 ppm in fat of red meat.

1979 A near miss: Leakage of PCB's from a capacitor occurred in a federally inspected hog slaughtering plant in Iowa. Quick action by observant officials of the firm avoided a massive potential contamination.

1979 Damaged transformers leaked PCB's into the waste system of an animal feed processor. In a common conservation measure, the wastewater was recycled with animal fats and processed into feed. Meat meal thus prepared became feed for poultry and livestock. Contaminated milk and eggs served as ingredients in soups and bakery items. Before this tragedy ended, destruction of food mounted to a toll surpassed only by the PBB incident in Michigan years earlier: 800,000 chickens, nearly 4 million eggs, 4,000 hogs, 74,000 different bakery goods, 800,000 pounds of animal feeds and feed ingredients. In the meantime, contaminated food was distributed to 19 states in the United States and to two foreign countries.

In one survey, PCB's were detected in 28 kinds of fish native to Lake Superior. They have been found in carp taken from Lake Pepin in Minnesota.

Problems of this kind obviously arise out of widespread application of a chemical compound to industrial goods—goods that most all of us accept and enjoy. PCB's have simply found too many "important" uses; plastics, carbonless copy paper, inks, adhesives, sealants, heat-transfer fluids, packaging materials, and in electrical transformers and capacitors. Prior to 1971, 40% of all PCB use was in products lost to the environment.

Prompted by the disasters and near disasters cited above, several United States regulatory agencies have proposed limitations on use of PCB's (see Federal Register, 1980c and 1981). Restrictions would limit concentration of PCB's for use either in food or nonfood processing applications. The chemical would be disallowed in heat exchangers used for making packages. Medicated pre-mixes and fertilizers would also come under control, along with other agricultural chemicals. Coupled with a vastly lowered production level of PCB's and also a new chemical method for detoxifying the compound, the risks from the contaminant could be eliminated—or nearly so—in 10 years.

In the meantime, milk of mothers over the world have been found contaminated with PCB's. Those regularly consuming fish from Lake Ontario yield milk levels of 5–10 ppm (see Yaffe and Waletzky, 1976). A nationwide survey in the United States puts average level in breast milk at 1–1.1 ppm on a fat basis. Sixth-day milk from 50 Swiss women averaged 2.0 mg/kg fat. The range in this study went from 0.3 to 13.3. That put 16% of the milk supplies in excess of the standard for PCB's in food products (2.5 mg/kg) (Schupbach and Egli, 1979). Levels of PCB's in milk of Polish women between the years 1975 and 1976 was found, in one quite extensive study, to range from 0.48 to 0.62 mg/kg fat. Dried whole cow's milk of that period of time yielded about tenfold less amounts, that is, 0.04–0.09 mg/kg fat. Raw cow's milk in Belgium has been found to average near 0.21 mg/kg fat. Infant food prepared with dried milk showed PCB's content of 0.25 mg/kg fat (Renterghem and Devlaminck, 1980).

As a general rule, just from the nature of the problem and the position of women in the food chain, one might expect somewhat higher levels of PCB's in breast milk than in the foods upon which mothers survive. Industrialized societies that regularly eat meat, poultry, fish, dairy and egg products, would also seem likely to show higher-than-average levels of this industrial pollutant. Already, and not unexpectedly, milk of older women (30–39) has been found to carry more PCB's than younger women (20–29) (Polishuk, et al., 1977). Yet it is significant that overall level of PCB's in food has been gradually trending downward.

Pentachlorophenols

As a category of pollutants these compounds might rightfully fall under pesticides. They are, in fact, used to kill certain pests, both slime-producing bacteria and fungi. Their most common use is as a preservative of wood. You might also find them in coatings for paper cartons and wrappers, and in adhesives used to seal food-packaging materials. It is these kinds of industrial and household uses that marks pentachlorophenols (PCP's) as potential industrial pollutants. Also, an increasingly frequent problem that stems not from PCP's themselves, but from commonplace contaminants of the products, one of which (dioxin) is among the most poisonous compounds known. It too has been detected in breast milk.

PCP reaches meat and milk through feed which has come in contact with wood. When animals lick treated wood or even rub up against it, contamination may occur. PCP also enters the animal body via inhalation. One problem case was ultimately traced to long-term confinement, where cattle breathed in the fumes of PCP-treated wood.

PCP itself has not been found carcinogenic to rats nor to cause reproductive problems in this species of animal at fairly high rates of intake. Two contaminants, however, are not only highly toxic but may be additive in their harmful effect. The chemical names of these compounds are dibenzofurans and dioxins. The latter are perhaps of greater significance, having also been found a contaminant of two widely used herbicides.

Dioxins

The abbreviation TCDD stands for 2,3,7,8-tetrachlorodibenzo-p-dioxin. This compound (or close chemical derivatives) has been found as a contaminant of PCP, the wood preservative, and of the herbicides silvex and 2,4,5–T. An estimated 7 million lb of the latter was used in the United States, mainly as tree and weed killer in power line right-of-ways, prior to an EPA ban for this kind of usage specifically. The ban was introduced upon evidence of larger-than-normal numbers of miscarriages of women near a spray area in Oregon. Evidence was taken over 6 years.

Dioxin(s), like many hazardous pollutants, is soluble in fat. It concentrates in the fat of animals, in the liver, and ultimately in the milk. University of Wisconsin scientist's found dioxin so toxic that the amount that causes harm must be measured in parts per trillion (ppt). Even single doses in parts per trillion cause death of animals. As little as 50 ppt causes an injurious response, the effects of which center chiefly on reproductive disorders. Some slight amount of the compound has turned up in dairy cattle; fish of some polluted waters have shown a degree of contamination (to 600 ppt in one badly polluted waterway). Levels of 10–40 ppt have turned up in breast milk, but only in a very limited survey (see Yaffe and Waletzky, 1976).

To make more of such findings than warranted is as inexcusable as it is to take them too lightly. Certainly, it is not suggested that women should not breast-feed as a result of evidence of this type. On the other hand, it is also far from reassuring to know that science offers no evidence of long-term effects of most of these compounds and that some of them, like the dioxins, are extremely toxic. Thus, I would prefer to leave this section, with whatever perspective it provides, as an overview of the ways in which pollution problems tend to creep up on us and as an expression of the need for continued vigilance. The use of pesticides, of course, must be weighed against the health of livestock and bounty of food. The risk of adding small amounts of contamination to mother's milk must share the stage with the risk of undernourishment. It is a situation somewhat different from industrial pollution. In that last, all of us can and should demand an environment free as possible of contaminants—and be willing to pay for it.

6

Infant Formula Composition, Formulation, and Processing

Most present-day infant formulas on the United States market are adaptations of the product designed by H.J. Gerstenberger and coworkers in 1915. On a fluid basis this early formula consisted of 4.6% fat (a homogenized mixture of both plant and animal fat), 6.5% carbohydrate, and 0.9% protein. Coined in 1919, the name for this product became Synthetic Milk Adapted (SMA).

Over the years the composition of infant formulas has been altered and adjusted, mostly in response to scientific evidence of need. The trend continues, as the 1977–1978 United States Department of Agriculture (USDA) nationwide food consumption survey attests (Pao, 1979). Compared with 1965, infant intake of food energy dropped significantly. Protein consumption went down 40%, from a mean intake of 39 g in 1965 to 25 g in 1977. Fat consumption declined even more, to 45% of the 1965 level. Calcium intake was down, sharply so, by 40%. All of these changes would reflect the use of infant formulas more nearly the composition of mother's milk—except for the amount of fat. At the same time, iron intake soared to twice the amount consumed in 1965. American infants are getting so much iron now that concern has been raised that mothers might overfeed this mineral. A mother might combine iron-fortified formula, iron-fortified infant cereal, and mineral (iron) supplements. This could pose some risk to certain infants.

The level of intake of certain vitamins dropped during 1965–1977, but not below recommended needs. One vitamin, riboflavin, fell 30% in usage but still remained at a level of intake 100% over need. Infant formulas have served an essential purpose. Their present formulation must surely serve better than early formulations the special needs of the hungry and malnourished. A look at their formulation and how they are (or will be) processed helps explain why.

THE NUTRIENT COMPONENTS OF INFANT FORMULA

Infant formulas can be categorized into four major types. These are: (1) milk-based, (2) milk and whey formulations, (3) soy-based, and (4) protein hydrolysates. Milk-based products consist mainly of fluid (or dry) milk ingredients, vegetable oils, and either lactose or corn syrup solids (or both) as a carbohydrate source. Various types of whey products, as sources of protein and/or lactose, become ingredients of (2). Soy-based formulas center on soy products as protein source. At one time soy flour was a major ingredient. However, because soy flour products tended to cause loose, malodorous stools, processors have recently shifted to soy protein isolates, that is, soy protein purified to 90% or higher protein content. Again, plant oils (with possibly some cow's milk fat) are used as sources of fat; corn sryup solids and/or sucrose are used as source(s) of carbohydrate. Protein hydrolysates are formulas in which the protein is broken down (hydrolyzed) into fragments of protein (called peptides) and amino acids. Casein (milk protein) and meat are the two most common sources of protein. Such formulas serve the needs of infants with various protein sensitivities. Because they are formulated without lactose, these products serve equally well infant victims of galactosemia (an inability to metabolize galactose, one of the carbohydrate components of lactose). Table 18 shows the major nutrient composition of the above types of infant formulas. They are designed for the essentially healthy, full-term infant. Special formulas (medical formulations) are designed for infants with more specialized needs—as for example those afflicted with (1) inborn errors of metabolism, (2) congestive heart failure, (3) steatorrheal disorder (requiring altered fat or carbohydrate intakes), and (4) enzyme or other deficiencies.

In addition to the preceding, formulas may be classified as either fortified or unfortified with iron. Iron-fortified formulas are usually recommended for healthy infants who are not being breast-fed. It is obvious that in shopping for

TABLE 18

Major Nutrient Composition of Various Types of Infant Formulas Designed for "Normal" Full-Term Infants[a]

Type	Use	Protein				Fat				Carbohydrate		
		Source	g/100 kcal	% kcal		Source	g/100 kcal	% kcal		Source	g/100 kcal	% kcal
Milk-based	Routine	Nonfat cow's milk	2.2–2.4	9		Vegetable oils	5.4–5.5	48–50		Lactose	10.5–10.9	41–43
Whey-adjusted	Routine	Nonfat cow's milk plus demineralized whey	2.2	9		Vegetable and oleo oils	5.4	48		Lactose	10.8	43
Soy isolate	Cow's milk sensitivity	Soy isolate	2.7–3.7	12–15		Vegetable oils	4.5–5.4	45–48		Corn syrup solids and/or sucrose	9.6–10.2	39–40
Casein hydrolysate	Protein sensitivity Galactosemia	Casein hydrolysate	3.3–3.4	13–14		Corn oil or corn oil and medium-chain tri-glycerides	3.9–4.2	35–36		Tapioca starch and glucose, sucrose, or corn syrup solids	12.8–13.1	51–52
Meat-based	Cow's milk sensitivity Galactosemia	Beef hearts	4.0	16		Sesame oil Beef heart fat	4.8	47		Tapioca starch and sucrose	9	37

[a] Adapted from Anderson *et al.* (1980).

infant formula one must be prepared to read in some detail the information on the label. As a guide, you may wish to browse Tables 19, 20, 21, and 22. Soy, milk, and milk and whey formulas are represented. Among them are certain similarities and some rather striking differences.

Proximate compositon of two formulas—one soy, the other milk—is shown in Table 19. Only protein (and perhaps mineral) level stands out as a major variation. The milk formula contains only 1.5% protein as compared with 2.5% for the soy product. In essential amino acid supply, the two may be fairly comparable, especially with methionine added independently in the soy formula (see Table 20). Milk protein, in this case made up of both casein and the whey protein lactalbumin, is of such high biological value that a smaller amount can serve equally the infant's needs. What appears to be a significant difference turns out to be artifact, for all practical purposes.

Table 20 enumerates individual ingredients of the two formulas shown in Table 19. Ingredients of two additional formulas are shown in Table 21. Note first the carbohydrate of the soy products. It stems either from the dextrose (glucose) of corn syrup solids or from a combination of sugar (sucrose) and corn syrup solids. Neither contains any milk sugar, or lactose. In both cases protein is a soy protein isolate. In the future a host of new, and in some cases better quality, proteins could supplant or add to soy products.

The fat of infant formulas may stem from a number of sources. In the soy products illustrated in Tables 20 and 21, soybean oil is found in both and serves the needs for a polyunsaturated fat. One of these formulas also combines coconut fat with soybean oil. Coconut fat is, of course, a relatively saturated (hard) fat. Other hard fats (cow's milk fat, specifically) could as well be used. The future will no doubt see more babassu and palm oil formulations. Certainly these oils will be exploited in those countries where these oil-bearing trees grow native to the land. They will also find use elsewhere. Currently, evidence would suggest that such oils are acceptable if they are combined with an appropriate level of unsaturated fats. Thus, the milk formulas contain both coconut and soybean oils. One formula also contains oleo and safflower oils, two additional sources of polyunsaturated fat.

All of the formulas, soy and milk alike, use lecithin as an emulsifier. Two of them also contain mono- and diglycerides, fats with one or two fatty acids missing. In all cases, these compounds are present to hold the fat in homogenous dispersion. To some extent, certain phosphates also have this ability. The Food and Agriculture Organization/World Health Organization (FAO/WHO) allowance for emulsifiers in infant formula recognizes only lecithin and mono- and diglycerides—the former to 0.5 g/100 ml, the latter to 0.4 g/100 ml ready-to-drink products (see Appendix 6).

TABLE 19
Proximate Composition of Soy-Based and Milk-Based Infant Formulas[a]

Component	Soy formula (% w/v)	Milk formula (% w/v)
Fat	3.4	3.6
Carbohydrate	6.8	7.2
Protein	2.5	1.5[b]
Minerals (ash)	0.5	0.25
Fiber	none	none
Calories (per 29.6 ml)	20	20

[a]Soy infant formula is a product of Mead Johnson Laboratories, Evansville, Indiana 47721. Milk-based infant formula is a product of Wyeth Laboratories, Philadelphia, Pennsylvania 19101. The figures presented are for use strength, that is, properly diluted liquid concentrates.
[b]Protein consists of 0.9% lactalbumin and 0.6% casein, for a 60:40 ratio of these two components.

If lecithin is common to these four infant formulas, so is carrageenan, a stabilizer and thickener. Only one formula, a soy product, adds a modified cornstarch to assist in this function. Using substances such as these and possibly certain of the mineral components, ingredients of liquid formulas (protein in particular) are held in dispersion and/or kept from forming a gel. See Appendix 6 for a list of stabilizers approved by FAO/WHO.

Both soy formulas add methionine, the limiting amino acid of soy protein. Neither milk formula needs this kind of supplementation. In one case, nonfat (skim) milk provides protein, which incidentally would contain both casein and whey proteins. The other milk formula supplements the skim milk with a specially prepared protein concentrate from whey.

All the preceding substances constitute the major ingredients of the four infant formulas shown in Tables 20 and 21. Soy products differ primarily in the source of protein and carbohydrate. Soy protein is the current protein of choice in nonmilk products. In the future any of a number of other proteins may serve equally as well. Nonmilk formulas generally replace milk sugar (lactose) with corn syrup and/or sugar (sucrose). Milk formulas derive some lactose from nonfat milk and also from the purified lactose added back literally as an additive. The only dairy ingredient lacking in the milk formulas shown in these tables is milk fat, or butterfat. All the butterfat, along with it the cholesterol (whether for good or bad), has been left out. In its place comes coconut oil (a fat of equivalent hardness, or saturation) and one or more sources of soft fat.

Look next at the vitamin sources in these products. Most speak for themselves. They are simply derivatives of the respective vitamins, and more

TABLE 20
Ingredients of Soy-Based and Milk-Based Infant Formulas[a]

Soy formula	Milk formula
Major ingredients and functional components[b]	Major ingredients and functional components[b]
Water	Water
Sugar	Nonfat (skim) milk
Corn syrup solids	Whey, demineralized (electrodialyzed)
Soybean oil	Lactose
Soy protein isolate	Oleo oil
Lecithin	Coconut oil
Carrageenan	Safflower oil
Amino acid source	Soybean oil
L-methionine	Lecithin
Vitamin sources	Carrageenan
Vitamin A palmitate	Vitamin sources[d]
Ergocalciferol	Vitamin A palmitate
dl-alpha-tocopheryl acetate	β-carotene
Sodium ascorbate	7-dehydrocholesterol (activated)
Folic acid	D-alpha-tocopheryl acetate
Thiamine hydrochloride	Ascorbic acid
Riboflavin	Folic acid
Niacinamide	Thiamin hydrochloride
Pyridoxine hydrochloride	Riboflavin
Cyanocobalamin	Niacinamide
Biotin	Pyridoxine hydrochloride
Calcium pantothenate	Cyanocobalamin
Phytonadione	Biotin
Choline chloride	Calcium pantothenate
Mineral sources[c]	Phytonadione
Tricalcium phosphate	Mineral sources[d]
Potassium citrate	Potassium bicarbonate
Dibasic magnesium phosphate	Calcium chloride
Potassium chloride	Calcium citrate
Sodium chloride (salt)	Potassium chloride
Ferrous sulfate	Sodium citrate
Cupric sulfate	Ferrous sulfate
Zinc sulfate	Sodium bicarbonate
Manganese sulfate	Zinc sulfate
Potassium iodide	Cupric sulfate
	Manganese sulfate

[a]The soy infant formula is a product of Mead Johnson Laboratories, Evansville, Indiana 47721. The milk-based formula is product of Wyeth Laboratories, Philadelphia, Pennsylvania 19101.

[b]Some of the mineral sources may serve a functional as well as nutrient purpose.

[c]Some mineral elements will also be derived from the soy protein isolate.

[d]Some vitamins and/or minerals will also be derived from the nonfat milk and whey solids.

TABLE 21
Ingredients of Soy-Based and Milk-Based Infant Formulas[a]

Soy formula	Milk formula
Major ingredients and functional components	Major ingredients and functional components
Water	Water
Corn syrup	Nonfat (skim) milk
Sucrose	Lactose
Soy protein isolate	Coconut oil
Coconut oil	Soybean oil
Soybean oil	Mono- and diglycerides
Modified corn starch	Soy lecithin
Mono- and diglycerides	Carrageenan
Soy lecithin	Vitamin sources
Carrageenan	Vitamin A palmitate
Amino acid source	Vitamin D_3 (concentrate)
L-methionine (plus soy protein)	Alpha tocopheryl acetate
Vitamin sources	Ascorbic acid
Vitamin A palmitate	Thiamin chloride hydrochloride
Vitamin D_3 (concentrate)	Riboflavin
Alphatocopheryl acetate	Cyanocobalamin
Phytonadione	Niacinamide
Ascorbic acid	Calcium pantothenate
Thiamin chloride hydrochloride	Pyridoxine hydrochloride
Riboflavin	Folic acid
Cyanocobalamin	Mineral sources
Niacinamide	Cupric sulfate (copper)
Calcium pantothenate	Manganous chloride (manganese)
Pyridoxine hydrochloride	Potassium citrate
Biotin	Zinc sulfate
Folic acid	
Choline chloride	
Mineral sources	
Calcium phosphate, tribasic	
Cupric sulfate	
Ferrous sulfate	
Magnesium chloride	
Potassium chloride	
Potassium citrate	
Potassium iodide	
Zinc sulfate	

[a]Liquid concentrates of Ross Laboratories, Columbus, Ohio 43216.

than likely more stable than the pure vitamin compounds. That is important, obviously. A vitamin altered during storage may lose its potency.

In the lists of vitamin sources, ergocalciferol and 7-dehydrocholesterol both function as vitamin D. Vitamin E is shown variously as alpha-tocopheryl acetate. Sodium ascorbate or ascorbic acid becomes vitamin C.

Cyanocobalamin is vitamin B_{12}, phytonadione is vitamin K. The other names are self-explanatory. Note that one of the soy formulas sports a longer list of vitamin additives than its milk counterpart. The reason has to do with vitamins found naturally occurring in milk; these number more than in soy products and in amounts adequate for needs in some instances. For example, if milk is eliminated, choline is also eliminated. In any event, vitamin additives of formulas are not equivalent in all cases. No harm is done in adding, for sake of consistency, vitamins found also in the major ingredients.

Mineral additives in soy formulas also often exceed in number those of milk-based products. In the two formulas shown in Table 20, the number of mineral ingredients is equal. There are, however, some differences in kind. As shown in Table 22, there are also quantitative differences. Calcium and phosphorus levels are much higher in the milk formula. Most mineral components are in fact present at higher levels; again this is because milk itself is a good source of these elements. The soybean, which is a good source of some mineral components, has simply been stripped of them in refining the protein isolate.

Differences do exist between formulas. They exist because each ingredient offers its own particular array of nutrients. In no case, however, need the infant be deprived of appropriate amounts and kinds.

INFANT FORMULA: ITS FORMULATION

Infant formula can vary in composition, but within fairly narrow and quite precise limits. In general, as a complete substitute for human milk, formula should provide protein (of appropriate biological quality) at 7–16% of calories, fat at 30–54% of calories, linoleic acid at 2–3% of calories, and the remaining calories from carbohydrate sources (NAS/NRC, 1980). For best fat absorption, it is desirable to have available a portion of mono-glycerides with palmitic acid in the 2 position (Nestlé, 1975). Both cow's and goat's milk fat represent sources of naturally occurring triglycerides with this fatty acid configuration. Vegetable fats have little or no such chemical entities. Nonetheless, a reasonable likeness of human milk fat is simulated through the use of various vegetable fats. Possibly corn oil is somewhat more acceptable because of its relatively high level of oleic acid. A complete replacement of milk fat is possible, or blends of milk fat and vegetable fat possibly serve even better. The state of scientific knowledge does not permit evaluation of the significance of cholesterol. Because many contaminants or pollutants of food are soluble in fat, specially refined fats and oils provide better control. To prevent conversion of *cis* to *trans* fatty acids, and loss thereby of essential fatty acids, low- (or ultra-high) temperature treatment

TABLE 22
Vitamin and Mineral Content of a Soy-Based and Milk-Based Infant Formula[a]

	Soy formula (per qt)	Milk formula (per qt)
Vitamins		
Vitamin A (IU)	1600	2500
Vitamin D (IU)	400	400
Vitamin E (IU)	14	9
Vitamin K_1 (mcg)	100	55
Vitamin C (mg)	52	55
Vitamin B_1 (mg)	0.5	0.67
Vitamin B_2 (mg)	0.6	1
Vitamin B_6 (mg)	0.4	0.4
Vitamin B_{12} (mcg)	2	1
Biotin (mg)	0.05	14
Niacin	8 mg	9.5 (mg equiv.)
Pantothenic acid (mg)	3	2
Folic acid (mcg)	100	50
Choline (mg)	85	130
Minerals		
Calcium (mg)	117	420
Phosphorus (mg)	78	312
Magnesium (mg)	10.9	50
Sodium (mg)	62.5	142
Potassium (mg)	109	530
Iron (mg)	1.9[b]	12
Copper (mg)	0.09	0.45
Zinc (mg)	0.78	3.5
Manganese (mcg)	0.16	150
Iodine (mcg)	7	65
Chloride (mg)	62.5	350

[a]The soy-based infant formula is a product of Mead Johnson Laboratories, Evansville, Indiana 47721. The milk-based infant formula is a product of Wyeth Laboratories, Philadelphia, Pennsylvania 19101.

[b]This product was not fortified with iron. Other soy infant formulas do come so fortified, to the same level as found in the milk formula. Products with and without added iron, both soy and milk base, are commercially available. The option is provided to accommodate to a variety of infant diets, which may or may not include some solid food or use of vitamin and/or mineral supplements.

must be used throughout processing. In addition, evidence exists to suggest a beneficial effect in fat absorption from presence of the amino acid taurine and the betaine carnitine. Human milk contains 26.6 μmoles/100 ml of the former and 59 nmol/ml of the latter. Cow (and beef) formulations are assumed to be equivalent or higher in content of carnitine, but soy formulas, lacking supplementation, could be considered deficient (Borum et al., 1979).

In human milk, the ratio of fat to protein is 2 (or more):1. This balance in formulas is likewise preferably kept within those limits.

Protein in milk-based formulas is best divided between whey proteins and casein in a 60:40 ratio. Of the major whey proteins is cow's milk, α-lactalbumin more nearly mirrors the whey proteins of mother's milk. Absence of the other major whey protein of cow's milk (i.e., β-lactoglobulin) eliminates a possibly significant allergen. Given 0.9% α-lactalbumin and 0.6% casein, a reasonable likeness of the protein profile of mother's milk is produced. Some researchers suggest the ideal protein composition of formula would be 1.0–1.2 g protein/100 ml, and made consistent with human milk in the levels of taurine and cystine (Lindblad et al., 1978). Moreover, certain glucosamines (of nonprotein nitrogen) may serve to stimulate growth of Lactobacillus bifidus. For this purpose, N-substituted D-glucosamines have been suggested (see The Bifidus Factor, Chapter 4), and also the co-enzyme A precursor, pantetheine phosphate. In addition, lactulose (4-0-βD-galactopyranosyl-D-fructose), a ketose derivative of lactose, has been shown to enhance growth of the organism. This is true even though the compound is not found to occur in raw (unheated) milk of either humans or cows. The formula in which the bifidus-stimulating phenomenon was originally noted consisted of 1.2 g lactulose/70 kcal, with lactose content of the diet held at 2.5 times the protein level. Further work by different investigators put the desired lactulose content at 1.2–1.5% of the diet. A heat-sterilized liquid infant formula causes conversion of between 1% and 5% of total lactose to lactulose (see Mendez and Olano, 1979).

Caloric density of infant formulas of 670 kcal/liter appears nearly optimal for normal full-term infants (AAP, 1976). The formulation should provide a calcium–phosphorus ratio of not less than 1.1:1.0 nor more than 2:1. The optimal ratio is near 1.5:1, at least through most of the first year of life. By 1 year of age, the appropriate ratio is more nearly 1:1 (NAS/NRC, 1980). Calcium should be of a chemical form that is biologically available and should be present to a minimum of 50 mg/100 kcal. Minimum phosphorus level is 25 mg/100 kcal. Minimum and maximum amounts of sodium, potassium, and chloride must also be observed. These levels are met within the ranges 6–17, 14–34, and 11–29 milliequivalents (mEq), respectively, in a formula providing 670 kcal/liter (NAS/NRC, 1980). One milliequivalent is equal to the atomic weight (in milligrams) of the element divided by valence. Osmolarity—in moles of solute/liter—should not exceed 400 mOsm (see Sodium, Potassium, and Chloride, Chapter 3). Some of these and certain other recommendations are shown in Table 23.

Major sources of protein for infant formulas include milk, whey, and soy. In the latter case, highly refined soy protein (soy isolate) is used in most instances. Nonetheless, various methods of purifying soy protein create

TABLE 23
Nutrient Levels of Infant Formulas (per 100 kcal)[a]

Nutrient	FDA 1971 Regulations minimum	1976 Recommendations[b]	
		Minimum	Maximum
Protein (g)	1.8	1.8	4.5
Fat			
(g)	1.7	3.3	6.0
(% cal)	15.0	30.0	54.0
Essential fatty acids (linoleate)			
(% cal)	2.0	3.0	—
(mg)	222.0	300.0	—
Vitamins			
A (IU)	250.0	250.0 (75 μg)[c]	750.0 (225 μg)[c]
D (IU)	40.0	40.0	100.0
K (μg)	—	4.0	—
E (IU)	0.3	0.3 (with 0.7 IU/g linoleic acid)	—
C (ascorbic acid) (mg)	7.8	8.0	—
B (thiamine) (μg)	25.0	40.0	—
B$_2$ (riboflavin) (μg)	60.0	60.0	—
B$_6$ (pyridoxine) (μg)	35.0	35.0 (with 15 μg/g of protein in formula)	—
B$_{12}$ (μg)	0.15	0.15	—
Niacin			
(μg)	—	250.0	—
(μg equiv)	800.0	— —	—
Folic acid (μg)	4.0	4.0	—
Pantothenic acid (μg)	300.0	300.0	—
Biotin (μg)	—	1.5	—
Choline (mg)	—	7.0	—
Inositol (mg)	—	4.0	—
Minerals			
Calcium (mg)	50.0[d]	40.0[d]	—
Phosphorus (mg)	25.0[d]	25.0[d]	—
Magnesium (mg)	6.0	6.0	—
Iron (mg)	1.0	0.15	—
Iodine (μg)	5.0	5.0	—
Zinc (mg)	—	0.5	—
Copper (μg)	60.0	60.0	—
Manganese (μg)	—	5.0	—
Sodium (mg)	—	20.0 (mEq)[e]	60.0 (17 mEq)[e]
Potassium (mg)	—	80.0 (14 mEq)[e]	200.0 (34 mEq)[e]
Chloride (mg)	—	55.0 (11 mEq)[e]	150.0 (29 mEq)[e]

[a] Adapted from Anderson et al. (1980).
[b] Modified from Committee on Nutrition (American Academy of Pediatrics, 1976).
[c] Retinol equivalents.
[d] Calcium to phosphorus ratio must be no less than 1.1 to 1.0 nor more than 2.0 to 1.0.
[e] Milliequivalents for 670 kcal/liter of formula.

significant differences in the composition of associated ingredients, particularly mineral components. All soy protein supplies should be carefully monitored, and the protein obtained from different suppliers should not be assumed to be identical. Chemical analysis will generally serve most monitoring and/or quality control functions. New protein sources (nonmilk, nonsoy) should undergo extensive metabolic and clinical studies prior to use.

Carbohydrate sources include lactose (or milk and whey products that contain lactose), sucrose, corn syrup solids (a source of glucose), and starch. Actually, modified starch is used not so much as source of carbohydrate as a stabilizer. Although there is no reason to believe that starch poses a digestive problem to infants, neither have studies been carried out to assess its relative digestability. However, generally more formulas are prepared without than with it.

Appendix 6 contains a listing, recommended by the Codex Alimentarius Commission (1976), of approved kinds and amounts of thickening agents, emulsifiers, antioxidants, and compounds for adjusting pH. Most of these agents have GRAS status in the United States. A recent ruling, however, failed to affirm "generally regarded as safe" (GRAS) status for D(-) lactic acid, DL-lactic acid, and their calcium salts for infant formulas. The action was taken because of insufficient evidence of no adverse effects on infants. For the α-isomer, no evidence of toxicity exists for persons of any age. Studies of the response of full-term infants to D(-) lactic acid and DL-lactic acid are apparently conflicting. Limited data taken on premature infants suggest some possibility of slowed growth and development of metabolic acidosis.

Conditions of use of additives in infant formula are regulated under the Code of Federal Regulations (CFR), Title 21, section 172.620 and section 180. Requirements vary, of course, by nation. The European Society for Pediatric Gastroenterology and Nutrition, Committee on Nutrition (ESPGAN, 1977) advises against the use of thickening agents in infant formulas for infants under 4 months of age.

Vitamin additives approved by FAO/WHO for use in infant formula are listed in Appendix 3. In some cases several different chemical forms of the vitamin or provitamin have approval for use. Processing requirements, availability, and/or stability in the specific food system will dictate which form(s) will serve best.

FAO/WHO also approves mineral sources for infant formula. This listing is shown in Appendix 6. At first glance, the list looks rather long and imposing. Yet a larger number of compounds are necessary to meet the varied demands of a vast array of different food systems. Suitability of any given mineral additive depends on composition and moisture level of the food product. Furthermore, each food imposes its own requirements for flavor and/or textural stability. Oxidative rancidity is an ever-present problem in iron and/or copper-fortified foods containing unsaturated fats. Gelation is a potential problem in concentrated liquid infant formulas. Reduced iron or electroytic iron, which serve well in dry foods, will settle out as a sediment in liquid formula. FAO/WHO also recognizes the need for acids and bases for making pH adjustments; however, these must then be accounted for in determining total content of any given mineral. In addition to the compounds listed in Appendix 6, other compounds pending approval (or deletion) by FAO/WHO for use as mineral salts are shown in Appendix 5. Still other salts are allowed only if (1) they provide technological and nutritional improvement, (2) the anion of the salt (or acid from which the salt is derived) is an approved food additive and would not, in application, exceed the Acceptable Daily Intake (ADI), and (3) the mineral has been shown to be biologically available.

One other fact should once again be repeated. Certain mineral compounds are needed in fairly large amounts in infant formula. Calcium and phosphorus are two examples. Other mineral elements are needed only in very small (trace) amounts (see Table 14). At these minute levels, these minerals are nonetheless essential. The difference in the amount that is needed and, for some nutrients, that which becomes toxic is very slim indeed. Thus, trace minerals in ingredients of infant formula must be considered, along with those that may be added in water supplies used to reconstitute various dry ingredients. Water supplies may or may not be treated for this purpose, depending upon the overall quality. Water quality should be monitored, however, along with the trace mineral content of finished formula.

In formulating mineral composition of dairy-based infant formula, certain factors should be kept in mind. They may be summarized as follows. The content of calcium in cow's milk varies somewhat on a seasonal and regional basis. The level of certain trace minerals—among them zinc, iodine, copper, sodium, manganese, and cobalt—vary to more or less an extent by the amount present in feed. The iron content of cow's milk seems uninfluenced by the intake of feed. Some amount of iron, copper, molybdenum, manganese, and magnesium is associated with the fat globule membrane and will be lost upon separation and exclusion of milk fat as an ingredient in formula. Perhaps a third of both calcium and phosphorus is associated with casein and remains with casein upon rennet coagulation. Most magnesium (about 75%) and essentially all zinc are complexed with casein. As they exist in milk, some amount of some mineral components will be lost to the permeate in milk or whey treated by ultrafiltration, reverse osmosis, electrodialysis, and other methods of concentrating protein. Of course, a certain amount of mineral depletion is necessary to provide a formula of appropriate osmolar strength. In the process, however, some amount of some trace minerals will be lost, for better or worse.

When trace minerals are added to formula, sulfate salts are commonly used. Acceptable levels of sulfate ions have not been specified, however (Anderson *et al.*, 1980). Because of the potential to cause methemoglobinemia, nitrate salts are usually not added to formula. Some small (safe) amount may occur in formula made up of vegetable products. Nitrates also occur, and occasionally at high levels, in some water supplies. Copper is another potentially toxic component of water. Soy products not adequately processed may contain goitrogens, necessitating the presence in formula of added iodine as a defense against goiter.

Minerals commonly added to formulas include calcium, phosphorus, magnesium, iron, copper, iodine, zinc, potassium, sodium, manganese, and chlorine (as chloride).

All in all, it is the low-mineral, high-globulin (albumin) requirements of milk-based formulas that pose the most difficult formulation problems. Yet present technologies make the problem one of choice of ingredients, not availability. The protein blend may consist of (1) skim or low-fat milk with various whey products, (2) modified (reduced mineral content) milk and various whey products, and (3) caseinates (sodium or calcium salts of casein) and various whey products. Some of those whey components represent immune factors. Thus, scientists now speak of the "humanization" of infant formula. What they mean is a product more closely approximating the true composition of human milk.

FORMULATIONS FOR PREMATURE INFANTS

For preterm or low-weight infants (under 2500 g), formulas are usually modified. Commonly protein and mineral content is raised somewhat. Lactose level may be lowered by one-third to one-half regular amounts, and the difference can be made up with corn syrup solids, a more readily absorbable carbohydrate source. Fat, calcium, and phosphorus must be available in readily utilizable form. Caloric density is raised to 800–1000 kcal/liter; 11% of calories come from protein and 50% from fat (see Foman, 1974; Anderson *et al.*, 1980). For infants weighing less than 1500 g at birth, nutrients may have to be provided by parenteral or enteral feeding. In limited work, a product with nitrogen osmolarity of 12.42 mOsm/liter (2.18 g protein/100 ml) and sodium plus potassium plus chloride osmolarity of 4.52 mOsm/liter appears not to overload the kidneys of infants in the birthweight range 1000–2500 g (Valjak *et al.*, 1978). In general, corn and soy oil appear reasonably well absorbed by premature infants. Some authorities (Naude *et al.*, 1979) caution against the use of soy formulas, which tend to raise serum alkaline phosphatase and blood urea levels in infants to higher levels than those fed cow's milk formulas.

SOME PROCESSING CONSIDERATIONS

Milk or milk and whey-based formulas must consider the need to alter the composition of natural cow's milk. There is the need to (1) lower protein content (without loss of biological quality), (2) raise carbohydrate content (compared with normal milk), (3) alter fat composition, and (4) lower mineral content. This is done usually through the use of an appropriate mixture of milk (or modified milk), whey components, vegetable fat, and corn syrup solids. The whey in this case provides albumins and globulins, though it is the former which is most needed. These proteins, however, must be added without adding significantly to the level of mineral nor greatly exceeding the amount of lactose found in human milk. Raising the carbohydrate level also reverts to a question of avoiding excess. Thus, a number of relatively new technologies find important application. Among them are electrodialysis, ion exchange, ultrafiltration, and gel filtration. Reverse osmosis also has use in concentrating dilute suspensions of nutrients, like whey solids. The important needs, though, are for reduction of mineral and lactose levels. Ultrafiltration, a modified form of reverse osmosis, both concentrates and provides for removal of various amounts of dissolved substances (lactose and minerals). Electrodialysis is especially useful in lowering mineral content. In this process, negatively charged ions (chloride, lactate, phosphate) are attracted out of the whey through a membrane permeable to anions. Sodium, potassium, calcium, and other positively charged ions are drawn off through a membrane selectively permeable to cations. Generally, whey is first concentrated to 25% solids. Then minerals and/or acids are removed by electrodialysis. To reduce lactose level, the electrodialyzed product is concentrated to 40–50% solids and cooled. A sizable amount of lactose crystallizes out of suspension upon cooling, and is spun off in a centrifuge. With electrodialysis it is possible to lower mineral content of whey by up to 90%. Mostly proteins remain, and these may then be spray-dried.

To separate various protein fractions, gel filtration may be applied. This process also provides a way of segregating protein from minerals. Whey is first pretreated to remove particles of leftover curd. It is then concentrated and lactose is removed by crystallization. The mother liquor is treated by gel filtration, as in a kind of molecular sieve. The gel, Sephadex in this case, forms a meshwork of tiny pores so small that only relatively small molecules are admitted. Larger molecules, like proteins, simply pass down the column more or less unimpeded.

Gel filtration is used to fractionate whey proteins into components useful in infant formula. Professor K.M. Shahani (1974) of the University of Nebraska passes whey protein concentrate through a column of Sephadex G-75. Proteins derived by this method include α-lactalbumin, serum albumin, immune globulins, and lactoferrin, all useful as formula ingredients. As a byproduct, β-lactoglobulin serves in other special dietary foods. This same researcher has also developed a special formula for infants born in need of cardiac surgery. The product, designed for fast weight gain, consists of maltodextrins, vegetable oil, whey protein concentrate, soy protein isolate, vitamins, minerals, and artificial flavor and color. In gross composition, the food contains 8.3% protein, 63.3% carbohydrate, and 28.4% fat. It provides 2528 kcal in 510 g. Electrodialyzed whey is the source of carbohydrate and part of the protein.

Carboxymethylcellulose (CMC) also serves as an ion-exchange medium for separating whey proteins either of acid or sweet whey. Pillinger and Langley (1978) report a method in which protein uptake on CMC is accomplished at pH 3.0. Protein fractions of varying α-lactalbumin to β-lactoglobulin ratios are then eluted from the CMC with increasing concentrations of sodium chloride.

Of course, the classical method of fractionating the two major whey protein components of cow's milk involve salting out from the whey the β-lactoglobulin with either ammonium sulfate or magnesium sulfate (see Jenness and Patton, 1959).

A number of processes and formulations of infant formula have been patented. As evidence of varying approaches, a few will be mentioned. One process calls for addition of sodium or calcium caseinates to liquid whey, along with minerals, vitamins, lysozyme, and a bifidus-stimulating factor. The mixture, as such, is simply homogenized and spray-dried. Another process passes milk through an ion exchanger to remove anions of weak acids. the deionized product is then combined with albumin, fats, vitamins, minerals, and lactose. Or, in a modified version, electrodialysis is used to reduce mineral level of the milk, and lactose and fat added to a level approximating human milk composition. Still other patents describe processes for hydrolyzing whey proteins to reduce allergenicity or inclusion of undenatured immunoglobulins as source of immune components. A low-sodium formula has been developed in which a "casein micelle" is formed from solubilized acid casein to which is added a potassium salt of an organic acid and/or potassium polyphosphate, and a calcium salt (at $<50°$ C). The pH is then adjusted to 6.2–6.8 and the "micelle" formed by heating to 65°

C. To this component is added fat, carbohydrate, and other nutrients. The product is then homogenized, pasteurized and concentrated (Nagasawa *et al.*, 1975).

Blending Ingredients

In processing either liquid or dry products, ingredients are first blended at warm temperatures (above the melting point of fats and oils) in tanks using some form of mechanical agitation. For processes in which intense preheat treatment is rendered, condensed skim milk or nonfat dry milk should be the "high-heat" type (Mulchandani *et al.*, 1979b). That is, heat treatment given these products during their manufacture should have been adequate to denature most whey proteins. If not, these ingredients will contribute to sediment formation during storage of the finished product. In evaporated products made from fresh milk, vitamin and mineral addition is usually delayed until after evaporation and just prior to retort sterilization (when this is the process used). Some loss of vitamins during forewarming and evaporation is thereby avoided.

The water supply used in reconstitution and blending of formula ingredients must come in for special attention. Treatment could consider the possible need to remove both organic and inorganic pollutants, that is, toxic components. Treatment should also consider the possible need to remove fluoride from fluoridated water supplies, and the need to standardize at some appropriate base level those same minerals with which the formula will ultimately be fortified. This latter requirement stems from the necessity to fortify formula to within rather narrow limits of mineral components, especially trace minerals. Untreated water supplies may vary daily in mineral content. Common mineral presence includes calcium, magnesium, manganese, zinc, iron, copper, selenium, sodium, potassium, chloride, and fluoride. Certain of these mineral elements pose some risk in overintake. Two of them, iron and copper, catalyze oxidative rancidity of fat. Common and known toxic minerals of water include arsenic, barium, lead (lead pipes being a serious source), calcium, and methyl mercury. Polluted water may also contain excessive levels of nitrates, the cause of a deadly blood malady (methemoglobinemia) in infants. The maximum allowable amount of nitrate in drinking water is usually set at 10 mg/liter. Municipal water supplies in the United States should meet this standard. Industrial, farm, and home ground or well-water supplies may exceed this level (though uncommonly). Both the blending water in the manufacture of infant formula and the water of reconstitution or dilution of finished formulas pose some hazard in this regard. Poisonings are recorded in breast-fed infants given drinking water high in nitrate content. Cows drinking such water will produce milk of potential hazard. Often the chemical waste of fertilizer processing plants is a source. Little more than 50 mg nitrate/liter must be considered a serious risk to infant health. A monitored, treated water supply is of profound importance in the manufacture of infant formula.

Processing Liquid Products

Infant formula is processed as ready-to-eat and concentrated liquids, and as dried products. To prevent spoilage during long-term storage, liquid products must be sterilized. Sterilization is the process of heating a food product to a specific temperature for a particular length of time needed to destroy all microbial life. A sterile liquid formula may be stored for 6 months to 1 year without undergoing spoilage or, more difficult to control, textural changes. Sterilized fluid milk products, like infant formula, are apt to alter in physical consistency over time. Sometimes these changes result in a sediment being formed. Other times the product may set up as a gel. Though microbial spoilage is not involved, such products are either less usable or, possibly, less nutritive. Prevention of these defects requires appropriate formulation, homogenization, and heat treatment.

A number of different processes may be applied to provide the heat treatment necessary to bring about sterility in liquid infant formulas. From a nutritional standpoint, the preferred method would be an ultra-high-temperature (UHT) process. Nutrient (vitamin) loss is minimized, as is the reaction (browning) between carbohydrates (reducing sugars) and lysine of protein, which lowers protein quality. As a general rule, UHT may be taken to mean temperatures ranging between 135 and 150° C for a time span of a few seconds to 1 second or less. The higher the temperature, the shorter the time needed to achieve sterility. However, the tendency of formula products to develop textural defects like sediment formation or gelation may make it necessary to hold the product for about 2.5 seconds even at the upper temperature of treatment. Furthermore, UHT treatment may have to be preceded by an intense preheat treatment to precondition the product. Gelation appears to be related to some extent to active enzymes, and pretreatment helps ensure their permanent destruction. Since some of these enzymes may be associated with bacterial contaminants of the original milk, only the highest quality milk (lowest bacterial numbers, especially of psychrophiles) should be used. (For a general review, see International Dairy Federation, 1972.)

INDIRECT HEATING METHODS

Both indirect and direct heating systems are used as sterilizing treatments for liquid formulas. Indirect heating units include plate heat-exchangers and tubular heaters. In the former, the product is raised to the temperature of homogenization ($82.2°$ C) in the regenerator section. The homogenizer itself then serves to pump the fluid to a final heating section. Either steam or hot water under pressure serves as the final heat source. A deaerator device placed just ahead of the final heating section will remove oxygen, which, in turn, decreases the loss of certain vitamins, particularly vitamin C and folic acid.

Tubular heaters are designed as single-, double-, or triple-tube types. Where more than one tube is involved, the tubes are placed inside each other. In double tube systems, the product is carried in the inner tube and steam in the outer tube. Three-tube systems position the product between the inner and outer tubes. Tubular systems are able to operate under high pressure, allowing homogenizer valves to be located on either the hot or cold side of the regenerator. Often, the homogenizer valves are separated, one operating on the raw, the other on the sterilized product. This last arrangement is particularly suited to products containing vegetable oil and aids considerably the stability of the finished emulsion.

DIRECT HEATING METHODS

Steam is the heating medium in direct heating systems. Either it is directed into the product (injection system), or the product may be directed through the steam (infusion system). The time and temperature of preheat treatment vary from 70 to $90°$ C for 10 to 30 minutes. Preheating is done by the indirect methods already mentioned. To avoid defects in texture, the product is usually homogenized after sterilization. This necessitates the use of an aseptic homogenizer. The product flow in injection systems is from the preheater to the steam injector. Steam is introduced; the product is taken to UHT temperature and then immediately directed through an orifice into a vacuum chamber at a temperature just above ($2°$ C) that of the product. A sterile centrifugal pump then moves the fluid stream to the sterile homogenizer. After homogenization, the product is cooled and either stored or packaged (aseptically) immediately.

For systems in which steam is directed into the product, the flow is essentially the same as the preceding. After preheat treatment (often at about $75°$ C), the food is forced into a steam-filled chamber through a spray-ball. In both direct and indirect UHT systems, the finished product may either be aseptically packaged at once or be stored (under aseptic conditions) for later packaging.

It is important to recognize the variety of heat treatments possible in the various systems used to process infant formula. Because heat treatment is directly related to the extent of loss of certain nutrients, a change in type of system or any significant change in processing conditions within the same system should be followed by extensive analysis of the finished product to ensure nutritional adequacy. In the United States, regulations proposed by the FDA would make such testing mandatory.

Age-thickening or gelation of UHT products may occur by a different mechanism than that which takes place in sterilized evaporated milk products. Several theories have been proposed. One suggests a fragmentation of casein by reactivated proteolytic enzymes. Another puts the blame on proteases that originate in bacterial contamination of the raw milk. In the latter instance, the preheat treatment may be used to destroy the enzymes, as mentioned previously. Research indicates that bacterial proteases are active at room temperature; their optimum pH is 6.5–7.0 (see International Dairy Federation, 1972).

Stabilizers may also help maintain an homogenous liquid state. Various starches, guar gum (obtained from seeds of the guar plant, *Cyamopsis tetragonolobus*), locust bean gum (from refined endosperm of leguminous seeds), and carrageenan (from red algae) are approved for use in infant formula (see Appendix 6). Maximum amounts are specified in all cases. Starches and carrageenan are probably most commonly used.

Generally speaking, above average homogenization pressures are needed to ensure the best physical stability during storage. Specific pressures, however, can only be considered within the context of other processing factors, including formulation. Overall, the stability of the finished product involves an appropriate integration of the homogenization pressure, salt balance, the type of stabilizer, and the heat treatment. The heat treatment includes both preheat and sterilization treatments. In UHT processes, the preheat may well be more important (to stability) then the sterilization process.

PROCESSING DRY INFANT FORMULA

Dried formula may be prepared either by blending dry ingredients as such or by drying an appropriate mixture of liquid (or liquified) ingredients. From a bacteriological standpoint, the latter is preferred. Both fresh and rehydrated dried milk (or dried milk products) can serve as ingredients. Fresh milk for the purpose is filtered, deaerated (to remove oxygen, which otherwise increases loss of certain vitamins during heat treatment), separated into skim milk and cream and pasteurized (74–77° C, 15–20 seconds). These fresh ingredients and/or rehydrated dried skim milk are then blended with vegetable oil(s). For this purpose the oil(s) is first warmed and may be metered into the blending tank. Emulsifiers, stabilizers, and possibly fat-soluble vitamins are added. For dried formula, vitamin or mineral fortification can be withheld until after the product is dried and cooled. This is generally not recommended, however, because of the difficulty in achieving thorough mixing. However, if vitamin or mineral concentrates are added prior to drying, some overages of heat-labile vitamins are required to account for losses during processing. Fat-soluble vitamins are perhaps best added prior to evaporation; water-soluble vitamins and minerals should be added after evaporation and just prior to drying.

Rehydration of dry ingredients can usually be accomplished at relatively low temperatures. To ensure a homogeneous mixture, special recirculating blenders may be employed, or the product can simply be cycled from a hopper, through a T and pump, back into the blending tank. Homogenization is used to stabilize the oil and water emulsion.

A concentrated product is prepared either by evaporation in vacuum pans or by blending ingredients to the appropriate solids level. As such, it may be placed in storage tanks from which the spray-dryer is fed. The total solids level of this concentrated product depends to some extent upon the type of drying system and the formulation. A formula high in carbohydrate content (lactose and/or corn syrup solids) is predisposed to sticking to the walls of the dryer at high temperature and/or high moisture levels (Sorensen, 1978). Since most infant formulas contain above-average levels of carbohydrate, suitable drying dictates one or more of the following: (1) low inlet air temperature, (2) low solids in-feed, (3) heating the concentrated milk prior to in-feed, (4) insulated or cooled-wall drying system. Generally, conditions for drying infant formula will require concentration to 45% (or possibly lower) solids and in-feed temperature of about 70° C. Inlet and outlet air temperature in the drying chamber approximate 160° C and 90° C, respectively. Two-stage drying is also possible. In this case the outlet air temperature may be lowered to a level at which a relatively moist powder emerges. The product then is dried to its final moisture content on a surface dryer. This process has the advantage of allowing a more efficient first stage of drying, that is, higher solids and higher inlet air temperatures. After drying, the product is cooled and either bagged in bulk or packaged into consumer size units. See Figure 1 for a flow diagram of the process for preparing dry infant formula.

Dry products in the hands of unknowing mothers, especially in areas of the world where water supplies lack microbiological purity, pose serious hazards

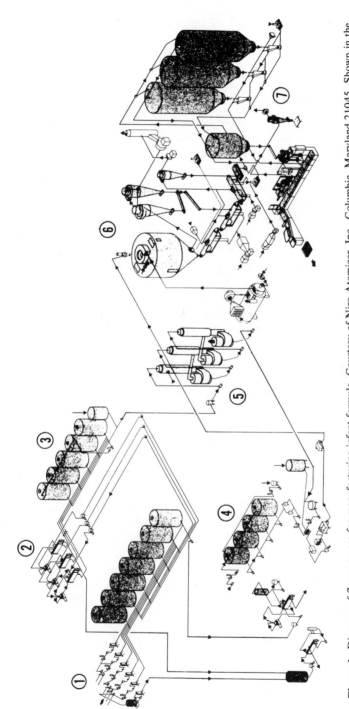

Figure 1. Diagram of flow process for manufacturing infant formula. Courtesy of Niro Atomizer, Inc., Columbia, Maryland 21045. Shown in the diagram are (1) milk receiving area; (2) milk separation and HTST pasteurization; (3) storage tanks for milk and cream; (4) blending tanks for ingredients of infant formula; (5) evaporators; (6) spray-dryers and instantizer; (7) powder storage, conveying, bagging, and packaging area.

to infant health. Liquid, sterile, use-strength formulas are one answer; though the cost is higher, it must be weighed against the value of life. Sterile, liquid formulas can be packaged in single-portion packets. This would seem the most foolproof method at present. Dry products might also be copackaged, though separately, with an appropriate amount of pure water for reconstitution purposes. Because the presence of water would add greatly to shipping costs of exported products, water supplies might better be purified and packaged in appropriate amounts in a relatively few, strategically located facilities in the country of use. This water, then, could be made available with single-portion packs of dry formula. Still a third possibility calls for a day-care center, hospital, or village processor to reconstitute dry formulas in boiled water in single-service bottles for use in-house or for delivery to points of need. Where the question of formula or water supply purity still exists, a small in-bottle pasteurizer might readily serve to pasteurize the reconstituted fluid product, again for distribution to nearby households. A pasteurizer of this type is described in a later section. The concept is interjected here because of findings of contamination of infant formula processed in Third World countries. The sophisticated technologies and rigid sanitation requirements make such problems difficult to overcome. Nevertheless, ways can be found to better ensure the safe use of these products. Aside from packaging or repasteurization considerations, more use might well be made of cultured products or dried products prepared with high levels of viable lactic acid cultures. However, this gets into the realm of immune-type formulations and is important enough to consider under a separate heading.

PROCESSING IMMUNE FACTORS INTO INFANT FORMULA

To better appreciate the potential and need to incorporate immune factors into infant formula, the reader might wish to review Chapter 4. Benefits of these kinds of improved formulations accrue to peoples of the Third World and industrialized nations. Soviet medical scientists have found marked positive effect and shortened hospital stays with the use of formulas supplemented with lysozyme for feeding infants (3 months to 1 year of age) suffering from anemia and pneumonia (Sarzhanova and Kudayarov, 1978). Czechoslovakian scientists (Dolezalek, 1979) have fermented lactic cultures into formulas for treating infant diarrhea. The more potent of these formulas contain *Lactobacillus bifidus* (*Bifidobacterium bifidus*), *L. acidophilus*, and *Pediococcus acidilacti* in a 45:10:45 ratio. Organisms are purposely picked from infant feces in order to ensure viability and activity in the human intestinal tract. Both mixed and pure cultures find use in infant feeding. Products of this type are aseptically packaged in single-service containers.

Italian scientists (Midulla *et al.*, 1976) likewise have added lactic cultures to dried formula or milk products as a preventive measure to lower risk of intestinal infection. Under testing conditions, such products were found to inhibit disease strains of salmonella. Both acid pH and nisin, an antibiotic elaborated by the growing organisms, are thought responsible for the observed effect.

A recent Japanese patent (Mutai *et al.*, 1980) covers a method for preparing a bifidobacterium culture for addition to infant food. Milk is inoculated with at least one oxygen-resistant and one obligate anaerobe of strains of bifidobacteria. The culture is incubated at 37° C for 20 hours, then freeze-dried. The presence of the oxygen-resistant strains allows the obligatory strain to grow under aerobic conditions in pure milk without the addition of growth-promoting substances.

Both N-substituted D-glucosamine and lactulose enhance growth of bifidus bacteria. The former has recently been prepared from chitin (B-$(1\rightarrow4)$-N-acetyl-D-glucosamine) extracted from crab and shrimp shells (Austin *et al.*, 1981). Lactulose is also a product of treatment of lactose with calcium hydroxide, other alkaline hydroxides, alkaline earth aluminates, or alkaline tetraborate. A number of processes of separation and isolation are applied, ranging from differential solubility to fermentation of unreacted lactose followed by filtration through silica and then deionization and evaporation (see Mendez and Olano, 1979). Olano (1979) developed a method for preparing and extracting lactulose from a methanol solution of benzyl-trimethylammonium hydroxide. But lactulose can also be prepared by heat treatment of lactose. This may occur as a natural result of the sterilization process of liquid formulas, or a formula may be pretreated specifically to yield some amount of lactulose, and processed to a dried product. A Polish patent (Kisza *et al.*, 1976) describes one such method. In this process 800 liters of milk are standardized for fat content, pasteurized at 85° C for 20 second, cooled to 3–5° C, and reheated to 105° C for 2 minutes. This latter heat treatment causes formation of lactulose from lactose present in the milk. The product is then evaporated to 45% total solids. This is followed by addition of casein hydrolysate, demineralized whey protein, cream, sunflower oil, lactose, and vitamins. The mixture is then homogenized and spray dried. A process for preparing a dried mixture of lactulose (78.2%) galactose, lactose, and bifidobacteria (*Bifidobacterium adolescentis* or *Bifidobacterium*) has also been patented (Ogasa, 1980).

Freeze-drying is the method most commonly used to dry cultures for use in infant formula. Cost and efficiency of drying are drawbacks, of course. Thus, research continues to find ways of spray-drying cultures while retaining their viability. Chilean dairy scientist Fernando Espina was able to recover 9.8×10^7 survivors per gram of solids of a *Lactobacillus acidophilus* culture obtained from an intestinal source. Drying conditions involved use of 25% solids and an outlet air temperature on a pilot spray-dryer of 75° C (Espina and Packard, 1979). In another process, Dutch scientists (Stadhouders *et al.*, 1969) spray-dried starter cultures by first evaporating to 22% solids, then drying to 9% solids using an inlet air temperature of 70° C. Further drying to 5% or less moisture was done in a vacuum chamber at 27° C with 1–2 mm mercury pressure. These scientists claimed little or no loss in bacteria count or activity.

Research goes on and methods improve for isolating and/or concentrating various immune factors such as lactoferrin and transferrin, lysozyme, lactoperoxidase, and, as produced by genetic engineering of bacteria, inferferon. Although isolation in a pure state has obvious advantages in many cases, concentrates also serve as sources of immune bodies. A concentrate of antibodies (human-type) from cow's milk, pioneered by Nestlé scientists (Hilpert *et al.*, 1975), will serve to describe one such process. Cows are first hyperimmunized with pathogenic strains of *E. coli* during the final 1 or 2 months of gestation. The cow produces antibodies to these specific strains of organisms, and these antibodies concentrate in colostrum. In the cow it is IgG_1 that predominates. All immunoglobulins of milk, however, locate in the whey fraction. The process by which they are concentrated goes as follows: skim milk is separated from fat in a mechanical separator at 37° C. Casein is removed by precipitation with rennin and citric acid (to pH 4.6), again at 37° C, followed by centrifugation. The serum (whey) is clarified both by centrifugation and filtration. Protein components are then concentrated by ultrafiltration and diafiltration. These processes remove most lactose and minerals. The protein concentrate—containing antibodies, lysozyme, lacto-peroxidase, lactoferrin and transferrin—is then sterilized by filtration and freeze-dried. On a dry basis the concentrate contains about 75% proteins (immunoglobulins, 40%; α-lactalbumin 15%; β-lactoglobulin, 35%; serum albumin, 2%; and other proteins, 5%). Lactose, mineral salts, and non-protein-nitrogen components still remain to levels of nearly 10, 5, and 5%, respectively. The whole concentrate, as such, is formulated directly into infant formula. At present, methods of further refining antibodies and lactoferrin are limited to laboratory fractionation devices based on immune adsorbent chromatography.

ADDING IRON TO INFANT FORMULA

Of all nutrient additives, iron has to be the most irksome. An iron compound that is generally well absorbed by the body may also be one that most readily induces off-flavors. Another that causes no flavor problems is apt to be low in biological availability. In the case of a third chemical form that satisfies both flavor and absorption requirements, the process itself (cooking or storage) may alter the iron form or tie it up some way so as to render it useless to the body. These are real and significant difficulties, and each food system poses its own unique set of obstacles to iron fortification.

First, some general observations:

1. Ferrous forms of iron are usually more readily absorbed by the body, generally more soluble (at least in certain infant foods) and more likely to cause oxidation of fat than ferric iron forms.
2. Processing may enhance or reduce bioavailability of a given form of iron.
3. Phosphates often used as food additives (Mahoney and Hendricks, 1978), egg solids, excessive protein, and certain chelating agents tend to reduce iron absorption.
4. Ascorbate (salt of vitamin C), certain amino acids, and binding of iron compounds to protein tend to enhance iron bioavailability (Lee and Clydesdale, 1979).

Of the many iron forms available, ferrous sulfate is likely most widely used in infant formulas. It is among those inorganic iron compounds thought to be most readily absorbed. Added to formula, it provides a source of iron adequate to meet an infant's needs. Generally speaking, ferrous forms of iron bind more readily to insoluble protein than do ferric forms. The amount bound goes up with an increase in the temperature of treatment, and with an increase in alkalinity. But ferrous forms of iron are also likely to cause oxidation of fat in whole milk if added prior to heat treatment (pasteurization). However, the compounds do not protect milk lipase, as do ferric iron forms. Therefore, lipolytic rancidity is avoided. Because fat oxidation is the more serious potential problem, ferric iron compounds are often used to fortify dry milk products. The nutrient source may be added to the dried product or mixed with either skim milk (prior to pasteurization) or concentrated milk prior to drying. Both ferric ammonium citrate and ferric chloride serve the purpose in nonfat dry milk products (which do in fact contain some fat and phospholipids, and are thus susceptible to oxidation). For drying whole milk, lipolytic rancidity must be considered. Ferric compounds are thought to provide protection for lipase(s) enzymes against denaturation by heat. To overcome the effect, heat treatment must exceed 79° C. Use of ferric ammonium citrate and 81° C pasteurization have been found to yield satisfactory results.

An iron-fortified syrup blend has also been found of use in making up infant formula. Compounds suitable for addition to the syrup include ferric ammonium citrate, ferric choline citrate, ferrous sulfate, and ferrous gluconate.

Latest research centers on more uncommon forms of iron. One compound has been found to be both more readily absorbed than ferrous sulfate, and to cause little or no discoloration, as does reduced iron, in infant formula. The chemical name is ferric-nitrilotriacetate (Fe-NTA). Ascorbic acid enhances uptake (of all iron sources). It makes nutritional sense, therefore, to include ascorbic acid, a nutrient otherwise lacking in cow's milk, to formulas supplemented with iron.

To enhance absorption, iron may also be bound to protein. Ferric polyphosphate and whey protein powder is one example. Ferric chloride and sodium polyphosphate are mixed with acid (cottage cheese) whey and dried. Of low bulk density, the product poses certain problems in handling and storage. Other proteins to which iron has been bound experimentally include wheat gluten, zein (corn protein), casein, soy protein isolate, and albumin (Nelson and Potter, 1979). Both ferrous sulfate and ferric pyrophosphate have been tried as iron sources. Compared to the former, the ferric compounds bind more readily to soluble protein and at acid pH. In addition, the temperature of treatment appears not to influence its binding capacity. Thus, while research is far from complete, it is apparent that both ferrous and ferric iron forms can be linked to a variety of protein sources. Doing so holds hope for improving iron bioavailability while avoiding adverse color, texture, and flavor changes. Mineral sources of iron approved by the FAO/WHO for use in infant foods are shown in Appendix 4. Of the phosphate compounds known to inhibit iron absorption, sodium pyrophosphate and sodium tripoly-phosphate appear more problematic than disodium phosphate or sodium metaphosphate (Mahoney and Hendricks, 1978).

PROCESSING OUT ALLERGENS

To overcome or reduce the allergy potential in formula products, several different approaches are possible. For one, products can be put together of protein sources other than milk. Where globulin and/or albumin fractions alone are the problem, casein might also be included in the formulation. Casein can also be modified to a nonantigenic protein or protein fraction.

Japanese scientists (Takase et al., 1979) have done so by predigesting casein with a mixture of enzymes. The mixture consists of pancreatin and two microbial enzymes, one obtained from Aspergillus oryzae, the other from Lactobacillus helveticus. After reacting casein with the enzymes, the nonantigenic fraction is isolated by gel filtration. With a food of this kind, the

Japanese were able to treat effectively stubborn cases of infant diarrhea caused by milk allergy.

Kuchroo and Ganguli (1980) report a process for preparing infant formula of low αs-casein content from buffalo milk. Calcium content of the original skim milk is first reduced by 50% by electrodialysis. Milk proteins, especially αs-casein, is then degraded by measured proteolysis with trypsin. To this product is then added a combination of milk fat and vegetable oil, and a lactose and vitamin mixture.

Preventing or minimizing browning carries with it two advantages, at least when the formula consists of some amount of β-lactoglobulin and lactose (or other reducing sugar). First, protein quality is ensured. Second, antigenic properties are minimized. Since browning occurs under the influence of heat, those processes that reduce heat damage serve best. For liquid formula products, this suggests use of UHT for very short holding times. However, some scientists (McLaughlin *et al.*, 1981) have reported a reduction in sensitizing capacity of cow's milk by heat treatment. The research was carried out on guinea pigs, not humans, but nonetheless might apply to humans. As temperature was increased or prolonged, both casein and β-lactoglobulin became less sensitizing. Boiling was found to be more of a desensitizing treatment for goat's than cow's milk. Various infant formulas also responded favorably to increased heat treatment.

In addition to processing out allergens, some value could be derived from processing into formulas certain antibodies and other immune factors like lactoferrin and lysozyme. Immune agents of these kinds serve to some extent as a barrier to uptake of various dietary antigens and microorganisms. Processing immune factors into formula carries a potential to prevent microbial disease and possibly to inhibit allergies.

STANDARDS OF QUALITY CONTROL

Composition control requires monitoring of each lot or batch for content of protein, fat, total solids, and total calories. Carbohydrate level is measured by difference. In addition, each lot should be analyzed for the amount of at least one vitamin or one mineral added in the vitamin and mineral premix to determine whether or not appropriate levels of micronutrients have been achieved.

To monitor the microbial condition in sterilized liquid formulas, sample containers are stored 2 to 3 weeks at elevated temperature, and then the contents are evaluated. No batch or lot should be released until after such tests are completed. Thereafter, microbiological quality and physical stability (tendency to gel or otherwise alter in texture) can and should be monitored for the shelf life of the product; the records of findings should also be maintained for future reference.

Such surveillance and control is essential to ensure that the formula itself does not become a vector of disease. Researchers in India (Singh *et al.*, 1980), surveying locally manufactured infant formulas and milk–cereal weaning foods, have found staphylococci of the kind able to produce enterotoxins A and B. *Bacillus cereus*, another disease agent, was also found. In one case, *S. aureus* and *B. cereus* counts were found to increase ten-fold in 3 hours when the reconstituted baby food was held at 37.5°C. The need for tight, continuous microbiological control remains an absolute necessity in the manufacture of infant foods.

Several United States regulations focus on process and quality control of infant formula. These include standards of manufacture, processing, packing, and holding of human food (21 *CFR* 110), processing requirements for low-acid foods packaged in hermetically sealed containers (21 *CFR* 113), and a temporary tolerance for polychlorinated biphenyls of 0.2 ppm (21 *CFR* 113). In addition, the Infant Formula Act of 1980 sets forth an entire protocol of testing and compliance. Major considerations follow.

INFANT FORMULA ACT OF 1980

Under the Infant formula Act of 1980, the FDA has proposed a complete regimen of sampling, testing, and analysis of products. Quality control would consider (1) an acceptance protocol for ingredients (to ensure conformity to specifications); (2) in-process control of ingredient addition, blending, homogenization, and standardization; and (3) finished product evaluation specifying sampling frequency and analytical format.

The original proposals have drawn considerable fire and most certainly will be altered before rules are finalized. Nonetheless, a brief coverage of their content seems in order if only to point the way. It is perhaps well to note only that, considering objections raised thus far (even from the American Medical Association and the American Academy of Pediatrics), future changes will likely come in the form of more simplified control procedures.

Ingredient Control

All ingredients shipped to the processing facility must be checked for damage to containers and for validity of label information. A code is applied to designate final disposition. Other than nutrient premixes, generally stable ingredients (corn sugar, for example), if certified and guaranteed, can be accepted as such. If an ingredient or a nutrient(s) of any ingredient is subject to shipping loss or alteration, a sample must be composited (using statistically randomized subsamples) from the lot, and a quantitative analysis must be made on the composite for each such nutrient.

A nutrient premix is defined as a combination of two or more nutrients, which is added as a single ingredient in the formulation (processing) of infant formula. Such premixes may come certified and guaranteed by the supplier or may be without such certification. In either case, a composite of subsamples must be analyzed. Where a guarantee accompanies a premix, it is necessary only to analyze for an indicator nutrient. Lacking certification, the composite must be tested for each nutrient present in the premix. Individual ingredients or nutrients are treated similarly. That is, lacking certification, quantitative analysis must be made of appropriately composited subsamples. In all cases, test methods must either be of recognized validity or originate in Official Methods of Analysis of the Association of Official Analytical Chemists (AOAC). The chemical method of vitamin D analysis is acceptable unless specifically excluded. Any lots of ingredients or nutrients found unsuitable are to be conspicuously marked as rejected and moved to a restricted area pending further disposition.

In-Process Control

In-process control starts with the blending of ingredients, including the basic macronutrients, premix nutrients, emulifiers, and stabilizers. As present in a single blending vat or tank, the mixture of ingredients represents an "in-process batch." Two or more such batches, blended and standardized for further processing and ultimate filling into finished product containers, constitute a "filling batch." A filling batch, therefore, reflects a finite number of packaged units when part or possibly all of the product is processed during a single shift of operation. A product produced within a single shift then becomes the largest single coding unit allowed. Thus, any one code must be traceable to a product processed during a single shift of work.

Records are kept on each in-process batch. The formulation must first be approved, checked, and signed by a quality control supervisor. The batch record will list each ingredient to be added, and the amount and place in the process where such addition is to take place. The batch record then proceeds with the product through the process. As ingredients are added, an operator enters an ingredient identification number and initials the fact of its addition (in kind and amount). Eventually the batch record is filed for possible further reference.

A base blend consists of various ingredients—including sources of protein, fat, and carbohydrate—mixed with potable water (of a quality mandated by the local public health agency). After thorough mixing, this blend is sampled, and a proximate analysis is made for protein, fat, carbohydrate, ash, and moisture. Each base blend is so analyzed.

Premix nutrients are analyzed (individually) prior to addition to the base blend, or these analyses are performed on filling batch samples taken from the holding tanks. The premix is added and product homogenized at the appropriate point in the process. At some suitable site, a sample is taken of this homogeneous blend. On this sample, analysis is made for indicator nutrients. These are individual nutrients known to be the most labile (readily destroyed) of the lot. For fat-soluble vitamins, the indicator nutrient is vitamin A. Vitamin C serves the purpose for water-soluble vitamins. Manganese is the indicator nutrient of choice for mineral premixes. Because certain nutrients are better preserved or product quality better served by separate addition at some specific point or time in the process, such nutrients may be added as the product requires. Following such addition, however, an in-process sample must be taken and an analysis made for the nutrient in question. Again, nutrient analyses will either be made on the in-process batch or on samples taken from the holding tank.

Once a filling batch has been assembled and thoroughly mixed, a sample is taken for analysis of composition and physical condition. Homogeneity, of course, determines the distribution of nutrients and is, therefore, as important as proper composition. This sample is analyzed for total solids content, homogeneity, osmolality, and sedimentation. In addition, indicator nutrients of premixes come under analysis, as well as protein, fat, and carbohydrate. If individual nutrient components have been formulated into the premix, if any nutrient has been added independent of the premix, and if analyses of these nutrients were not made on the in-process batch, the amount of each is now determined in the filling batch. During the time analyses are being made, the batch is held from further processing. Found acceptable or found inadequate and subsequently corrected for any deficiency (as determined by further analyses), the batch is then released for heat sterilization or drying.

Finished Product Analysis

In essence, finished product analysis becomes a program of statistical quality control, with statistically representative sampling, and composition and physical condition are assessed by means of statistically determined upper and lower control limits. Because some nutrients are regulated both on minimum and maximum amounts (see Table 19), both upper and lower control limits come into use. Given an average target level for any one nutrient, warning limits are set at two standard deviations above and below this value. The control limit—the point beyond which the nutrient level is unacceptably high or low—is taken as three standard deviations from this average.

One set of control samples consists of three containers taken randomly over each 2-hour period of filling. Such sampling must be made from each packaging line. The product from these three containers is composited and subjected to "immediate analysis" for (1) total solids, homogeneity, osmolality, and sedimentation and (2) indicator nutrients. These latter might consist of vitamin A, vitamin B_1, vitamin B_6, or vitamin C.

At the same time the first set of control samples are being taken, replicate samples of containers are also taken for more extended analysis. Sampling must come from the first of every ten filling batches or on a semimonthly basis, whichever comes first. The product from these containers is then subjected to "extended analysis." This includes testing for the content of reducing sugar and all nutrients specified in the regulations and declared on the label, except linoleic acid, vitamin D, vitamin K, choline, inositol, biotin, tryptophan (if necessary because of declaration of niacin equivalents), and indicator nutrients analyzed in the "immediate analysis."

Replicates of samples collected from each filling batch are also held for later "progressive analysis." These samples will be tested at 3-month intervals to determine if changes in composition or physical properties have taken place, changes that would render the product unfit for consumption. During each 3-month interval, samples taken from a new filling batch are tested for solids, homogeneity, osmolality, sedimentation, and for all nutrients declared on the label. For this purpose, allowance is made to analyze for vitamin D by chemical methods—except at the 6-month interval. At this latter testing time, vitamin D is to be assayed by the appropriate AOAC bioassay. Protein Efficiency Ratio (PER) must also be determined at 6-month intervals. Current official methods call for rat bioassay for both vitamin D and PER.

For regulatory purposes, the manufacturer of infant formula is allowed to set acceptable limits for solids, homogeneity, osmolality, and sedimentation. Range in nutrient content, however, must not exceed the minimum and maximum levels set by regulation. The target value, therefore, will always be predetermined at some higher or lower level than the minimum and maximum limits. In this way, process and testing variables, which would otherwise range above and below the limit, are accounted for.

As long as nutrient composition remains within acceptable limits, no action is needed. When the level falls between the warning and rejection limits, corrective action is called for. If three consecutive tests on filling batches show a trend away from specified ranges of nutrient content, steps must be taken to determine the cause and to implement appropriate corrective measures.

Separate and additional control procedures take place whenever minor or major changes are made either in ingredient or processing conditions. Minor changes might include an increase or decrease in some nutrient level to bring the nutrient more nearly into the appropriate range. It might also include a change in supplier and in some unique nutrient component(s) of the new supply of nutrients. A change in water supplies would also fall in this category. Whatever the minor change, a testing protocol must be undertaken. This involves the taking of three composite samples representing the first, middle, and last of the filling batch of each of ten separate batches. These samples must be analyzed prior to shipment to note the impact of the change(s). In addition, composite samples from the first and tenth filling batches, and two composites from batches two through nine, likewise come under analysis for all nutrients that might be expected to be affected by the change(s). Needless to say, a nutrient might constitute a variation in and of itself or might induce a variation in the level of some other nutrient. Analysis must account for any and all expected variations in nutrient content.

Major changes are considered to be those that involve a major change in ingredients (for example, the exchange of soy flour for soy isolate) and major changes in processing conditions. The latter might include a conversion from indirect to direct heating methods, or significant changes in preheat treatment. They would include changes in mixing times or temperatures, or in holding times or temperatures of sterilization. In the event of these kinds of alterations in ingredients or conditions of processing, analysis for all regulated nutrients and for PER must be on composite samples taken from the first and tenth filling batches, and from any two others representing batches two through nine. If filling batches one and ten show adequate levels of linoleic acid, vitamin D, vitamin K, choline, inositol, biotin, PER, and tryptophan (as required for declaration of niacin), these nutrients may be excluded in analyses made on samples taken from batches two through nine.

Coding

Clear, legible codes are placed on each container of the finished product. The code identifies the specific establishment where the formula was packed, the product itself, the year and day on which packing took place, and the period (the working shift) during which the formula was packed.

Records

Records of all pertinent analyses, as described previously, must be kept for at least as long as the shelf life of the finished product.

New Formulations

New formulations require prior notification to the FDA of compliance with all testing procedures described in this section and of the presence of regulated nutrients at appropriate levels. Such notice is rendered 90 days in advance of the first day of processing of the new formulation. The format for making notice is a stated, standardized form.

Reformulations

Prior notice to the FDA is required when reformulations, as defined by regulation, are made. The notice must precede the first batch to be processed.

Other Requirements

In addition to requirements thus far mentioned, manufacturers of infant formula must also supply the FDA with one label from each formula produced (whether for commercial or charitable distribution). In the event of knowledge of a failure of compliance of a formula already in the marketplace, the FDA must be notified, directly, by phone.

LABELING INFANT FOODS

In the United States any infant food made up of two or more ingredients must be labeled with the common or usual name of each ingredient. That includes spices, flavoring, and coloring. Nothing should be left out, and all sources of plant or animal food, however masked in the finished product, must be made clearly known. Labels of infant formula specifically must also bear the percentage by weight or volume of the content of moisture, protein, fat, available carbohydrate, ash, and crude fiber. Caloric load of a unit of ready-to-eat formula should also be declared. The label should acknowledge the presence and amount of those vitamins and minerals both natural and added shown in Table 24. Minimum amounts (per 100 kcal) are specified, and these are also given in Table 24. If the product fails to meet these standards, a statement must note that fact. The label must then indicate the amount necessary to make up the difference.

The importance of protein is recognized by a number of specific mandates in the labeling of this nutrient. The phrase "this product should not be used as the sole source of protein in the infant diet" must accompany any product in which content of protein (of quality equivalent to casein) is less than 1.8

TABLE 24
Vitamin and Mineral Requirements for Labeling
Purposes of Infant Foods[a]

Vitamin and mineral	Minimum amount (per 100 cal)
Vitamin A (IU)	250
Vitamin D (IU)	40
Vitamin E (IU)	0.3
Vitamin C (ascorbic acid) (mg)	7.8
Vitamin B_1 (thiamine) (mg)	0.025
Vitamin B_2 (riboflavin) (mg)	0.06
Niacin (mg equivalents)[b]	0.08
Vitamin B_6 (mg)	0.035
Folacin (mcg)	4.0
Pantothenic acid (mg)	0.3
Vitamin B_{12} (mcg)	0.15
Calcium (mg)	50
Phosphorus (mg)	25
Magnesium (mg)	6
Iron (mg)	1
Iodine (mcg)	5
Copper (mg)	0.06

[a]Adapted from *Code of Federal Regulations* (1978).
[b]The term *niacin* is taken to include niacin (nicotinic acid), niacinamide, and 1 mg equivalent for each 60 mg tryptophan in the food.

g/100 kcal available. The same phrase is required when the biological quality of protein is less than 70% that of casein; that is, the PER is less than 1.8, given casein at 2.5. Finally, the declaratory phrase must be used when protein quality and quantity are such that the food fails a simple mathematical relationship. That relationship is expressed as the biological quality of the protein, taken as a fraction of the biological quality of casein, times the amount of protein in 100 available kilocalories. The result must not fall below 1.8. Here's an example: Assume a protein of PER 2.0. As a fraction of casein PER, the expression becomes 2.0/2.5, or 0.8. Assume then that 100 kcal supply 2 g protein. Then $0.8 \times 2 = 1.6$. The protein quality and content thereby fail to meet the requirement. The declaratory phrase is called for.

The level and quality of fat must also be considered for labeling purposes. If the food supplies less than 15% of total available calories as fat, or less than 2% of calories as linoleic acid (present as a glyceride), the label must indicate the need to seek one or both, as the case may be, from other sources. Manufacturers of all infant foods except whole milk and evaporated milk must comply with these labeling requirements. Whole milk and evaporated milk need show only a lack of of ascorbic acid, vitamin D, and iron. Lack in this case is taken as less than 7.8 mg, 40 IU, and 1 mg 100 kcal, respectively, of these three nutrients.

Other facets of infant formula labeling are also being considered. In the United States, the Infant Formula Council is proposing to place a dilution symbol on concentrated liquid products to better distinguish them from ready-to-use products. The symbol in this instance would be a white spot encircled by a dark border. Pictograms depicting appropriate proportions of formula and water would be uniformly designed and applied to liquid and dry products in which water addition is necessary. A similarly styled and located pictogram would indicate, where appropriate, that a product requires no dilution. Or a symbol implying such a fact may be designed and applied. Other possibly helpful labeling practices might include a declaration of nutrient levels in terms of a common measure, that is, quart or liter or kilocalorie. Lastly, over and above label information per se, products of similar types are expected to be packaged in similar kinds of containers, but containers that differ from those used for different kinds of formulations. Concentrated liquid formulas would come in 13 fluid oz cans. Ready-to-eat formulations would come in a variety of glass and metal containers, but none in 13-oz sizes. Powdered formulas would come in cans but cans shaped differently from those used for liquid products. Powdered formula might also come in individual serving packets. These are proposals, at any rate.

7

Human Milk: Extraction, Processing, and Storage

A lactarium, or milk bank, is a place where human milk is stored for later use. Hospitals often serve this function. Just as proper controls are essential to high-quality infant formula, so are similar controls needed to ensure best quality human milk. Needless to say, spread of disease through human milk is as readily possible as through cow's milk or infant formula. So great are potential risks that some pediatricians refuse to feed anything but sterile (microbe-free) or pasteurized (disease-free) human milk; however, some heat treatment is necessary to achieve these states of purity, and some loss of immune factors occurs as a result.

STANDARDS OF BACTERIAL QUALITY

Some percentage of samples of expressed, raw (unheated) human milk can be expected to be sterile. A larger percentage will show the presence of bacteria, but generally of types considered not to produce disease. Still other samples of human milk will contain known pathogens. Percentages in each of these three categories will vary greatly depending upon the health of the individual and sanitary conditions under which milk is expressed, packaged, and stored. Examples taken from reports from two British hospitals serve as comparison. One hospital was able to obtain 49% of milk samples in the "sterile" state. Another was able to procure only 3% of samples in this state of purity. In the former, 38% of bacteria counts were under 10,000/ml milk; 8 and 5% yielded counts of 10,000–20,000, and over 20,000/ml, respectively (Ikonen and Maki, 1977). The latter, a survey of 207 samples representing 70 women in a hospital environment (Carroll *et al*., 1979), yielded 82% of samples with presence of what were presumed to be nondisease-producing bacteria. Some 15% gave evidence of the presence of pathogens. These latter were divided between *Staphylococcus aureus* (6%), enterobacteria (7%), and Group B streptococci (2%).

Breast milk may be contaminated in the breast prior to expression. Studies in one hospital in the United States led to diagnosis of acute mastitis in 2.5% of mothers (Marshall, *et al*., 1975). *S. aureus* was the causative bacteria in 23 of 48 samples. The evidence of Polish studies suggests that infections of this type are not uncommon. Of milk samples taken from 100 women selected at random, 63 were found to harbor strains of *S. epidermis* or *S. aureus*. Over 82% of *S. aureus* were found to produce toxin (Nowakowski *et al*., 1976). Though untested in this study, strains of *S. epidermis* cannot be considered to lack the potential to produce toxin. Other common pathogens of human milk include *S. albus* and *Bacterium anitratum*. *Escherichia coli*, *Pseudomonas aeruginosa*, and β-hemolytic streptococci are also frequently found. Human milk can also be a carrier of germs that cause typhoid or paratyphoid fever, scarlet fever, septic sore throat, polio, diphtheria, dysentery, hepatitis, and other viral diseases. Salmonellosis has also been occasioned by feeding breast milk (Ryder *et al*., 1977). Thus, human milk may pose a threat to infants no less serious than contaminated cow's milk or infant formula.

Human milk may be fed for one or more of several reasons. Often it is simply the food of choice of either mother or pediatrician. Though a debate over adequacy still continues, human milk is often suggested (with supplementation, possibly, with phosphorus or other nutrients) for premature infants. It is also the food of choice for infants suffering the zinc deficiency disease acrodermatitis. Demand for human milk, therefore, runs high. Practices and criteria of feeding have taken on added significance.

The literature contains a wide range of opinions on the quality (bacterial purity) of human milk considered appropriate for infant feeding. Some authorities (Kende and Bekesy, 1977) state unequivocally that no raw (unheated) milk should be fed, irrespective of numbers and kinds of bacteria. Others would feed only raw milk found on bacterial analysis to be sterile. Still others would feed raw milk if it were found free of pathogens (Carroll *et al*., 1979) or both free of pathogens and containing no more than 20,000 bacteria/ml of "nonpathogens" (Ikonen and Maki, 1977). The reason for the quotes around the word *nonpathogens* is to note a certain difficulty in proving the presence of only harmless kinds of microbes. Rarely are sufficient numbers of tests made to make this determination irrefutably. One Swiss report (Roten, *et al*., 1978) provides standards as follows. One ml of sample is taken and incubated in a Urotube for 16 hours at 37° C. If the resulting count is less than 10,000 bacteria/ml, the milk is considered safe to use without heating. At counts of 100,000/ml, heating is mandatory. For milk used within 48 hours, refrigerated (4° C) storage is deemed adequate. For longer storage, freezing must be applied.

Obviously, criteria of quality for human milk for infant feeding varies among health professionals. Concern over pasteurization focuses entirely on loss of immune factors, and for this reason, subminimal treatment is sometimes employed. Lacking anything but complete pasteurization, though, the bacterial quality of human milk will reflect primarily the sanitary conditions under which it is expressed and stored. Taken aseptically, the milk can and most often will be free of pathogens except for those that originate in infections of the breast. If no infections are present, a sterile milk is possible to obtain. To do so, however, requires exacting control on the part of the mother or donor. Some suggestions for sanitary practices follow.

TIPS FOR DONORS

First, any prospective donor should consider her previous history of disease, diet, and drug intake. Women who have had tuberculosis (TB), venereal disease (syphilis), or hepatitis should not serve as donors. No woman who is ill should provide milk for at least 24 hours following that illness. Any sign of breast infection (redness, hardening of the breast, pain) should signal withholding of milk. Most drugs are forbidden. Nothing other than vitamin or mineral supplements and food should enter the body while milk is being extracted for infant feeding. Generally, both nonprescription as well as prescription drugs are excluded from use. In some cases milk may be withheld for 48 hours or more after a drug is taken (or administered to the donor), and then once again be used. During this withholding period, milk is regularly expressed, as always, in order to maintain yield and to clear the breast of the drug. The milk, however, is discarded. Some drugs persist for periods of time exceeding 48 hours. The donor should always consult her medical advisor whenever any drug is being considered.

It is always best to assume that some amount of any drug taken by mouth, injection, vaginal or anal suppository, or even possibly as skin cream or ointment, may end up in the milk supply. Antibiotics are administered by all these routes and likely pose the more common threats of contamination. But no drug should be discounted, no matter how it is taken. Donors should also refrain from smoking, either tobacco or, worse, marijuana.

Finally, a donor should eat a balanced diet. Coffee intake should be limited to 1–2 cups daily. Intake of other sources of caffeine and artificial sweeteners must also be limited. Soft drinks are likely sources of each. Intake of gas-producing foods as well, such as onion, garlic, cabbage, sauerkraut, and pickles must be moderate (Applebaum, 1976). Certain volatile oils from these foods are transferred to the milk and may cause colic (stomach distress) in the feeding infant. Excessive intake of chocolate, nuts, berries, and citrus fruits have also been implicated as causes of colic. Whether breast feeding or donating breast milk, the best dietary advice is: Eat moderately of a variety of foods.

SANITARY EXPRESSION OF MILK

This section outlines a safe, clean procedure for the donor to follow in the expression of milk. First, make sanitation a watchword. Always assume that the skin harbors bacteria, some of which may cause disease. Cracked nipples shed *Staphylococcus aureus* more often than healthy nipples (Belcheva, *et al.*, 1966). Before handling the breasts, always scrub the hands thoroughly. Wash them in hot detergent or soapy water for at least 1 minute. A hard-bristled scrub brush can be most helpful. Wash the hands as though preparing for surgery. It is that important. Fingernails, too, come in for special attention. Remember that the water supply itself can be a source of bacterial contamination and infection. If there is any question of purity, boil the water before use. Since warm water is often used to rinse off the breast and stimulate milk let-down, water purity becomes doubly important. Other ways of stimulating milk let-down include a warm shower or drinking some warm milk or tea. If difficulty persists, the hormone oxytocin (Syntocinon) may be administered as a nasal spray (Applebaum, 1976). Check with your medical counselor for advice on use.

After washing the hands, dry them on a clean towel (or, preferably, a sterile, disposable towel). Pat the breast dry with a clean (sterile is best) towel. Cloth towels can be sterilized by boiling for 20 minutes. Towels (or washcloths), especially those used previously, are prime sources of microbial contamination. Dirty clothing or soiled bras are likewise important sources. Once hands are washed and sanitized, do not touch anything except possibly the milk pump, if one is used. Both hand and electric pumps are available. Hand pumps are only used after first being sterilized. Commonly this is done by boiling for 20 minutes. Pumps are washed and sterilized *after each use*. This must be done without fail. Breast attachments for electric pumps either come presterilized or must be sterilized before and after each use.

Always discard the first few expressions (5 ml) of milk. This milk literally washes the duct through which milk flows. It is commonly the milk of highest bacteria count (West *et al.*, 1979). Even under sanitary conditions, first milk will generally show higher bacteria counts than the milk that follows. In a

California study (Asquith and Harrod, 1979), comparisons were made of 20 donors who had previously been advised on measures for thoroughly cleaning hands and breasts. Donors were asked to segregate the first 5 ml of milk from the remainder. Milk samples thus taken were frozen, held 1–7 days, then thawed overnight. Bacterial numbers by standard plate count averaged 3,500 colonies/ml on first milk, 700 colonies/ml on later milk.

In expression of milk, the breast is clasped between the hands. Thumbs slide down the breast to the edge of (but not onto) the alveolar (dark) area. The breast is then compressed (forced back) against the chest, and milk flows. The process is repeated, working around the periphery of the alveolar region.

If milk is expressed by hand, do so directly into a *sterile* container. If a pump is used, pour milk from the sterile collection container into a sterile shipping container immediately following milking. Some hospitals provide previously sterilized collecting vessels. These vessels should remain sealed, with lid or closure in place, until the donor is ready either to express milk into them or to transfer milk to them. Always place the lid on a clean, sanitary surface while working with the sterilized container. Do not touch inside surfaces with the hands. Replace the lid immediately after the container is filled (usually to 3/4 full).

To sterilize the cup, boil it for 20 minutes. Cups or holding containers are sometimes sterilized with a hypochlorite solution (Lucas and Roberts, 1979). Effective concentration is 200 ppm. Contact time at this strength is 1 full minute; that is, every part of the surface that will or may come in contact with the milk must remain in unbroken contact with the chlorine solution for at least 60 seconds. This assumes, of course, that the cup or container has previously been thoroughly washed and is free of soil deposit. Even the thinnest film of soil can protect bacteria from the killing influence of the sanitizer. No doubt boiling is generally the more fail-safe sterilizing method.

Some authorities recommend plastic containers only. Stored in glass, human milk loses "active" leucocytes to the glass surface, where they tend to adhere (Avery, 1976). Both clear glass and clear or opaque plastic admit light. Light causes a direct, irrecoverable loss in vitamin B_2 (riboflavin) and, to a lesser extent, vitamin A and pyridoxine. Loss of vitamin B_2 may reach 70% by no more than 2 hours of exposure. Sunlight is by far the most damaging source, but fluorescent and incandescent light also cause significant losses. Even diffused light destroys vitamin B_2. It is essential, therefore, either to use lightproof containers or to store milk in darkness. It is equally important to keep milk from absorbing light both in the home following collection or en route to the milk bank.

Breast shields or cups are available for those women whose breasts tend to leak milk. If used, these devices should be sterilized. As a general rule, however, any milk collected in this manner should be discarded. The only exception might be very fresh milk, within the last 15–30 minutes.

STORAGE OF MILK

Once milk is collected in a sterile vessel, cool it (or freeze it) quickly. If the milk is refrigerated, take the milk rapidly to a temperature of 1–2° C. Preferably, freeze milk at −17 to −20° C. Unfrozen (refrigerated) milk should be delivered to the milk bank daily. Frozen milk should not be held more than 7 days prior to delivery (Lucas *et al.*, 1979).

The necessity for quick-cooling or freezing milk cannot be overemphasized. *S. aureus*, the disease agent discussed elsewhere, can grow from very low initial counts and produce measurable amounts of toxin within 3–7 hours at body temperature (37° C) or thereabouts. It thrives well in the range of 10–44° C. (Other germs likewise develop rapidly at these temperatures.) Toxin, once produced, is not destroyed by further heat treatment. Even sterilization temperatures (121.1° C for 15 minutes) will not completely destroy the poison(s). However, the growth of staphylococci is slow in unheated milk treated properly. In fact, the growth is slower in unheated (unpasteurized) milk than in heated milk.

Prior to use, frozen milk should be thawed quickly; the milk should be gently shaken to redisperse fat and other components that are swept to the surface in the cream layer. Some small amount of protein may also be noted to have coagulated into very fine flakes, but less so in high quality milk. Gentle agitation will disperse any of this component that may have begun to settle out. Although quick thawing is preferred, care should be taken not to use excessive heat if the milk is intended for use in the raw state or if there is any concern over protection of immune factors. Vigorous agitation (aeration and foaming) of raw *cow's* milk also induces hydrolytic rancidity (a splitting off of free fatty acids from milk fat). If this also occurs in human milk, the author is unaware of research to that effect. Absence of, or very low levels of, short-chain fatty acids (C_4–C_8) in human milk would minimize off-flavors that evolve from this process, which is catalyzed by naturally occurring lipase(s) of milk. Immediate feeding of thawed, mixed milk would obviate the problem, which may take 30 minutes or longer to develop, depending upon the extent of agitation involved. Storage of unused milk, following feeding, might well provide the time necessary for fat breakdown to occur. The rancidity reaction is also triggered by cooling, rewarming (to 16–37° C), and recooling of raw milk. This treatment would occur if refrigerated milk were warmed for feeding purposes, and leftover milk re-refrigerated. Prompt, single-use feeding of raw human milk would avoid any such potential problems. Since pasteurization destroys the lipase enzyme(s), no rancidity should take place in milk of this kind, irrespective of physical abuse.

PASTEURIZATION OF MOTHER'S MILK

Ordinarily the task of preparing human milk for infant use is undertaken by professional staff of hospitals. Yet it could be done by mothers in the home. Lacking laboratory tests, however, only pasteurized milk would serve this interest. Even then, very real precautions would need to be taken to guarantee freedom from postpasteurization contamination. The concept is brought up at all only because of the resurgence of interest in feeding breast milk, and because one firm distributes a kind of home milk-bank kit (Gazzard and Lee, 1979). Equipment consists of a hand breast-pump, a pasteurization tank, and plastic milk bottles. Facilities for freezing the milk are also needed. It is recommended that milk be expressed before the morning feeding (some milk from each breast, or from one breast during this first feeding). Milk could be taken while on maternity leave, if necessary, and on weekends after work is again taken up. Such milk could serve as a supplement to fresh milk.

Any milk taken and used in the home should be pasteurized to kill any disease-causing germs. Home pasteurizers are available from commercial suppliers, or pasteurization can be readily accomplished by heating milk in a double boiler to 74–77° C for a few seconds, and then quickly cooling. Accurate thermometers are needed, and the thermometer itself should remain immersed in the milk throughout the heating period. Any containers used to store such milk should be thoroughly cleaned and sanitized (preferably in boiling water), and every precaution should be taken to prevent postpasteurization contamination. Storage containers should be covered at all times, or, preferably, milk should be stored in sterilized, capped, infant bottles. Refrigerated (4° C) storage is essential. Because pasteurized milk may still contain microbes that can cause spoilage, quick use is strongly advised. Pasteurized milk could also be frozen in plastic infant bottles, if somewhat longer holding times are needed.

IN-BOTTLE PASTEURIZATION

Postpasteurization contamination is the single greatest risk in feeding pasteurized milk, whether human, cow, goat, or other species. For this reason, in-bottle pasteurization can serve a useful purpose. In this process, milk is heated in a capped (waterproof) container immersed under water. No need exists to transfer the pasteurized milk to another container, thus postpasteurization contamination poses no problem. Milk can be heated in quart glass jars of the kind used in home canning, or it can be heated directly in infant bottles.

In the hospital environment there is need to control time and temperature relationships precisely, whether or not subminimal pasteurization treatment is given. The lowest possible temperature that still maintains the process at a temperature above the minimum being rendered provides to the extent possible for the survival of certain immune factors. Tight control has its advantages, therefore. It was for this reason that an in-bottle system was developed around modern electronic control devices.

Before considering the design of this equipment, however, some definitions are in order. As used in this discussion, *pasteurization* is taken to mean that heating process that renders milk free of disease germs. *Sterilization*, however, is a process resulting in the destruction of *all* microbial life. Sterilization is a much more severe treatment, therefore. Considerably more nutrients are lost; no immune factors of note would be expected to remain viable. However, depending strictly on the kinds of microorganisms present, milk could conceivably be rendered sterile by a pasteurization process. Very high quality milk might even be rendered sterile by a heat treatment less than full pasteurization. Certainly it is possible that a high quality milk product could be rendered *disease-free* by a treatment less than full pasteurization. It is on this latter possibility that some pediatricians recommend heating to 60° C for 10 minutes (Siimes and Hallman, 1978), or 56° C for 30 minutes, or other subminimal pasteurization temperature–time relationships. Research suggests that some level of immunoglobulins survive the treatments cited. Minimal full pasteurization, however, calls for 62.8° C for 30 minutes, or, as often used commercially, 72° C for 15 seconds.

Truly, no one should consider anything less without extensive laboratory services for evaluating microbial purity of the finished product. To guarantee proper treatment, pasteurization (or other heating process) should be carried out in equipment that provides exacting control of temperature and time. Such a system has been developed by Martinez-Suarez and Packard (1981) for in-bottle treatment. A diagram is shown in Figure 2. Although originally designed for quart containers, the system would as readily accommodate containers of smaller volume. Major components include a tank, immersion water heater, submersible pump (for circulating water), temperature probe, and temperature controller. The heart of the system is the controller. In Martinez-Suarez's design, a Model 76 FD 4320-003-10-BO (Partlow Temperature Control, Inc.) served this purpose. Sensitivity was such as to guarantee control of milk temperature at 62.8° C with the water temperature (as maintained by the controller) at 64° C $\pm$ 0.5°. The controller alters heat input by an amount proportional to the magnitude of change required and in an appropriate direction to restore or maintain temperature. As the tempera-

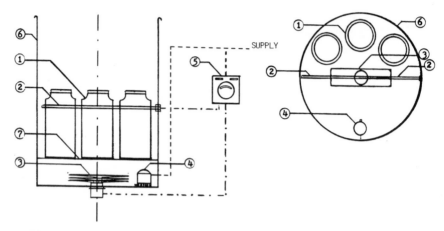

Figure 2. Schematic of an in-bottle fluid milk pasteurizer with a capacity of six quart bottles. The pasteurizer is powered by 3000 W and can attain a temperature of 93.3° C. The electrical supply is 120 V, single phase, 60 Hz. Numbers indicate (1) bottle, (2) probe, (3) heater, (4) circulating pump, (5) controller, (6) tank, (7) screen. Control line indicated by –·–·–; supply line by –––.

ture moves closer to the predetermined target value, the controller continuously adjusts on a proportional basis. As a safeguard to ensure desired heat treatment, the controller times the process and—should temperature fall below target level—shuts down until that temperature is once again achieved. Then the timing is automatically reset for the full time initially established. Control charts can be attached to record temperature–time treatment.

The system can be sized for a variety of process volumes. The protocol unit held six quart bottles. For this size, a 3000 W, 120 V heater sufficed. The submersible circulating pump was a one-phase, 120 V, 140 gal/hour unit. The temperature probe was sheathed, type 316 stainless steel, 3/16 inch outside diameter, 12 inches in length. Purposely, all equipment was derived of readily available commerical sources, easily replaceable and low in cost. Pasteurized milk should always be cooled quickly to 1–2°C or frozen at −17 to −20°C.

HEAT TREATMENT, NUTRIENTS, AND IMMUNE POTENCY

Any significant heat treatment will result in some loss of nutrients and immune potency of milk. Of the two, immune factors seem most sensitive. Use of low temperature pasteurization (62.8° C, 30 minutes) perhaps reduces vitamin C content by 20%. Lacking supplementation, such loss could be significant. Thiamine (vitamin B_1) and vitamin B_{12} content drops about 10%, likely not a serious threat (Causeret, 1977). Considering the total nutrient load, little harm would appear done by minimal, long-hold pasteurization. Were nutrients alone at issue, few objections could be raised to such treatment. Immune factors are another matter. Here it is possible to draw only from limited research. Nonetheless, one point is clear: Even minimal pasteurization—even minimal heat treatment—causes some loss. Leucocytes may be totally destroyed. Freezing alone does as much (Goldman, 1977). Researchers report a 20% drop in IgA activity. Most IgM is apparently destroyed (Ford *et al.*, 1977). According to one source, 60% of lactoferrin fails to remain active following pasteurization. Another source, however, cites no loss whatever of this iron-binding protein. Lysozyme(s) seems to survive unscathed. Also surviving is the binding agent that fastens to folic acid and keeps it from being utilized (and thus lost) by bacteria (Ford *et al.*, 1977). Lactoperoxidase appears to be denatured and, therefore, no longer active as an immune agent.

   In one of the more extensive studies on the effect of heat on immune globulins, Hungarian scientists (Frank and Dobias, 1976) evaluated 1420 samples of human milk. Prior to heating, one sample was found to contain no IgA and no IgG. This would have to be considered very unusual, but it is mentioned as indication of the wide variation in composition and immune potency that one might expect in the milk of the population as a whole. Both IgA and IgG were found in below-average amounts in 9 samples. In 24 samples heated to 60° C for 10 minutes, all but 1 still evidenced presence of active immunoglobulins (Igs). Raising the temperature to 75° C for a similar length of time caused the complete loss of Igs in 22 of 24 samples. Extending the time from 10 to 30 minutes at both 60° C and 70° C produced little change in Igs activity of the former, but it dropped the latter from 13 to 2 samples of 24 still showing some Ig activity. Moreover, a division of samples by the level of protein showed, at similar heat treatment, more extensive loss of Igs in milk of low protein content (900 mg/100 ml) as compared with that of average protein content (1300 mg/100 ml).

   Thus, the end result of either pasteurization or even subminimal pasteurization treatment appears to be a mixed bag of surviving immune factors. Important ones like IgA and lysozyme are still present in significant quantities.Of course, the total or drastic reduction of the disease potential of the milk lessens accordingly the need for some given level of immune potency. One should not willingly yield up a single unit, but loss of immune agents must be weighed against destruction of those germs that otherwise call them to action.

COLD (CHEMICAL) STERILIZATION OF MILK

This prospect must await further scientific study. Yet it is well to note that at least one scientist (Reiter, 1978) is working on a process of sterilizing milk without heat. It is conceived of the lactoperoxidase–hydrogen peroxide–thiocyanate system that performs so well as an immune factor in mother's milk. The enzyme itself is present in high concentrations in milk (whey), and the other two components are common chemical compounds. Hydrogen peroxide (followed by catalase treatment to remove residual peroxide) is used alone as a treatment for milk to be used for cheesemaking in certain special processes, and has known bactericidal efficiency. It is quite possible that appropriate mixtures of enzyme, hydrogen peroxide, and thiocyanate could be assembled to serve as a "chemical" sterilization process—at least for those milk supplies not heavily contaminated. Again, laboratory proof of sterility would be essential.

REDUCING LACTOSE CONTENT

Although mother's milk is the food of choice, there are still disease states of the infant that demand a milk free, or nearly so, of lactose. The level of lactose of human milk runs very high, nearly the highest of all mammalian species. Chapter 9 considers this component of milk and commerical reduction or removal by crystallization and/or enzyme hydrolysis. Only one process will be considered here; it was developed by Danish scientists (Edelsten et al., 1979) for production of lactose-free mother's milk for jaundiced infants being treated by phototherapy. The technology uses a yeast, Saccharomyces fragilis, and fermentation of lactose into carbon dioxide and ethanol. In 4-liter batches, milk is first sterilized. Then 200 ml of yeast culture are added, and the fermentation is carried out, with stirring for 48 hours at 31–32° C. The product is concentrated in a rotary evaporator, and carbon dioxide and ethanol come off in the process. Next, distilled water is added to bring the concentrate back to its original volume. After adjusting pH to 6.7, yeast cells are spun off by centrifugation at $500 \times$ gravity, 3 minutes. The milk is then homogenized at 200 kg/cm^2, and sucrose is added to 7%. The mixture is heated to 75° C for 2 minutes, cooled, and stored at $-20°$ C. Osmolarity of the finished food is unchanged from the original, the lactose content runs less than 50 mg/liter, and the milk is free of galactose. In feeding trials, infants showed no symptoms of lactose intolerance.

8

Infant Food:
Use and Misuse

The scientific literature is replete with honest disagreement regarding the "facts" of science as related to infant feeding. If true consensus exists on any one aspect, it is that mother's milk is the food of choice. Yet we cannot stop at that point. For a variety of reasons many women either cannot or, far more frequently, choose not to breast-feed. This is true in industrialized societies, and it is increasingly the case in Third World countries. To state such fact is not to encourage it. But to ignore the fact is to place infant life in some state of health less than what it might be. There is always the need to make of infant formula—of any infant food—the very best substitute for mother's milk possible. There is equal need to see to its safe use. At the same time, no mother should assume breast milk to be absent of all risk to the breast-feeding infant. Thus, one other fact seems clear: Whether breast feeding, bottle feeding, or both, the informed mother will best see to her infant's needs. This chapter assesses the advantages and disadvantages and the risks and benefits of the various foods commonly used in the feeding of newborn infants.

BREAST MILK

The Advantages of Breast Milk

A number of components of human milk differ from milk of other mammalian species, and from formula products. Are these differences significant, or to a great extent unimportant? Although science is very good at measuring differences, it is much less exacting as an interpretive tool.

187

Therefore, I feel it is wiser to assume the significance of certain components of mother's milk when the fact itself is unproven. Some of the biochemical factors in human milk that may to some extent provide positive benefits for the infant include:

1. a somewhat different casein system than milk of other mammals that differs in proportion of various subunits, produces a finer (possibly more digestible) curd;

2. an unusually high level of the free amino acid taurine, which is thought to play a role in brain development, management of cholesterol, and uptake of certain nutrients from the intestines;

3. a composition and physical structure of fat predisposed to good absorption and adequate in essential fatty acid content;

4. carnitine, a compound thought to aid absorption of fat;

5. a "generally" appropriate level of vitamins and minerals;

6. iron-binding properties that ensure good iron absorption of whatever iron is available;

7. zinc-binding compound(s), like picolinic acid, to ensure good uptake of zinc;

8. a composition appropriately balanced in electrolytes;

9. certain hormones, like thyroxin and prostaglandins;

10. good bioavailability of all nutrients;

11. a passive immune system with potency toward a number of disease bacteria and viruses, and possibly an aid in prevention of allergy;

12. a composition generally (though not necessarily always) less disposed to cause allergy;

13. a component(s) favoring growth in the intestines of *Lactobacillus bifidus*, a bacterial species able to produce acid to a level inhibitory to many disease bacteria (see Chapter 4).

Some of these components can more or less be duplicated in infant formula. Obviously, though, an appropriate chemical–nutrient composition is a major advantage of mother's milk. So is immune potency. The milk itself is a source of ready-to-battle immune bodies. These factors, overall, can be of immense importance, especially in early infancy during the time that the infant lacks an active immune response of its own. Nonetheless, in considering the advantages or disadvantages of any infant food, the nutritional potency takes precedence over the immune competency of the food source. Mother's milk provides both nutritional sustenance and a passive immune response, the latter to some extent geared to combat those infections prevalent generally in the environment in which the infant is raised.

Fortunately, although malnutrition in the mother lowers the output of certain immune bodies, it does not necessarily cause the milk to be greatly lacking in nutrients and immunity capability. Immune activity remains as high or possibly even higher in the milk of undernourished mothers, as compared with well-nourished mothers. One must distinguish, however, between undernourished and more serious cases of starvation or malnourishment. The more severe the condition, the worse the impact on both the nutrient and immune composition of the milk.

Another possible benefit of breast feeding is the biological control of new pregnancies. At least one-third of women who nurse their infants continuously for 9 months fail to menstruate during that time; the norm for these lactating women, however, is 3 months. It is usually, but not always, shortly thereafter that the first egg is released; ovulation can also occur before menstruation. In no case is the nursing of a baby a fail-safe method of contraception, but it is true that new pregnancies overall are delayed.

Another benefit of nursing is the bond cemented between mother and child that comes from the mere act of breast feeding. It is a bond all mothers and offspring should enjoy if possible. However, a mother who is unable to breast-feed should not feel great distress; fondling, love, and attention will unite the two as surely.

An obvious advantage of nursing is that cost of breast feeding is less than formula feeding—unless possibly one considers the cost of keeping the mother at the extra high caloric intake required for nursing. Those extra calories amount to about 500 per day (NAS/NRC, 1980). That is about the same total caloric need of an infant from 0 to 2 months of age (as given by the Protein Advisory Group of the United Nations). In formula alone, however, that many calories would have taken 55% of the income of an Ethiopian family, 66% of Malawi's income, or 28% of an Egyptian's. These are 1975 figures based on income for menial labor. But, of course, a difference exists between extra caloric needs for a mother and the caloric needs of an infant. A mother lacking the financial means will simply go without food, will use more of the cheaper food native to her homeland, and will provide whatever milk her body allows.

The Disadvantages of Breast Milk

Shortcomings of mother's milk might be summed up as follows:

1. inconsistency in nutritional content;
2. a nutrient content dependent to some extent on dietary habits and food availability;
3. a production rate dependent on food (caloric) intake;
4. generally lower potential than formula to maximize growth rate (weight gain);
5. transfer of drugs taken by the mother to the feeding infant;

6. transfer of environmental pollutants from the mother's food or other environmental exposure to the milk and thence the feeding infant;

7. staphylococcal infections of the breast, with production of toxin;

8. transmission of certain viral diseases (hepatitis B and cytomegalovirus).

None of the preceding need necessarily be considered greatly limiting of breast feeding generally. Still, vitamin content of mother's milk does depend, in specific instances, on vitamin intake of the mother. Malnourishment may reduce to deficiency levels both vitamins A and C in human milk. Riboflavin content likewise follows a similar pattern. In a study of Gambian mothers, specifically, riboflavin content of milk was found comparatively lower than standard levels even during the season of the year when food intake was generally higher (at 1600–1750 kcal/day) than during the season of short food supply (Prentice, 1980). Generally speaking, supplementation of the mother's diet will raise appropriately the level of the respective vitamin in the milk supply. This is true at least for most water-soluble vitamins. As an example, Belavady (1980) noted prolonged high levels of both riboflavin and ascorbic acid in milk of low-income Indian women supplemented with 3.0 and 200 mg daily of riboflavin and ascorbic acid, respectively. Vitamin A levels in milk could also be raised and maintained, but only with supplementation with *emulsified* suspensions of the vitamin.

Both amount of zinc and copper in milk may be less than adequate for breast-feeding infants of some malnourished mothers (Prema, 1978). Normally, for reasonably well-nourished women, level of neither of these minerals in milk is greatly influenced by supplementation of the mother's diet. Calcium and iron content of milk may actually be lowered by supplementation with these minerals (Belavady, 1980).

The most serious impact of undernourishment most likely is generally in a reduction of milk yield. On diets of 1350–1450 kcal/day, milk output of Gambian mothers was found to be 40% less than that of women consuming 1600–1750 kcal/day (Prentice, 1980). Average yield of milk among a group of malnourished Egyptian women has been put at 714 ml as compared to 914 ml/day in a well-nourished control group (Hanafy, 1980). In still another study, pattern of milk yield was observed to change dramatically under conditions of undernourishment. Chavez and Martinez (1980) noted a sudden drop in production of milk after 2–3 months of reasonably abundant output among one-half of a group of rural Mexican poor. The other half of this particular group were simply unable to increase milk yield commensurate with infant demand. By 8 months of age, infants of all of these women weighed significantly less than those of a similar group whose diet had been supplemented throughout lactation with vitamins, minerals, protein (20 g/day), and calories (300/day). The evidence, therefore, appears quite clear: Undernourishment not only increases the percent of underweight (less than 2.5 kg) infants, but tends generally to cause poor lactation performance. By 3 months, protein content may become limiting in mother's milk. The milk may also lack appropriate levels of certain vitamins; it may be deficient in calories. Scientists of the London School of Hygiene and Tropical Medicine suggest energy to be limiting to breast-fed infants before protein (Waterlow and Thompson, 1979). Where undernutrition is prevalent, these authorities would recommend supplemental infant feeding at 2–3 months. Supplemental feeding of mothers is perhaps another alternative, though not necessarily effective in increasing yield in all cases (Belavady, 1980). Concerning physical growth of the infant, Leichtig and Klein (1980) suggest that supplementation of the lactating mother's diet is most important during the infant's first 6 months of life, but supplementation of the infant's diet per se becomes more important during the second 6 months.

In extreme situations, where death of the infant commonly occurs, level of fat (therefore energy) may be found wanting in mother's milk. Amounts of 1% or less have been recorded (Crawford et al., 1977). Infants, especially those beyond 3 months of age, succumb from lack of calories. Or if they survive, they become one of many whose growth is severely stunted (Whitehead, 1976). This malady, the result of undernutrition generally, has been cited as foremost among populations of China and other Asian countries, and certain African and Latin American countries. For infants of about 3 months of age, infant formula might well serve its most beneficial function. For although many weaning foods may be used, few even approach the nutrient load of fortified formula. All, unless properly treated and handled, are no less potential vectors of disease.

In a study of 11 different cultures throughout the Third World (U.S.A. Human Lactation Center, 1978) lack of supplemental food beyond 3 months of age has been reported to be the major cause of infant death, irrespective of whether or not infants are breast-fed. In addition, those groups and subgroups of populations in which breast-feeding reaches its highest rate of practice are always the poorest of the poor, and it is this stratum of society that likewise spawns the highest rate of infant death (U.S.A. Human Lactation Center, 1978).

Women of means, however, may not necessarily provide as abundant a supply of breast milk as the poor over extended periods of time, that is, beyond 6 months of lactation. Given the option, these women may breast-feed only on an irregular basis. This practice, in turn, tends to lower the concentration of the hormone, prolactin; milk production then falters (Rajalakshmi, 1980; Edozien, 1980).

Such facts are important in view of the findings and conclusions of scientists at Johns Hopkins University (Ahn and MacLean, 1980) who suggest that breast milk alone of healthy mothers should suffice for most infants for the better part of the entire first year of life. These researchers found merit in providing food supplementation for the mother rather than the infant under Third World conditions. Not all authorities would agree, at least for the second half of the first year (Belavady, 1980; Leichtig and Klein, 1980).

An advantage to supplemental feeding over and above nutrition itself may derive from variety alone. That is, exposure to flavors and textures of other foods may help build lifelong patterns of nutritious eating. Assuming generally adequate nutrient intake from either breast milk and/or infant formula, focus falls on introduction of various kinds of foods, less on amount. It must be remembered that many tastes are in fact acquired tastes, and that monotonous diets ultimately place life at risk of nutritional deficiency. Indeed, narrow desires or, as more frequently arises in the Third World, limited choices of food, lead literally to boredom of food intake and refusal to eat even of available food.

Few studies suggest anything but more rapid weight gain on formula than breast milk. Not all authorities consider weight of most breast-fed infants to be less than adequate. Some do, however (O'Connor, 1978), and report a higher failure of breast-fed than formula-fed infants in achieving an ideal rate of gain in weight. Again, the critical time frame usually occurs at 3–4 months, when energy (calories) becomes a limiting factor.

Some pediatricians, however, would readily risk underfeeding than risk any food source other than breast milk. Others though, cite the advantage of proper nourishment in the battle to resist infections, and would encourage use of food in supplementation to mother's milk, especially where exposure to infection runs high (Waterlow and Thompson, 1979). The debate continues in this respect and has centered of late on whether it is best to supplement the mother's diet or the infant's—and, if the latter, when supplementation should begin. Those who recommend additional food generally call for its use about the fourth month, among healthy women and infants. At this point, risk of food allergy has been greatly reduced. Even on infant formula exclusively, need for beikost appears unnecessary and possibly risky prior to this time (Droese et al., 1978).

Though viewpoints differ, there appears to be little movement away from nutrient supplementation of the infant, usually with vitamins A, C, and D, and fluoride and iron. If formula use and/or nutrient supplementation have significant merit, it is as a safeguard against deficiency in face of rather widely differing needs and circumstances.

Becoming overweight is a problem both of breast-fed and bottle-fed infants, and the one source of food need not necessarily prove significantly worse than the other in this regard. If there is a common determinant in the milk of breast-feeding mothers of obese infants, it is perhaps an above-average level of fat. However, milk of lower amounts of fat is also associated with overweight infants, and occasionally at niggardly levels of 2–3%. In most instances, the problem is overcome by feeding less, that is, 5–7 minutes duration (Lazarev, 1976).

Drugs are a possible contaminant of mother's milk. Little more need be said, except that all breast-feeding mothers should be aware of the problem and prepared to seek counsel. Environmental pollutants pose an unknown health risk to the breast-feeding infant. Compared to formula, breast-milk will usually be found to be more heavily contaminated by environmental pollutants, with the possible exception of lead. Not uncommonly, breast milk contains levels of contamination of organic pollutants higher than the standards set for cow's milk and, therefore, formula prepared of this ingredient source.

Breast infections pose a risk of loss of some or all productive capacity, but this is only one disease state that hinders adequate production of milk. Heart disease can also force a mother to a substitute for breast milk. A history of hepatitis or cytomegalovirus disease may do likewise. "Active" tuberculosis, which is still common around the world, is another disease that makes of breast feeding a needless risk.

Some women also find their milk supply gradually giving out. The reasons offered are diverse: excessive work at home, bad housing, belief that one has nursed for a long enough period, and family conflicts. In one survey of 1970 women (Cvengros and Stadtruckerova, 1978), over 14% found themselves losing milk production for one or more of the preceding reasons. No matter what the true basis is, the loss of milk yield was nonetheless real. Mothers also switch to bottle feeding out of fear that the child is not getting adequate amounts of food, which may or may not be the case. Some mothers suggest that their own milk appears "thin"; although this may be true in comparison to milk of cows, it is the natural state for the most part. A mother's foremilk (the very first milk from the breast) is especially thin.

With proper training and with adequate numbers of dedicated health professionals, most of the shortcomings of breast feeding could be readily overcome. Yet this ideal is rarely met, either in industrialized societies or in the Third World. Thus, supplemental feeding continues to be a widespread need.

INFANT FORMULA

The Promises of Infant Formula

The advantages of infant formula are several. Well-made, fortified formulas offer

1. consistency of nutrient content;
2. monitored quality;
3. generally low level of contamination with industrial or agricultural pollutants;
4. a variable composition as might be needed to treat certain specific nutritional maladies;
5. a potential for the incorporation of a wide variety of immune factors, from antibodies specific to infant intestinal diseases to nonspecific immune factors such as lysozyme, lactoperoxidase, the bifidus factor (or acid-producing cultures as such), and, in the future, interferon.

Fortified infant formula provides a consistent and balanced source of all nutrients known to be essential to the infant. Quality is usually extensively monitored. Comparison of formula with mother's milk often shows the former to contain lower levels of most food and environmental contaminants. Lead is the major exception. Formula also offers versatility. Specialized nutritional needs can be met by formulation and use of specialized formulas. Though allergy to ingredients in formulas pose the most general risk, "nonallergenic" formulas have been prepared and found successful in many instances. That fact notwithstanding, allergy to common formulas remains a signficiant problem, especially in families with a known history of allergies.

On balance, formula can serve an infant's basic nutritional needs better than any other known food. Research suggests that it will serve better in the future, either in lieu of or as a supplement to mother's milk, whichever needs or desires dictate. In the immediate future, more formula may come fortified with taurine, carnitine, and zinc-binding agents. Where research indicates a worthy component in mother's milk, formula can usually be so adapted. One constant need is the improvement in bioavailability of nutrients. Though no apparently serious risks prevail, formula cannot match mother's milk in general availability of nutrients.

The most significant advances in infant formulas are in the area of immune potency. In this respect, it seems worthy of note that pH in the form of an acid environment is a common preservative function applied to food systems. Acidity alone is a formidable opponent of disease agents. Acidity within the intestinal tract, as represented by presence of L. bifidus, L. acidophilus or other lactic cultures, provides a stable, consistent form of passive immunity as yet scarcely considered as an ingredient in infant formula. Coupled with other immune agents derived of animal or other sources (including genetically altered species of bacteria), a quite "natural" arsenal of weapons can be built into formula. Lysozyme and lactoferrin are already used. Lactoperoxidase use will likely expand. "Immune-type" IgG of cow's milk will do for infants much of what IgA of mother's milk does. As food, food supplement, or weaning food, formulas of this type offer real hope in the control of infectious diarrhea, a major enemy of infant health. To the extent that immune agents to diseases common to the hospital environment can be built into formula, protection is offered against germs to which even mother's milk may fail. To the extent that "natural" immune agents might be used instead of antibiotic or other treatment, the infant's own fledgling immune system is better protected. These are the possibilities present research portends.

The Risks of Infant Formula

In underdeveloped countries, ignorance and poverty may cause some serious risks in the use of infant formula. Without clean water to mix with and reconstitute a powdered formula or liquid concentrate, without adequate fuel for boiling water for this purpose, and without fuel for washing and sanitizing feeding bottles and other utensils, mothers put their infants in danger of contracting any number of waterborne or filth-related diseases. Any one of these diseases, coupled with a constant state of malnutrition, can be deadly. They are just as deadly whether formula or some other gruel of local formulation happens to be the source of food at weaning time. Research done in Keneba, New Gambia, showed 96% of samples of traditional cereal-based weaning food to be bacteriologically unsuitable for feeding 8 hours after preparation. Local practices promoted such lengthy storage. As a scientific observer pointed out, the gruel itself was a very poor nutritional substitute for infant formula (Lackey, 1978).

Part of the answer to serious nutritional maladies lies in the fortification of weaning food. Addition of vegetable protein or milk to cereal-based products can add considerably to the nutrient profile. In addition, of all nutrients, vitamin A supplementation seems perhaps most necessary, if only as a means of preventing blindness. A number of countries have tried fortification of weaning foods, albeit with varying benefits. The National Academy of Sciences recommends the addition to cereal-based weaning food of ten nutrients: vitamin A, thiamine, riboflavin, niacin, pyridoxine, folacin, iron, calcium, magnesium, and zinc.

Of potential germs spread from water to food, pathogenic coliform are among the most dangerous. Other waterborne pathogens include those causing typhoid fever, diphtheria, poliomyelitis, and infectious hepatitis. Still other pathogens may be specific to the local habitat. Just as important, certain infectious agents survive longer in water and are more resistant to chlorine, the usual chemical purifier, than others.

Statistics show the first few days of life to be the riskiest; in most poor nations other periods of risk are the third or fourth month and the second year

(Cameron and Hofvander, 1976). Onset of disease appears to correspond roughly with inadequate milk yield (in comparison to the infant's needs and/or with the introduction of food in addition to breast milk. No doubt these factors are related.

The major killer in these periods of risk is diarrhea. The question arises: Is formula to blame? Among the many causes of diarrhea are those related to food: misformulated or infected formula; contaminated food, even that of local preparation (Lackey, 1978); improperly cooked beans; and spicy foods like chili. Illnesses such as malaria, pneumonia, and ear infections (Cameron and Hofvander, 1976) and poisons such as staphylococcal toxin of infected breast milk are known to cause diarrhea. No one at this time has determined just how significant this last problem is, especially in populations seriously at risk because of bad sanitation conditions. Malnutrition itself is also a cause of diarrhea, and diarrhea occurs more frequently in undernourished infants. Finally, allergies can lead to diarrhea. Despite the prevalence of diarrhea, only 20% of such cases can be diagnosed as to cause(s) (Cameron and Hofvander, 1976). The great majority (80%) go unspecified. Thus, to condemn formula alone is without foundation. Because adequate nutrition promotes the body's own defenses, some authorities would even recommend formula, particularly at weaning time, as a preventive to diseases. Studies by the World Health Organization have shown sharp drops in diarrhea (in a community setting) when appropriate food supplements are properly administered (Scrimshaw et al., 1968). A healthy body simply fights infection more vigorously.

From a technological standpoint, no serious obstacles prevent packaging of use-strength liquid formula in single-service, one-feeding units. German processors provide such servings in 0.2-liter Tetra Pak cartons or plastic feeding bottles. An offshoot of this technology has also been developed by the International Center of Diarrheal Disease Research in Bangladesh for supplying Oralyte, a mixture of glucose and salts, as a home remedy for infant diarrhea (Pearson, 1980). The product is marketed in the dry state, however, and therefore must be mixed with boiled water prior to use. The concept has proven exceedingly helpful in the treatment of infant diarrhea. Expense is a major detraction of packaging liquid formula products in this manner. However, dried formula could be provided possibly at less cost and possibly with added viable cultures of lactobacilli. Other immune agents could as well be added.

With dried products, mixing the wrong amount of water for reconstitution does indeed pose a constant threat. If too much water is added, the nutrient load is proportionately weakened. If not enough water is added, such concentrated milk may cause kidney failure. In this latter instance, the infant's kidney (renal) system may simply be taxed beyond its capacity. If the renal solute load becomes too great, the immature kidneys cannot handle it; dehydration may occur, or the renal system may fail altogether. It can happen in 5 days from feeding undiluted (full-strength) evaporated milk. It could happen as quickly by feeding overboiled skim milk, or improperly reconstituted commercial powdered milk (or baby formula) in dry (powdered) or concentrate form. The use of regular whole milk (undiluted) is also to be avoided, even as weaning food. Less than 1 liter of such milk per day has been found associated with gastrointestinal bleeding. Such occult blood loss is serious enough in and of itself, but it also leads to iron deficiency. Risk in this instance carries through to the time the infant's immune system reaches a fair degree of maturity, usually not until or near the end of the first year. This does not imply that nonformula milk products cannot be used, only that they should never be used full-strength. Even then there are risks, and precautions should be taken to reduce those risks to the extent possible. These considerations follow.

PREPARATION AND USE OF NONFORMULA MILK PRODUCTS FOR INFANT FEEDING

When necessary, nonformula milk products in diluted form can serve an infant's needs. The poorest of the lot, for use only in extreme emergency, are sweetened, condensed products. Note the word *condensed*. This word is used to distinguish the food from evaporated milk, which is also a concentrated milk product, but one that has no added sweetener (and is sterilized by heat). Condensed milk products come both as skim milk and whole milk concentrates. Without fortification, the former will be badly lacking in fat-soluble vitamins (A, D, K, and E). Both will have a sugar content near 45%. In no case should they be used full-strength. In no case should they be used except as short-term, stop-gap measures in times of great need. For that purpose, however, both products may be diluted with seven parts of clean (boiled, if necessary) water to one part of condensed milk product.

Skim milk powders alone are as about as unfit for infant feeding as condensed milk products. Again, extreme need should dictate use and extent of use. Keep in mind that skim milk, as such, will lack vitamins A and D. In dried form, with no added vitamins, the food will still be lacking. It will also be deficient in vitamin C, vitamin E, essential fatty acids, and iron. In the United States, most skim milk powder (called nonfat dry milk) comes fortified with vitamins A and D. It would serve emergency needs somewhat better than unfortified powder. As infant food, it is still lacking in fat and lactose, and thus calories (at usable strength). Addition of fats or oils of local origin could upgrade energy (caloric) value, but could not be counted on to add adequate amounts of fat-soluble vitamins (vitamins A and D being particularly critical). Fats and oils are also not sources of vitamin C or iron.

Of several milk products available, regular milk (liquid whole milk) full-fat (whole milk) powder, and evaporated milk are perhaps most adaptable to an infant's needs (if nothing more suitable is available). When water purity is in doubt, only boiled water should be used for dilution purposes. If raw (unpasteurized milk) fluid milk is the source of food, it must always be heated to destroy germs. Lacking thermometers and other controls, this can be done simply by bringing the milk to a boil. Extended boiling should be avoided.

Tables 25 and 26, adapted from the United Nations Manual on Feeding Infants and Young Children (second edition) (Cameron and Hofvander, 1976), give dilution and other information needed to modify a variety of milk products for infant feeding purposes. Two things must be remembered, however: (1) The extent of dilution depends upon the age of the child and (2) the amount of the prepared milk product that is to be fed depends upon the weight of the child. The object is to feed as much as needed without overloading the infant's kidneys. Age and weight are the two critical factors. Note also that sugar may be added to adapt the product to infant use. With skim milk powder, both sugar and fat improve nutritional value. Of all nonformula cow's milk products, canned evaporated milk has probably seen most widespread use. It usually comes fortified with vitamin D; it may also be fortified with vitamin A. The level of fortification is usually placed at 25 international units (IU) per fluid ounce (29.6 ml) (79 IU/100 g) of vitamin D and 125 IU/fluid ounce (29.6 ml) (396 IU/100 g) for vitamin A. Overall nutrient content of evaporated milk is shown in Table 27.

INFANT BOTULISM

Botulism is the name of the disease state caused by a spore-forming bacterium called *Clostridium botulinum*. The Food and Drug Administration's Center for Disease Control identified 139 cases of infant botulism between 1978 and 1981. *C. botulinum* survives widely in nature. Soil is a common habitat; 25% of soil samples taken at 50-mile intervals across the continental United States have been found positive for the organism. The presence in soil puts the organism in contact with various vegetable and other crops grown for food. Home-canned string beans, corn, beans, spinach, and asparagus account for perhaps half the botulinum poisoning cases occurring in the United States in recent times (Institute of Food Technologists, 1972).

Soil, however, is only one source. *C. botulinum* is also present in bottom sediment of streams, lakes, and coastal waters. Fish and shellfish ingest it, and thus, the intestinal content of aquatic life becomes a source. Even household

TABLE 25
How to Prepare Various Milk Products as Food for Infants up to 3 Months of Age[a,b]

Treatment	Cow's milk (boiled)[c]	Evaporated milk	Whole milk powder	Skim milk powder[d]
Dilution				
Milk[e]	100 ml (½ cup)	50 ml (2 tbl)	14 g (1½ tbl)	10 g (1 tbl)
Water (boiled)	50 ml (¼ cup)	100 ml (½ cup)	150 ml (¾ cup)	150 ml (¾ cup)
Add				
Sugar[f]	10 g (2 tsp)	10 g (2 tsp)	10 g (2 tsp)	10 g (2 tsp)
Oil	—	—	—	5 g (1 tsp)
Calories	70	75	75	75
Protein (g)	2.2	2.3	2.4	2.4

[a]Adapted from Cameron and Hofvander (1976).

[b]Average weight of infant is 4.6 kg (10 lb). Product, as prepared, is fed at a rate of 150 ml/kg (2½ oz/lb) body weight at 4-hour intervals, 5 times daily.

[c]Or pasteurized.

[d]To be used only in extreme emergency, especially so if unfortified with vitamins A and D.

[e]As given, "tbl" means tablespoon, level measure.

[f]As given, "tsp" means teaspoon, level measure.

TABLE 26
How to Prepare Various Milk Products as Food for Infants 3–5 Months of Age[a,b]

Treatment	Cow's milk (boiled)[c]	Evaporated milk	Whole milk powder	Skim milk powder[d]
Dilution				
Milk[e]	175 ml (¾ cup)	80 g (3 tbl)	25 g (3 tbl)	20 g (2 tbl)
Water (boiled)	1–2 tbl	120 ml (½ cup)	200 ml (>¾ cup)	200 ml (¾ cup)
Add				
Sugar[f]	10 g (2 tsp)	10 g (2 tsp)	10 g (2 tsp)	10 g (2 tsp)
Oil	—	—	—	5 g (1 tsp)
Calories	105	100	110	105
Protein	3.5	3.7	4.3	4.8

[a]Adapted from Cameron and Hofvander (1976).

[b]Average weight of infant is 6.7 kg (14.7 lb). Product, as prepared, is fed at 150 ml/kg (2½ oz/lb) body weight.

[c]Or pasteurized.

[d]To be used only in extreme emergency, especially so if unfortified with vitamins A and D.

[e]As given, "tbl" means tablespoon, level measure.

[f]As given "tsp" means teaspoon, level measure.

TABLE 27
Nutrient Content of Evaporated Milk[a] (per 100 g)

Nutrient	Handbook 8-1	Average literature values	Range of literature values	Percentage loss Process	Percentage loss 1-year storage
Total solids (g)	25.96	26.1[d]	25.09–27.30	—	—
Protein (N × 6.38) (g)	6.81	6.7[d]	6.54–7.35	—	—
Fat (g)	7.56	7.9[d]	7.14–8.24	—	—
Carbohydrate (g)	10.04	10.1[d]	—	—	—
Calories (kcal)	134	138	—	—	—
Vitamin A (activity) (IU)	243	369	342–464	0	0
Vitamin D (IU)	79[b]	79[b]	—	0	0
Vitamin E (mg)	0.22[c]	0.26	0.22–0.30	0	0
Ascorbic acid (mg)	1.88	1.1	0.4–1.8	50–90	5
Thiamine (mg)	0.047	0.056	0.04–0.08	20–60	15–50
Riboflavin (mg)	0.316	0.38	0.28–0.48	0	28
Pyridoxine (mg)	0.05	0.07	0.055–0.137	36–49	0(?)
Vitamin B$_{12}$ (μg)	0.163	0.14	0.10–0.19	90	0(?)
Folacin (μg)	8.0	1.40	—	0	0
Niacin (mg)	0.194	0.20	0.18–0.23	0	0
Panthothenic acid (mg)	0.638	0.70	0.58–0.80	0	0
Calcium (mg)	261	258[e]	—	—	—
Phosphorus (mg)	202	199[e]	—	—	—
Iron (mg)	0.19	0.09[e]	0.08–1.90	—	—
Copper (mg)	—	0.03[e]	0.009–0.150	—	—

[a]Adapted from Owen and McIntire (1976).
[b]Fortified product.
[c]From Wyoming Agricultural Experiment Station (1965).
[d]From Webb and Whittier (1970).
[e]From Webb and Johnson (1965).

dust may be carrier. Honey may also be a carrier, as so could a variety of ingredients of foods prepared for infants. A large number of infant foods including infant formula are under study and remain potential sources. A very small number of corn syrups have been noted to yield *C. botulinum* spores, but the number of such contaminated supplies is so small as to appear of little or no concern. Lacking further information, honey has been spotlighted as a probable source, and mothers are thus forewarned. With household dust a potential carrier, contamination could even take place in the home. Other potential sources are canned fruit, fruit juice, fresh cooked carrots, cow's milk, nonfat milk, sugar, and dry cereals.

Most often botulinum poisoning results from the growth of the organism outside the body, that is, in a food product. Growth takes place only in the absence of oxygen. When multiplication occurs, a toxin is produced. Upon intake, the poison is absorbed through the intestines. Food *intoxication* results; symptoms appear within 8 to 72 hours. This is the usual manner in which botulinum poisoning occurs; the infant form, however, appears to be of an infectious nature. When the bacterial cells are ingested, they grow and multiply in the intestines and, in so doing, produce toxin. It can happen in ways possibly unrelated to the growing or processing of infant foods.

Symptoms of the disease may be mistaken for polio. Breathing is difficult. There is general weakness. Swallowing becomes both difficult and painful. Chest muscles tighten. Other signs, however, may be no more unusual than those of a stomachache or of constipation. In any event, professional diagnosis is not especially difficult, and symptoms alone provide a fairly good basis.

Botulinum poisoning occurs very infrequently and can, in fact, be termed rare. Although it is a most serious disease, it is often treatable if caught in time.

9

Lactose: At Weaning and Beyond

Sooner or later an infant must obtain succor from food sources other than mother's milk. This process or transition is called weaning. It may take place precipitously, as when a mother's milk supply suddenly gives out or becomes unacceptable, or slowly over a long period of time. The process may begin after a few weeks or as late as 6 months. It may end soon, with mother's milk withdrawn shortly after birth, or may carry on for 2½ years or more. Commonly, weaning is a gradual process, with mother's milk supplementing other foods for a fairly lengthy period. The start of weaning, at whatever point, is indeed a critical time. It is far more critical for those who are short of food, particularly food of high protein value.

The importance of breast-feeding to the impoverished is a means of maintaining a milk supply, a supply that may never be in more need than at weaning time. As a supplement to foods low in nutrient content, as a supplement to whatever meager amounts of food are available, mother's milk has no equal. Formula, of course, could serve as well—if it were affordable available, and used properly. Any of a number of foods might, in fact, be used in the weaning process. Like formula, however, they too must be handled and stored in a sanitary manner, or risk becoming contaminated. Early weaning only lengthens the duration over which this kind of risk, and the risk of underfeeding, is spread.

For an excellent reference to various kinds of weaning foods and their preparation, the reader is referred to *Manual on Feeding Infants and Young Children*, a publication of the Protein-Calorie Advisory Group of the United Nations (Cameron and Hofvander, 1976).

Under normal circumstances weaning goes on through the first year of life. If there is a choice, formula serves better than the natural milk of most animals, even if weaning does not commence until the fifth or sixth month. It may well begin sooner, however. Most pediatricians recommend formula and/or other weaning foods to begin at between 4 and 5 months of age. The critical point is this: The earlier weaning is begun, the more important it is to feed formula rather than natural milk, for reasons cited elsewhere (see Chapter 3). By the end of the first year, infants can handle most adult food. Weight can be used as an indication of feeding adequacy. Weight of males does differ from females in this respect. A general rule of thumb puts weight at 5 months at double the birth-weight. At 12 months, it is three times the weight at birth. As a measure of protein-calorie malnutrition, the circumference (distance around) the arm may be used. From 1 to 5 years of age this distance remains fairly constant at about 16 cm. Normal arm-size at birth is about 10 cm. The arm expands rapidly in size up to 6 months, when it should approach 15 cm. Such measurements are not precise indicators of shortage of protein and calories. They serve, however, as rough screening methods for this deficiency state.

Thus far an assumption has been made that, with breast milk, evolution has done for humans what they might not otherwise have done for themselves. Even so, anomalies exist, one of which crops up at weaning or sometime thereafter. What for the infant was a nutrient in the form of milk sugar, for much of the human race may become the source of an upset stomach. Not that it will, and not as a universal occurrence by any means, but the malady exists. Orientals, blacks, and certain other races, in fairly high numbers, show an inability to digest lactose as readily beyond infancy. Stomach cramps, gas, and in some cases, diarrhea are symptoms of the problem. One way to overcome the difficulty is through the use of milk-like foods formulated without lactose (or from which lactose has been removed). "Formulas" of this type, though prepared chiefly for infants, have been discussed in previous pages (see Chapter 6). Such foods can as readily be prepared for children and adults. Some processes, like cheesemaking, also serve well this very same function. In this case, the technology itself results in the removal of lactose. Fluid products, too, can be made. Soy milk is one approach. Using a variety of other milk ingredients, other types of lactose-free milk are likewise possible. The food will not be milk, as such, but rather a modified or rebuilt food that looks and tastes like milk.

How did this digestive disturbance come to be? Is it appropriate to assume that nature did not intend that humans should drink milk beyond weaning? Did evolution, adaption, or genetic change make it possible for certain members of our species to go on consuming milk through old age, while others—the great majority of humankind—should be more or less impeded in so seemingly natural a process as the ingestion of food ingredients suckled as an infant from the breast of one's own mother? This is the question we shall examine at this time. A brief, though speculative, history of what has come to be termed "lactose intolerance" may yield some worthwhile insights.

THE VERY FIRST MILK DRINKERS

To begin, consider the chemical makeup of lactose, the major carbohydrate (and major food solids component) of milk. It is a disaccharide; that is, it consists of two discrete simple sugars, glucose and galactose, bound to each other by chemical bonds. It is found in all mammalian milks, though in far lesser amounts in the milk of seal, sea lion, and walrus. Scientists believe that the evolutionary process of these animals in the frigid Arctic seas favored more fat in milk, thus more energy, to the eventual exclusion of "low-energy" sugar. Thus, there is a precedence for the apparent intercession of nature in the scheme of things that would formulate the makeup of that first food to enter mouths of the newborn. Cow's milk contains lactose to about 5.0%. Human milk contains lactose to an average level of around 6.9%. It can perhaps be presumed that the inference nature is trying to put across is her intention to feed certain infant mammals some lactose. We repeat (with added emphasis): *infant* mammals. Was it nature's intent, however, to go on feeding milk to her offspring throughout life? Certainly not mother's milk, obviously. In a manner of speaking, nature tends to beg the question. She tears the child from its mother's breast at a very early age and literally commands it to go out and feed itself henceforth (with mother's teaching) on whatever seems to agree with it. Whole ecological systems of mutually beneficial eating habits (notably in the few unspoiled wilds of Africa and the Arctic ice caps) grew out of this stern, irrevocable injunction.

As the early human species evolved and its brain grew in size, its whole being was forced, nonetheless, to concentrate on the attainment of food. Then about 11,000 years ago one group of the human species learned to herd animals as a means of relieving themselves of the daily burden of chasing sustenance. These people inhabited what is now northwestern Europe. They were also Caucasians, but that is only coincidental. What happened, if indeed it happened at all, has no racial distinctions. One theory holds that these people banded together, herded animals, and began the regular practice of drinking milk. Persons of all ages, not just preweaning children, gradually indulged the habit. We may perhaps assume that this had never happened before. The human body, which heretofore had been exposed to milk only for a short span of life very early in childhood, now was asked to nourish itself on this food throughout its entire natural existence. Could it do so? Would it?

LACTOSE DIGESTION AND UPSET STOMACHS

The answers to the two questions call for a very casual understanding of the digestive process, that is, the process by which living animals convert food to useful, usable nutrients. In the case of lactose (as in the case of most life processes), an *enzyme* is involved. An enzyme is a protein entity capable of entering into brief, though intimate, contact with a particular food component or metabolic substance and, without itself being used up in the process, swiftly causing a reaction to take place. Enzymes build chemical units. They also tear them down. There are many dozens of enzyme systems at work in the human body, each one peculiarly specific to both the reaction and the chemical substance with which it contracts to perform a job. Generally speaking, one enzyme cannot substitute for another. If you lack any one, you are in fact a wounded being; some exceedingly specific chemical reaction taking place naturally and easily in other human bodies is totally blocked in yours. Even if your body has some of the enzyme, the reaction may be partially blocked if there is not enough of the enzyme to handle all of the nutrient or metabolite presented to it during the time it must function.

The net result may be a serious handicap, as in babies born missing the enzyme to break off phenylalanine from protein in food. These infants cannot even digest milk protein. The affliction may also not be so serious, but the body (mind) goes on blithely unaware of its sputtering engine. In between these two extremes, the human system may simply get a bad case of indigestion. In fact, this is what could happen to the majority of us when confronted (challenged) with significant quantities of milk (lactose) in the diet at some point following weaning. This means only that an enzyme, the one needed to split lactose into its component parts (glucose and galactose) is lacking to more or less degree. The greater the lack, the worse the digestive upset. Change the *o* to *a* in the word *lactose*, and call the enzyme *lactase*. Your ability to split, and thereby digest, milk sugar depends on whether or not you have this enzyme, or to what extent your digestive system (intestinal mucosa) can manufacture and secrete it. If you cannot, if this mechanism is totally or even partially blocked, a significant amount of lactose remains intact within the intestines. By osmosis, its presence draws water from the surrounding intestinal tissues. Some of it may be fermented by ever-present bacteria. Organic acids and the gases carbon dioxide and hydrogen are formed (Newcomer, 1979). The result, as evident from what has taken place, is gas, bloating, cramp pains, and, with all the water, diarrhea. This condition, the inability to digest lactose properly, has become known as "lactose intolerance."

It is intriguing to speculate how this digestive problem came to be remedied in a segment of earth's population. For whatever light it may shed on the question of food sources in relation to human nourishment, a speculation is offered here. Since the capacity to digest lactose readily in the adult years appears to be an almost unique ability of Caucasians of northern European descent, and since the majority of our species to this day is hampered in this digestive process, we can reasonably presume that the function was not prescribed by nature in our ancestral history. In earlier times, food for the race probably did not routinely consist of milk after weaning. The need, therefore, to digest milk sugar did not exist, and the body simply stopped producing as much of the enzyme required to break it down. This was "normal" for early humans. It is still "normal" for most of us even now. If lactose digestion beyond childhood may be considered an abnormal or newly gained function, it probably came about by one of nature's laws at work; it was a mutation of some sort, that is, a change in the genetic makeup of some members of the race, which could then be passed on and dispersed through a mass of the population.

Suppose for the moment that a mutation that resulted in a prolonged capacity to produce lactase, thus a "tolerance" for a daily diet of milk did take place. For such a mutation to establish itself, two conditions are almost essential. First, milk must be readily available; it must be a food to which a hungry person, cramps or diarrhea notwithstanding, will turn. Second, when the mutation occurs, when some one or several newborn infants come wailing into life with a chromosomal oddity providing for milk digestion into later life, this genetic quirk must be given opportunity to reproduce itself within the clan. The two predisposing conditions, then, are: availability of milk for the diet and a kind of species life-style that favors transmission of a genetic aberration through a sizable cross-section of the population.

Further interpretation of what might have happened will consist of a merger of two theories developed recently by two different groups of scientists. The first is an evaluation of Simoons (1978): the second is the product of a team of scientists headed by Allan C. Wilson of the University of California, Berkeley.

The Simoons analysis is an attempt to explain why lactose tolerance confines itself chiefly to northwestern Europeans and their descendants. It suggests that this came about, possibly some 11,000 years ago, when the inhabitants of that area commenced herding animals as a regular practice and that the practice probably grew out of a desire to keep a food source nearby. These people (tribes, clans) became herders, and very likely in times of need, which may have been most of the time, they took to a diet of milk. Eventually, by writ of mutation, some of them found it possible to drink milk without suffering the consequence of upset stomach. To complete the cycle, these persons had only to pass this nature-given trait on to their children. Did conditions favor that?

Professor Wilson's team would likely say yes. In an extensive study of genetic differences in 1230 species, these scientists sought to determine why mammals—breast-feeders—have evolved ten times more rapidly than other vertebrates. Why have not frogs and lizards, for example, come along at the same rate of speed? These scientists suggest that mammals owe their success to the habit of forming close-knit groups. They congregate, and they stick together. When one mammal, with nature's help, pops up with a new trait, the probability that it will be passed on is very great. Mammals are in-breeders. They tend to come together in clans and pass on to offspring the character-istics of their evolutionary process. Herders of animals, who had the good fortune to bear children of genuine lactase potency, would be reasonably well assured of the continuance of this attribute. Their habits favored it. Lending weight to their viewpoint, the Berkeley scientists note how, even among various mammalian species, the slowest to evolve are those with great mobility (such as bats and whales), which can literally put distance between themselves. Those mammals that approach the human's rate of evolution are apes, rodents, and horses; these are species tending to congregate in small, though reproductively efficient, clans. For better or worse, as genetics would have it, "human needs" now tend to make more certain the passing on to future generations the imprint of any chance alteration in chromosomal messages. Thus, while some persons may gain an ability to digest milk sugar more readily, with equal assurance some will lose their capacity to metabolize an essential amino acid (phenylketonurics). It is written in the immutable laws of nature.

One theory now holds that lactose tolerance is passed on as a gentically dominant trait. If one parent carries the gene, the children will be so endowed. On the other hand, lactose intolerance may be a recessive genetic process in which the characteristic (intolerance) is transmitted to the children only if both parents are intolerant to lactose (Lisker et al., 1975; Newcomer, 1979). These facts being the case, the situation should ease over time; that is, more persons should gain the ability to digest milk sugar more readily. Curiously enough, those mammals whose milk contains little or no lactose are themselves intolerant to it. No doubt male and female seals, sea lions, and walruses both carry recessive genes. What if it were an adaptive process? Then, of course, exposure to the compound would be essential. That all humans (except for very rare cases of congenital deficiency) for a part of their lives are in fact able to digest lactose, would lend credibility to the hypothesis of adaptation. The ability to digest lactose later in life resulted from a forced extension of a digestive process already acquired but never before sufficiently challenged to promote its acquisition, through natural selection, among a large group of people (Anonymous, 1972). Those persons whose bodies were able to adjust survived to pass on this digestive advantage (where milk drinking was a necessity) to future generations.

Speculation is useful only as it lends insight into food sources as they relate to human nourishment now and the future. The question of whether or not lactase activity is inherited, acquired, or a case of genetic adaptation remains as yet unresolved.

Through racial integration and interbreeding of persons more or less capable of digesting lactose, a whole range of tolerance levels (from little to 100% ability to digest the sugar) seems to have evolved. Some persons assimilate it handily; others have some or much difficulty in doing so (under certain conditions). Estimates of incidence of low lactase activity (lactose intolerance) vary from 15% for Scandinavians and persons of western and northern European extraction to 60–80% for Greek Cypriots, American Indians, Arabs, Askenazi Jews, Mexican-Americans, and American blacks and to 90% for African Bantus and Orientals (Luyken, 1972; Jones and Latham, 1974; Sahi, 1974).

THE ROLE OF LACTOSE IN THE DIET

Having made a case for at least questioning milk (lactose) as a natural nutrient source for most adult humans, let us hasten to balance the ledger with scientific evidence of its possible metabolic roles, that is, its value in the diet. As a constituent of mother's milk, lactose can certainly be considered the carbohydrate of choice for the newborn infant. Why? What, if any, special role does it serve the infant (or later on, the adult)? There are several possibilities (in various states of scientific understanding):

1. For the infant, lactose provides galactose, a compound needed in the formation of galactolipids, a major component of the brain. However, preformed galactose is apparently not essential to the diet (Dairy Council Digest, 1974).
2. Lactose aids calcium absorption (Condon et al., 1970; Ambrecht and Wasserman, 1976).
3. Lactose aids absorption of other minerals (cations): strontium, magnesium, barium, radium, and manganese (Lengeman, 1959; Morris et al., 1963; Dairy Council Digest, 1962).
4. Lactose promotes the growth of a variety of intestinal bacteria, which, in turn, are able to synthesize the vitamins biotin, riboflavin, folic acid,

and pyridoxine. The function may properly be considered a vitamin *sparing* role; if intestinal bacteria can manufacture vitamins that must otherwise be provided from without, the level of intake of these vitamins can perhaps be reduced by a like amount (Dairy Council Digest, 1962).

5. Lactose helps prevent the late onset of rickets and osteomalacia (softening of bones in persons deficient in vitamin D), for example, where (or when) sunlight is in short supply. Some scientists believe this to be indicative of lactose's ability to promote calcium absorption (Dairy Council Digest, 1974).

6. Lactose may aid protein absorption and possibly the less digestible proteins of plant sources. This is a conclusion suggested by research on hogs as test animals (Dairy Council Digest, 1974).

7. Lactose may help control obesity, a predictable possibility as evidenced by studies with rats (Dairy Council Digest, 1974).

8. Lactose, as a fermentable sugar in the intestinal tract of lactose-tolerant persons, promotes proliferation of certain kinds of bacteria at the expense, possibly, of others. Those bacterial species found in the intestinal tract when lactose is missing tend to be those that interfere with intestinal absorption (Dairy Council Digest, 1974). Can it be assumed then that lactose assists the digestive process generally in this manner, and that lactose-tolerant herders of old would have a distinct survival advantage over less fortunate neighbors and kin, especially as might relate to availability of vitamins to the individual (see the third item above)?

Taken together, these or other possible metabolic roles provide reason to be cautious at least in making dietary recommendations against use of milk because of its lactose content. Any advice must always be tempered by considerations of the status of the eater. Where malnourishment runs endemic and surplus milk is available, failure to recommend its general use is to favor slow death in lieu (possibly) of a gassy stomach or bellyache. The only exception is for persons suffering severe diarrhea. This has prompted the Food and Nutrition Board of the National Academy of Science (NAS) to state, "It is highly inappropriate . . . to discourage programs for improving milk supplies or those that encourage milk consumption in either the United States or foreign countries because of the fear of milk (lactose) intolerance" (NAS, 1972).

This statement is supported and was at least in part prompted by the concerns of the Protein Advisory Group (PAG) of the United Nations (1972). The PAG would go one step further and attempt to avoid confusion and misunderstanding by indentifying various degrees of lactase deficiency, thus its impact on the consumer of milk. By their definition, lactase deficiency becomes low lactase activity (less than 2 units lactase activity/g wet mucosa); Mucosa is the tissue (cellular) site where lactase is formed. Lactose malabsorption refines out as "reduced absorption of lactose, (as) a consequence of low lactase activity, *determined by lactose tolerance tests.*" (The emphasis, which is my own, points out the objective approach.) Finally, the PAG would restrict the term "lactose intolerance" specifically to individuals showing "clinical signs" of digestive distress following administration of a standard dose of lactose in water, and then *only to those persons* previously proven (as defined above) to evince lactose malabsorption. (Again, the italics are mine). The PAG would rule out conjecture, which is not a bad idea in the battle against ignorance, to say nothing of the war against hunger.

A lactose tolerance test, therefore, becomes an essential aspect of diagnosis and treatment. The test itself is simple enough. After fasting, the subject is fed a standard dose of lactose. Blood glucose levels are then measured. If the level fails to rise above 20 mg/100 ml, a degree of lactose malabsorption is indicated. If the individual also experiences symptoms of digestive upset (abdominal pain, gas, bloating, and diarrhea), the diagnosis becomes "lactose intolerance." It is possible for persons to be malabsorbers, or poor absorbers, of lactose without undergoing clinical signs of distress. By this definition, persons of low lactose activity are not necessarily lactose intolerant.

If lactose intolerance is diagnosed, should such persons be directed to exclude milk from the diet? Should otherwise healthy children be taken off milk? What about infants and children (or adults) suffering some form of digestive upset? Would the burden of diarrhea only be worsened by feeding milk? Answers to these questions distinguish lactose intolerance or malabsorption from "milk intolerance." It is a distinction of importance. It also calls for some further definition, not to split hairs, but to assess the nature, extent, and distribution of the problems involved.

Garza (1979) of Baylor College of Medicine defines three categories of lactose intolerance: congenital, primary, and secondary. "Congenital intolerance" indicates that the condition is present at birth. Infants suffering this malady could respond adversely to mother's milk itself, or any lactose-containing formula, and do so prior to weaning. Fortunately, this condition is rare. Far more prevalent are the other two classes of lactose intolerance; these are the ones with which mass feeding recommendations must deal. "Primary intolerance" is defined as a condition existing without sign or history of presence of other gastrointestinal disease state. Intolerance simply exists as an affliction unto itself. Onset appears at weaning or beyond. "Secondary intolerance" presumes some other gastrointestinal disease, either in the past or the present. A disease state alters the present ability to digest food. A serious disease of the past could be responsible for present impaired ability to digest lactose. Whatever the cause, secondary factors introduce certain specific complications. They determine, for example, the course of action in feeding children or adults who are suffering any of a number of gastrointestinal disturbances or diseases.

Lactose intolerance and lactose malabsorption differ by definition. One is an expression of clinical symptoms, the other concerns the specific uptake of glucose. This difference is true following identical levels of intake of lactose based on body weight (or surface area). Either lactose intolerance is congenital (a rare state), or it is primary or secondary in its outgrowth. Under these definitions, researchers find an incidence of lactose intolerance in about 18% of blacks and Latin American children aged 2–5 years (see Garza, 1979). By 10–14 years of age, incidence among these populations climbs to 56%. Among American Indians, lactose malabsorption ranges between 63 and 74% at ages 5 through 8 years. Of these persons, some ¾ are also lactose intolerant. Note, however, that these conditions presuppose a measurable or observable response at precise levels of lactose intake. This level is commonly set at 2 g lactose/kg body weight (or 50 g/m^2 body surface area), up to a maximum of 50 g total (given as a 20% solution in water). These are the test conditions, precise enough, but also arbitrarily selected. The test dose is actually realistic only for infants. This last fact and the maximum level given explain how lactose came into much debate and controversy.

PRACTICAL IMPLICATIONS

How did lactose find its way to the center of controversy? Or better yet, how does any food component *avoid* controversy these days? In truth, none can. The reason is that any and all food components taken in overdose will cause an adverse response, up to an including death. That statement bars nothing whatever presently considered food or any part thereof. Thus, in the case of lactose intolerance the real question is, If people do differ in their ability to handle lactose, how much is too much? Can persons exhibiting an "intolerance" response by actual test consume some, any, or a lot of milk without (or with) minimal symptoms occurring?

Answers come in part from the research work that first demonstrated the problem to be fairly widespread. In that study (Bayless and Rosenweig, 1966) 50 g lactose (in solution) were given test subjects, all of whom were in the fasting state. In practical terms, the test groups got the equivalent of nearly a liter of milk taken all at one time on an empty stomach. Such intake is far from common, obviously. Still, the research dose of 50 g was set at such levels to gain insights into the occurrence of one kind of digestive upset. What of the practical consequences? In general, most people who react against lactose at high levels get by without trouble at lower levels of intake. Although a quart of milk on an empty stomach might be too much, a glassful at a time causes little or no upset at all.

This is the gist of most recent research. It seems to apply to both adults and children. In fact, lactose in amounts equivalent to 300 ml (about 1¼ cups) of milk on an empty stomach was found in one case to cause no symptoms among persons previously diagnosed as "lactose intolerant" (Garza and Scrimshaw, 1976). Another study in India, where the incidence of this problem runs very high, found children quite readily able to take in milk at levels of 200 ml without any sign of "intolerance" symptoms (Reddy and Pershad, 1972). Similar results were noted in a study of habitants of northern Thailand (Flatz *et al.*, 1969), where incidence of lactose intolerance was put at 100%. Researchers concluded that levels of milk intake up to 300 ml (just under 1¼ cups) at any one time were acceptable "for all age groups." This amount of milk provides the equivalent of 14 g lactose. Other studies seem to confirm this level as reasonable; that is, as much as 15 g lactose can be ingested either without any onset of symptoms, or at worst only mild symptoms, among persons previously diagnosed as lactose intolerant. Not all researchers would agree that such a rule of thumb would cover every individual. However, the consensus appears to support that belief generally.

In the United States, researchers Cutberto Garza and Nevin Scrimshaw (1976) observed the response of both black and white children to dietary lactose. They concluded that earlier work, designed to determine the extent of the problem, involved unrealistic test conditions, that is, the feeding of overly large amounts of the sugar. These scientists fed levels the equivalent of up to two 8 oz glasses of milk (475 ml). Though half the black children over 6 years of age were known to be lactose intolerant, neither group, white or black, showed symptoms of stomach upset. Just to be certain that results would not be biased by a child's occasional normal dislike for milk, equal amounts of lactose were secreted away in peanut butter sandwiches.

No doubt this and other work like it is the reason why international agencies hasten to encourage the use of milk and milk products overseas, even among nations and peoples known to have difficulty digesting lactose. As one field-worker reports, protein of milk can be and is digested altogether satisfactorily in those persons having problems with lactose. Furthermore, research suggests the good probability that not only protein but milk fat, vitamins, and minerals likewise find their way into the body (Calloway and Chenoweth, 1973; Bowie, 1975; Debongnie *et al.*, 1977). Most of the nutrition of milk is available, therefore, even among sufferers of low lactase activity. This brings up the last important distinction. Lactose intolerance or low lactase activity is not synonymous with intolerance to milk. Again, for sake of definition, some arbitrary level of intake must be imposed. In this case, a cup of whole milk taken on an empty stomach would seem realistic and appropriate. Given that level and symptoms of digestive upset as the measure, true milk intolerance may run somewhere between 0 and 8% of the population. This is the conclusion of Garza (1979), a foremost researcher in the field. He observes further that primary lactose intolerance in no way impairs the ability to digest and absorb protein or fat. In studies of secondary lactose intolerance, only 1% of dietary problems with milk could not be explained away as "milk" intolerance.

Thus, milk intolerance—the inability to consume and derive nutritional benefits from reasonable levels of milk intake without upset—appears to be a relatively rare condition. Low lactase activity may not be the sole criterion of its development. The important point is, few serious problems have arisen from feeding milk to children recovering from protein-calorie malnutrition. At best, lactose-free milk finds optimal use in earliest treatment of severe undernourishment. If this is not available, unmodified milk will also serve needs. Incidence of true "milk intolerance" (of adverse response to intake of a cup of milk at regular intervals) appears slight. Diagnosis of lactose intolerance offers no sure guide to occurrence of milk intolerance. These are the findings of note. Moreover, protein needs can and likely will outweigh other factors in cases of severe protein-calorie malnutrition. It is estimated that milk protein is three to six times as effective in improving nitrogen balance (a measure of the state of protein nourishment of the body) as is the addition of energy (as carbohydrate or fat). Because human needs for protein may have been underestimated by reliance on data taken at submaintenance levels of protein intake, the situation is perhaps more critical than otherwise appears. Milk proteins offer great potential to enhance the quality of plant protein in supplemental feeding programs. There is no question of this; only the precise amounts needed to ensure reasonable health are not known. In this regard, milk intolerance—true milk intolerance—is only a minor matter.

Furthermore, keep in mind that not all stomachaches derive from milk or lactose intolerance. A hundred other factors could just as well be at the root of a digestive upset. Moreover, intolerances to sugars other than lactose are also known. One such sugar is maltose; another is sucrose, or cane sugar. Still others are as common as a plate of beans. One researcher (Latham, 1977) summarizes the situation with the question, "Are we all legume intolerant because beans cause some increased gas?" Yes is the answer. However, we do not call it intolerance, and we do not look upon it as a major digestive problem. It derives from the very same general process as does distress to lactose. The body simply lacks enzymes to break down the sugars found in beans. For that reason, intestinal bacteria come into play; in their activity, gas is formed. The amount of gas or the amount of general distress is as varied as the intestinal flora of different individuals. It is lactose intolerance all over again in many respects, and it represents a major obstacle to greater use of one of the world's most productive sources of protein, the soybean. So bad is the problem that scientists refer to its source as an antinutritional factor. It stems from the body's inability to break down stachyose and raffinose, two sugars common to this legume. They are found in amounts far less than lactose in milk, 3.8% and 1.1% respectively. As mentioned earlier, sucrose is the other major carbohydrate for which intolerance is also known. Sucrose averages about 5.0% in soybean meal.

In summary, lactose intolerance is fact. In rare instances, it occurs as a congenital ailment, a genetic lack of the ability to produce lactase. It may be caused as a side effect of infections and/or other agents known to produce injury to the intestinal mucosa. Most often it results from a lowered ability to produce lactase beyond a certain age. For the great majority of lactose-intolerant persons, old and young alike, symptoms can be controlled by limiting intake of milk to 1–1¼ cups at a time, preferably taken with other food at mealtime. Severe diarrhea is the only major constraint. Even where lactose intolerance is fact, the body is able to utilize other important milk nutrients, that is, protein, calcium, and phosphorus.

TECHNOLOGY: A PART OF THE ANSWER

Technology was in the picture long before the condition of lactose intolerance came to light (in 1901). Over the years, one process in particular has served needs most well, doing so by depleting the dairy product of lactose. That product, of course, is cheese. Data in Table 28 show the amount of protein and lipids in a variety of cheese products. Cholesterol content is also included. Most of the cheeses contain no detectable lactose. Except for cottage cheese, they contain ample amounts of calcium.

Other dairy products may likewise offer nutrients while minimizing the symptoms of digestive upset caused by lactose. Fermented products, in particular, have been found helpful (Goodenough and Kleyn, 1976; Kilara and Shahani, 1976; Gallagher *et al.*, 1975; Sandine and Daly, 1979). Yogurt, buttermilk, cottage cheese, and other similar foods could well contain large numbers of viable organisms, some of which produce lactase (the lactose-splitting enzyme). Found in these cells taken in with the milk product, this lactase may serve the needs of lactose digestion in much the same manner as lactase formed within the body. One species of bacteria of apparently high lactase content is *Lactobacillus acidophilus* (Sandine *et al.*, 1972; Speck, 1976), the culture used to make acidophilus milk. This fermented food was first made famous as an elixir of longevity by the Russian writer Metchnikoff in 1908. Ever since, the interest in cultured dairy foods has waxed and ebbed on this pivotal question. Almost every nation has its own brand of fermented milk tonic: kumiss in Mongolia, kyr in Iceland, kefu in Balkan countries, mazum in Armenia, and leken in Egypt. Russia has its acidophilus milk and a handful of centenarians to offer up as a living evidence of this wellspring of youth. Research over the years suggests a number of side benefits: (1) a means of overcoming lactose intolerance, (2) an enhancement of galactose digestion, (3) a quick way to restock the intestinal pool of microbes following antibiotic treatment (Shapiro, 1960; Sandine *et al.*, 1972), and (4) antitumor activity (Bailey and Shahani, 1976).

As a matter of interest, most yogurt does not contain *L. acidophilus* bacteria. Instead, it is cultured with a combination of *Streptococcus thermophilus* and *Lactobacillus bulgaricus* (somewhat poorer sources of lactase). If *L. acidophilus* bacteria is added to yogurt during fermentation, these other two cultures quickly overpower it and wipe it out. However, so strong is the interest in *L. acidophilus* itself that some processors simply add the culture after the fermentation is over. Because pasteurization of milk kills it, a freeze-dried culture of the organism is sometimes added to regular whole milk following heat treatment. This creates the relatively new product called sweet acidophilus milk, which could indeed serve at some point as weaning food.

More recently, technologies have evolved for putting together milk-like beverages, excluding lactose, from a number of nutrients. Commercial processes also provide for reacting lactose with the enzyme lactase (β-galactosidase). It is done in two ways: (1) by use of "immobilized" enzymes placed on a reactor column similar to ion exchange (see Figure 3) and (2) by treating fluid milk with lactase. For the former, silica beads (30–45 mesh size) become the solid to which lactase (stable to acid) is attached (Anonymous, 1980a). Lactase itself is derived from a bacterial source (*Aspergillus niger*). Coupling is brought about by treatment with silane and gluteraldehyde. In the method used for splitting lactose of whey, protein and minerals are first removed. Solids level is taken to some point under 20%, pH adjusted to 3.5, and the temperature raised to 35° C to start. Gradually, the temperature is increased to 50° C. After being pumped into the top of the enzyme column, the product passes through. Galactose and glucose drain off at the bottom. For increased capacity, several columns may be placed in parallel. Hydrolyzed products may then concentrate to a syrup of 60% solids or higher. Columns can be cleaned and sanitized by back-flushing with dilute acetic acid.

Lactose in milk can also be hydrolyzed by adding lactase enzyme directly. The enzyme may be derived from numerous sources (Shukla, 1975). It is

TABLE 28
Protein, Total Lipids, Fatty Acids, Cholesterol, and Lactose Content of Selected Cheeses[a,b] (amount of nutrient per 28 g edible portion)

| Cheese | Protein[c,d] (g) | Total[e] lipids (g) | Fatty Acids[e] | | Cholesterol[f] (mg) | Lactose[d] (g) |
			Saturated (g)	Unsaturated (g)		
Blue	6.03	8.29	5.35	2.55	21.06	N.D.[g]
Brick	6.55	8.23	5.04	2.80	N.A.[h]	N.D.
Camembert	5.47	7.31	4.59	2.38	20.17	N.D.
Cheddar	6.96	9.18	5.66	3.00	28.67	N.D.
Colby	6.67	8.62	5.43	2.74	26.57	N.D.
Cottage, creamed	3.49	1.12	0.73	0.34	3.89	0.17
Cottage, uncreamed	4.85[i]	0.11	0.06	0.03	1.88	0.13
Cream	2.10	9.46	5.94	2.97	30.52	0.48
Edam	7.21	7.81	5.07	2.32	24.99	N.D.
Mozzarella, low moisture, part skimmed	7.72	5.43	2.86	1.42	15.13	0.11

Neufchatel	3.25	6.78	4.31	2.16	N.A.	0.29
Parmesan	10.82[i]	7.42	4.70	2.32	20.49	N.A.
Provolone	7.27	7.28	4.62	2.27	19.28	N.D.
Ricotta						
Part skimmed	3.11	2.41	1.45	0.76	N.A.	0.40
Skimmed	3.27	4.09	2.60	1.26	N.A.	0.41
Swiss	8.14	7.73	4.93	2.46	24.05	N.D.
Pasteurized process American	22.47	8.09	5.04	2.66	N.A.	N.D.

[a] Adapted from Dairy Council Digest (1975).
[b] Calculated from data based on nutrients per 100 g edible portion.
[c] Total nitrogen $\times$ 6.38.
[d] Source: Feeley, Criner, and Slover (1975).
[e] Source: Posati, Kinsella, and Watt (1974).
[f] Source: Lacroix, Mattingly, Wong, and Alford (1973).
[g] N.D.—none detectable.
[h] N.A.—not available.
[i] Average of values for long- and short-set types.
[j] Source: National Cheese Institute. Unpublished data.

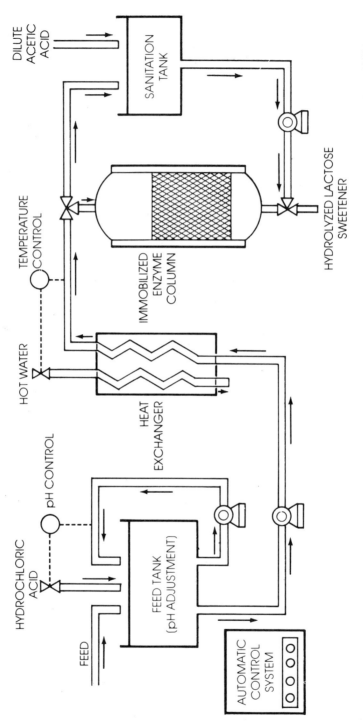

Figure 3. Diagram of immobilized enzyme technology for hydrolyzing lactose. (Courtesy of Corning Glass Works, Corning, New York 14830.)

capable of acting at refrigeration temperatures (4° C), making it possible to incubate milk in the range in which spoilage bacteria do not readily develop. The process runs to completion within 24 hours. Because glucose and galactose are sweeter than lactose, a lactose-hydrolyzed milk product tastes sweeter than normal milk. Desirably enough, it contains no greater caloric load.

Cultured dairy products can be processed from milk in which the lactose has been hydrolyzed. Yogurt is made from it, using 4% added milk-solids-not-fat and a milk with lactose treated to 40% hydrolysis. Sweetness becomes a flavor advantage. The organisms assist to a degree in lactose digestion. Incubation time (to pH 4.6) can be reduced by 40 minutes for a yogurt in which 90% of the lactose has been hydrolyzed (Gyuriscek and Thompson, 1976). One advantage is enhanced sweetness without added calories.

LACTOSE AND CATARACTS

The headlines read: Milk Sugar Causes Cataracts. It was no slipup at the laboratory bench. That was the finding when rats were fed huge quantities of galactose, one of the breakdown products of lactose. Nonetheless, the headline at best was grossly misleading. The amounts of galactose fed were excessive, as is usually the case when the response to a given substance, nutrient or otherwise, is being tested. Such bizarre results, therefore, are not uncommon. Test conditions may in fact promote the rare and unusual. Just as vitamins A and D are required at specific levels for good health, both are most toxic at exaggerated levels of intake. Nevertheless, cataracts have been found to occur in rats fed very large amounts of galactose. Some scientists believe that, for this specific nutrient, rats serve as a poor model for humans (Moore, 1978). Pigs may serve better, and research on these animals gives no evidence of cataract formation. Yet the above findings stand.

Clearly, one must read beyond most headlines. Another example may be useful. Not long ago a study was conducted to determine if some factor in cheese whey might aid in overcoming the symptoms of lactose intolerance (see Anonymous, 1973). To test the hypothesis, a group of 20 rats were fed a diet of casein (milk protein), yeast, a mixture of salt, and a large amount (70% of the diet, by weight) of either lactose or galactose. On this diet only 6 rats survived to 5 weeks. Of the 6, 4 had developed cataracts. By addition of a whey cocktail (0.4 ml whey per rat per day) to the basic diet, 18 of 20 rats of a second grup survived, none had cataracts, and the body weight of survivors increased by 142% during the experiment (it had only increased 78% for survivors of the first trial). Following this, the researchers went on to try to pinpoint the component(s) of whey that was responsible for the improvement in lactose tolerance. As for the point being stressed here is concerned, it is only necessary to suggest that any of a number of inter-pretations could be assigned the results of this work. This includes the obvious interpretation that a diet heavily concentrated in milk sugar caused the *death* of 14 of 20 test animals.

Epilogue

This book could perhaps as well be ended at this point, yet to do so without a concluding statement on the infant formula controversy would seem to leave this work in some important way unfinished. Of course, as a dairy products specialist, the subject of infant formula interested me, but it was because of the widespread debate over the use of formula that I undertook the task of writing this book.

At first it was small curiosities that led me into the subject. I wondered, for example, about the amount of cholesterol in human milk. Over the years, the dairy industry has been concerned with this issue because of research relating cholesterol to heart disease. Are breast-fed infants exposed to some, a little, or a lot of the compound?

As discussed in Chapter 1, what I found was that the level of cholesterol in human milk is just about the same as in cow's milk. I cannot tell you, however, whether exposure to the compound in infancy is healthful or not. The literature is not clear in that regard. Obviously, it is a question of some import. Infant formulas, formulated as they often are with vegetable oils, are essentially cholesterol-free. On the other hand, mother's milk, obviously the most appropriate food for most infants, comes stocked with a quite liberal amount of cholesterol.

The question of cholesterol content led me to check to see just how much more polyunsaturated fat is in human than cow's milk. When I found the answer, I understood why vegetable oils, particularly corn oil, are used in infant formula. Not only was corn oil appropriately unsaturated, but it carries a relatively high content of oleic acid, a fatty acid found in sizable quantities in human milk fat. But cow's and goat's milk fat also have chemical and physical characteristics that make them desirable ingredients in infant formula. The situation is not strictly either/or. There is good reason, perhaps, for combining animal and vegetable fat.

221

I next looked for data on the amount of lactose (milk sugar) in human milk. I learned that breast milk of the lactating human female held just about the largest store of this carbohydrate of any mammal—nearly 7%! This surprised me after all I had read about "lactose intolerance" (which, of course, expresses itself in sensitive individuals only at weaning and beyond). With mother's milk such a rich store of lactose, why are certain infant formulas formulated without it? Did an infant do as well on such formulas? It seems so, because several reputable scientific bodies give approval to lactose-free formulations.

What about the protein of human milk? The literature claims that there is about one-third as much protein in human as in cow's milk. In fact, the very high level of nonprotein nitrogen in mother's milk led one to believe that some literature values, at least those derived mainly from total nitrogen, might be, if anything, excessively high.

Mother's milk is thin in this respect, and biological implications suggest that it should be. I was aware, then, why infant formulas are now prepared with relatively low protein content. I also found out why lactalbumin casein formulas of a 60:40 ratio more nearly simulated the protein quality of breast milk than other ratios or other formulas that include as a protein ingredient β-lactoglobulin (see Chapter 1).

β-lactoglobulin was important because of research that seemed to indict it as a common allergen. Allergic responses to infant formula seem to be a quite common occurence, but I wondered if any controlled studies had been run to determine just how common.

Indeed, there had been, and the percentage of allergic reactions of infants to cow's milk has been put at anywhere from 0.3% to 7.5% (Bahna, 1978). This rather wide range is understandable in view of the difficulty in diagnosing food allergies. Of course, allergies to soy protein formulas exist, and even to breast milk (Kulangara, 1980). The latter has been found particularly problematical when the mother's diet consists largely of wheat. Antigens migrate into human milk, and this fact should not be overlooked in diagnosis of infant illness.

Nor should we forget that human milk is not a food of consistent composition. This is especially true of water-soluble vitamin content, and a whole host of factors enter in, not the least of which is the mother's eating habits. Thus I viewed with alarm a paper concerning a case of vitamin B_{12} deficiency in a breast-fed infant in California. The mother in this instance was a strict vegetarian. That was one of my first inklings of concern for Third World mothers, many being vegetarians, of course, by circumstances. This deficiency occurs because animal foods are often the primary source of vitamin B_{12}. I continued to research that topic at some length. However, my jury—the scientific literature—is still out.

The same may be said about the hypothesis of Australian researchers that "crib death"—the mysterious syndrome that snuffs out infant lives all around the world by the tens of thousands each year—might in some cases be linked to biotin (a B vitamin) deficiency. Mild stress (possibly a *minor* infection, one missed feeding, a little too much heat or cold) could perhaps trigger the deadly chain of events. Lack of biotin both in human milk *and* commercial baby food could lie at fault. These researchers have hypothesized that stress alone on the mother could possibly lower the biotin level in her milk.

Today, of course, other factors influence the vitamin content of human milk. I virtually stumbled across the fact that nursing mothers who have been on the "pill" for some months prior to pregnancy are apt to produce milk low in content of vitamin B_6. That was news to me.

It was of real concern, too, to read of an "outbreak" of alkalosis among a number of formula-fed infants. Because mineral imbalance probably is involved, my attention was turned to mineral content of human milk and infant formula. Up to that point, I had not realized that the overall level of minerals in mother's milk was so low. One thing a formula manufacturer has to do, therefore, and do with precision, is to balance the right amount and kinds of mineral components. There is little room for error. Both pH of body fluids and load on the infant's developing kidneys are at stake. For this reason, it is dangerous to feed an infant undiluted cow's (or other specie's) milk instead of formula. Even today this seemingly innocent practice causes an occasional infant death. In the same context, it becomes apparent why dry infant formula must be reconstituted to proper strength. Failure to do so either results in too high a concentration and an overtaxing of the infant kidneys, or, too weakly diluted, a deficiency of required amounts of nutrients. Lacking vitamin A, for example, a child goes blind! This is a compelling reason for the use of fortified formula when a substitute or supplement is needed. Ready-to-use formula is the best alternative to the dry product, but cost is prohibitive for many mothers.

While investigating minerals, I became interested in the iron-binding properties of mother's milk and in what way the infant formula industry managed to add an available source of iron to formula without the product becoming oxidized (rancid). I was even more intrigued by the proposed zinc-binding agent of human milk, picolinic acid, and I am wondering now if it is appropriate to consider adding it (or some similar zinc-binding agent) to infant formulas—just to ensure better zinc uptake. This is another of those issues that remains to be researched.

It was a controversy over fluoridation of drinking water supplies that caused me to check out a question in that regard. Would content of fluoride in drinking water influence fluoride content of mother's milk? The answer appears to be no (see Chapter 3). What, then, of lead, the poisonous heavy metal? If a nursing mother in a poor neighborhood drank water delivered through a lead pipe, would that lead contaminate her milk supply? In this case, it appears so. But, generally speaking, infant formula might be expected to add slightly more lead to the infant diet. The same appears to be likely for mercury, and, possibly, cadmium. In the event of a nuclear leak (or worse), radioactive isotopes in food and feed would reach both human milk and cow's milk. For the latter, though, (and therefore formula) technologies have been developed for the removal of such contaminants. Not so for PBB's and PCB's however. These industrial pollutants have also been detected in human milk. PCB's have been found at a level two to four times the allowance set by FDA for cow's milk!

Of course, DDT continues to be detected in breast milk—and just about everything else. The problem is that humans are at the very top of the food chain. I wondered if some mothers might not wish to use formula now and then to spread the risk? That could easily be done in the developed world. In the Third World it would not be so easy, however, and in some of those nations DDT is still approved for use. Thus you find intake of this insecticide in breast-fed Guatemalan infants far in excess of the acceptable daily level (see Chapter 5). Recent reports hint strongly of massive misuse of pesticides in some Third World nations. Certainly this is an issue with which our world must grapple in its pell-mell struggle to achieve food sufficiency.

Even formula cannot be guaranteed to be entirely free of such compounds. I only can tell you that some contaminants are routinely monitored, and regulations often limit the amount permitted in infant formula. Then, too, you can find statements by pediatricians in which risks to infants from some of these contaminants are generally played down in preference to what are considered the benefits of breast-feeding. In my job, though, I must be cautious in my use of "statements" and try to evaluate the source. Thus, where contaminants are concerned, I am unable to come to any one incisive recommendation.

Drugs pose a similar, though not identical, problem. Are mothers generally aware that Valium, possibly used to ease the tensions of motherhood (and thereby introduced into breast milk), can cause jaundice, lethargy, and weight loss in breast-feeding infants? Are they aware of what happens when lithium, the antidepressant, is used, and laxatives, and sedatives, and pain-killers like Darvon?

How about cocaine? and LSD? If there was anything specific in the literature regarding these latter drugs, I overlooked it. But I can tell you, in all sincerity, that scarcely any drug taken into the body—and by any and all routes of administration—fails to reach the milk supply. Women who smoke will yield milk with nicotine in it, and their infants actually become sick from it. Marijuana smokers not only add the active ingredient of that drug to their milk, but also some 50% more cancer-causing compounds than tobacco smoke. Alcohol is not good either, the literature warns. And coffee drinkers will have caffeine in their milk.

Antibiotics are also carried into the milk supply. So frequent has their use become that we are perhaps in danger of overlooking them as a source of contaminants in human milk. Yet they are necessary medications, and often are used to combat infections of the breasts, which is in turn a leading cause of lowered milk yield.

Consider infections for a moment. Scientific literature identifies a particularly virulent species of bacteria, the one that seems to predominate in human breast infections, known as *Staphylococcus aureus*. (The literature on research of *S. aureus* is sparse, but I finally found a Polish study to serve my purposes). *S. aureus* secretes a toxin when it grows. Breast-feeding infants may come down with what in fact is a form of food poisoning. Possibly, serious infections of this type are not too prevalent. However, the figure for Polish women was far higher than I would have anticipated based upon the general level of education in that nation, and the relatively high standards of sanitation. (I noted that treatment for ailing infants involved nothing more than feeding formula. The success rate was given as 100%.) I was driven, then, to search out the incidence of infections in Third World nations where, for many, sanitation in our terms is just about nonexistent. As sometimes happens, my search in this instance was fruitless.

Again I moved on, but now, in contrast, I found an abundance of information on the topic of immune agents of breast milk. The evidence was unmistakable: Human milk simply has a lot going for it, and particularly for infants reared under the stress of an infectious environment. Mother's milk even contains tailormade immune factors for her breast-feeding infant. And mild undernourishment actually seems to heighten the milk's immune potency!

Hence, mother's milk packs a potent passive immune response. That much is clear. Still, there are always a large number of women who cannot nor will not, for any number of reasons, breast-feed. Was there any way to improve the immune potency of formula? Was there any way to produce a formula with specific immune defenses against pathogens of the hospital environment?

The answer to that last question carries a significance perhaps not readily apparent. Hospitals tend to harbor an uncommonly broad spectrum of infectious agents. To the extent that a mother's exposure to a specific disease may be essential to generation of antibodies in her milk supply against that disease, even human milk may lack the most appropriate immune factors. Was it possible, then, to produce and process formula with antibodies specific to any of these human pathogens? For the breast-fed infant who might contract a given disease, such formula would offer hope as a kind of "natural" medicine, one which would not in itself pose a risk to healthy development of the child's own immune system. For the bottle-fed infant, a formula of this type would serve as a "natural" defense in exactly the same way as human milk serves.

Clearly, the evidence cited in Chapter 4 gives promise of an infant formula that can match or even surpass in some respects the immune potency of mother's milk. Scientists have already induced cows to yield a milk with defenders against human strains of enterpathogenic coliform—the first or second most common cause of infant diarrhea! You can also expect to find certain nonspecific immune agents in formula. It is likely, the literature suggests, that *L. acidophilus* might serve in lieu of *L. bifidus*, the helpful bacterial organism that seems to generate itself almost spontaneously in the intestinal tract of breast-feeding infants. Or bifidus-stimulating compounds per se can be added to formula. With recombinant genetics there is hope even of achieving a formulation with, as additive, "human" interferon, the virus killer.

I finally came to focus on Third World issues, the core of which I shall now sum up. First, the major impact of malnourishment and/or underfeeding on lactating women is a reduction in yield of milk. Breast infections, too, lower production or force a mother to stop breast-feeding altogether. Failure to get a good "let down" response likewise withholds milk from an infant. The latter may occur if a mother becomes anxious about her ability to breast-feed, or is worried that she might not have enough milk for her infant. Failure to produce milk can also occur because of the stress of life in the squalor of big-city slums, from family squabbles, or from anxiety over the health of siblings of the newborn—in short, because of the myriad of anxieties in human existence.

Need for providing infants with supplemental food, therefore, is great among Third World nations. Formula, of course, is one alternative. Local foods are another. Formula is often criticized because of the need to train women in its proper use. The same need, however, is apparent for the preparation of local foods as well. Furthermore, methods of preparation of such foods cannot be overlooked as an essential requisite of their use. Cassava, a major staple (and weaning food) of Africa generates cyanide poisoning in the body unless properly fermented. Peas of the genus Lathyrus, a common food of India, cause permanent paralysis unless boiled for at least 30 minutes.

Not only are there obvious hazards in the use of some local foods, none match formula in nutritional quality. Both local foods and formula contain precisely the same venomous infectious agents when diluted with polluted water. If it comes right down to it, an infected formula is a better substitute for mother's milk than an infected food of any other kind. A formula at least comes fortified with every nutrient needed for survival of normal infants. A child has a better chance of warding off disease with that kind of nutritional punch. Although a dry infant formula can be incorrectly reconstituted, so can a bean gruel that is made into a feedable slurry.

For infants born prematurely, or underweight, the situation becomes even more critical. Pre-termers are a special case. Some are too weak to suckle. Even if they can suckle, their nutrition needs are different from full-term infants.

Because of poor maternal nutrition, incidence of premature births in Third World nations is significantly higher than elsewhere. And of all foods, formula has seen most widespread use for this feeding purpose—in developed nations anyway. Note, however, that the debate goes on: Some pediatrician researchers are arguing in favor of formula, others in favor of breast milk. The question has to do with whether or not mother's milk has adequate amounts of protein (and certain other nutrients) for this specialized need. For formula products, this is not a problem. You can readily tailor-make the food with more or less of any given nutrient. You can, in fact, prepare formula products to meet a number of specialized needs of variously afflicted infants.

But what, then, is the major disease state that causes death around the world, and to what extent might infant formula share the blame? To the first part of that question, the answer is diarrhea. That is *the number one* condition causing infant death in Third World countries today, and 80% of all cases of diarrhea go undiagnosed as to cause! (See Cameron and Hofvander, 1976). I found that last figure somewhat startling, mainly because I had gotten the impression, based on various statements, that infant formula contaminated with polluted water was the leading cause of death. No one doubts that this or any other food so contaminated could result in a diarrhetic condition, but what else might produce the disease state?

In answer to this question, the scientific literature comes through in profusion, and alas, just about everything under the sun causes diarrhea. Malnutrition in a variety of forms causes the condition. Undernutrition—starvation—produces diarrhea. Dozens of different infective agents transmitted in a hundred different ways cause the disease state. Bathing in polluted water, washing clothes in polluted water, washing eating utensils in polluted water—all spread diarrhetic diseases. The mixing of bad water with food, therefore, is but one manner of contamination.

S. aureus, we now know, will cause diarrhea in breast-feeding infants. These germs are everywhere, of course, on the skin, in pimples and boils, in fecal matter. Ear infections also cause diarrhea. Even the feeding of chili beans causes diarrhea. Would a Third World mother resort to that? Indeed she might if she had little or no choice. But what, then, is the nutrient content of chili beans? Does this food in any way compare at all favorably with vitamin/mineral fortified formula? Are there not serious nutritional risks to consider over and above the tendency of this legume to cause diarrhea?

All in all, it should not be surprising, perhaps, that the major nutritional problem worldwide is stunted growth. Both lack of food and lack of certain specific nutrients are given as reasons. Neither should it be surprising that the major infant killer in 11 different Third World cultures has been found to be a lack of supplemental food—*whether or not the infant is breast-fed!* This fact does not detract from the significance of surveys that find generally *fewer infant deaths* among breast-fed than bottle-fed infants! But caution is needed in interpreting such data. Too often surveys of this kind become a basis for condemning use of formula generally. What these surveys do not prove, however, is equally revealing. They do not prove, nor even imply, that foods other than formula, similarly tested, would fare better than formula. No food would, and it seems necessary to emphasize that fact. Neither do these surveys identify the death rate among infants whose mothers were *unable* to breast feed and who did *not* have access to infant formula. Data of that kind are not available. You get an ominous notion of what might happen, however, by evaluating the situation that exists among the poorest of the poor. For this stratum of society, the cost of infant formula puts it beyond reach; breast-feeding, of necessity, reaches its highest rate of practice, *and it is among this group that infant mortality exacts its highest toll of all.*

I am not recommending bottle-feeding in lieu of breast-feeding when mothers are able and desirous of nursing infants, or where conditions predispose its improper use. What I am suggesting is that if a substitute or supplement to breast milk is necessary, infant formula is the best equivalent; to deny this option of feeding—for whatever reason—is to condemn that many more infants to malnutrition or death.

Appendixes

APPENDIX 1
Composition of Human Milk

Component	Amount
Gross composition (% w/w)[a]	
Water	87.5
Calories	70.0
Protein	1.03
Fat	4.4
Carbohydrate (lactose)	6.9
Ash	0.2
Vitamin (water-soluble) (per 100 ml)[a,b]	
Vitamin C (ascorbic acid) (mg)	5.2
Thiamine (vitamin B_1) (μg)	14.0
Riboflavin (vitamin B_2) (μg)	37.5
Niacin (μg)	183.7
Vitamin B_6 (μg)	11.4
Pantothenic acid (μg)	230.0
Vitamin B_{12} (μg)	0.046
Biotin (μg)	0.8
Folic acid (μg)	5.2
Choline (mg)	9.0
Inositol (mg)	45.0
Vitamin (fat-soluble) (per 100 ml)[a,b]	
Vitamin A	
Retinol Equivalents (μg)	64
IU	241
Vitamin D (IU)	0.42
Vitamin E (mg)	0.56
Vitamin K (μg)	1.5
Mineral (per 100 ml)[a]	
Calcium (mg)	33
Phosphorus (mg)	14.4
Magnesium (mg)	3.1
Sodium (mg)	17.5 (7 mEq)
Potassium (mg)	52.6 (12.8 mEq)
Chloride (mg)	39 (11 mEq)
Iron (mg)	0.031
Zinc (mg)	0.175
Trace mineral (select) (μg/100 ml)	
Copper	15–105
Iodine	4–5
Manganese	1.8–2.5
Fluoride	5–30
Selenium	2–3
Boron	8–9
Protein and other selected nitrogenous components	
Protein, total (g/100 ml)	1.06
Nitrogen, total (g/100 ml)	0.14–0.21
Casein nitrogen (% of total nitrogen)	35

APPENDIX 1 *(continued)*

Component	Amount
Whey protein nitrogen (% of total nitrogen)	40
Whey proteins (g/100 ml)	0.30–0.80
α-Lactalbumin	0.15
Serum albumin	0.030–0.040
Lactoferrin	0.10–0.20
Transferrin	0.005
Lysozyme	0.04
Immunoglobulins, (select)	
IgA	
colostrum	0.41–0.47
3–4 weeks	0.036
IgG	
colostrum	0.006–0.021
3–4 weeks	0.006
IgM	
colostrum	0.010–0.049
3–4 weeks	0.004
Nonprotein nitrogen (% of total N)	25
Nonprotein nitrogen (select components) (g/100 ml)	
Urea[c]	0.027
Creatinine[c]	0.021
Glucosamine[c]	0.111
Free amino acids (μ moles/100 ml)[d]	
Taurine	26.6
Aspartate	5.4
Threonine	12.6
Serine	12.9
Glutamine	58.4
Glutamate	146.7
Glycine	11.7
Alanine	20.6
Valine	6.2
Cystine	5.6
Methionine	0.4
Isoleucine	1.0
Leucine	3.1
Tyrosine	1.6
Phenylalanine	1.9
Ornithine	0.5
Lysine	2.1
Histidine	2.1
Arginine	1.1
Ethanolamine	0
Citrulline	0
α-NH_2-butyrate	1.3
Total free amino acids	321.8

(continued)

APPENDIX 1 *(continued)*

Component	Amount
Amino Acids (protein-bound) (mg/100 ml)[a]	
Tryptophan	17.5
Threonine	47.5
Isoleucine	57.8
Leucine	98
Lysine	70.2
Methionine	21.7
Cystine	19.6
Phenylalanine	47.5
Tyrosine	54.7
Valine	65
Arginine	44.4
Histidine	23.7
Alanine	37.2
Aspartic acid	84.6
Glutamic acid	173.4
Glycine	26.8
Proline	84.6
Serine	44.4
Fat and other related components[a]	
Fat, total (% w/w)	4.4
Triglycerides (% w/w)	98
Diglycerides (% w/w)	<1.0
Free fatty acids (% w/w)	<1.0
Sterols (% w/w)	<1.0
Cholesterol (mg/100 ml)	14
Carnitine (nmol/100 ml)	590
Fatty acid (g/100 ml)[a]	
Saturated	
4:0	—
6:0	—
8:0	—
10:0	0.062
12:0	0.27
14:0	0.33
16:0	0.95
18:0	0.30
Total saturated	2.07
Monounsaturated	
16:1	0.134
18:1	1.53
20:1	0.04
22:1	trace

APPENDIX 1 *(continued)*

Component	Amount
Total monounsaturated	1.7
Polyunsaturated	
18:2	0.38
18:3	0.052
18:4	—
20:4	0.031
20:5	trace
22:5	trace
22:6	trace
Total polyunsaturated	0.52

[a]Data from U.S. Department of Agriculture (1976).
[b]Data from Causeret (1977).
[c]Data from Nishikawa, *et al.* (1976).
[d]Data from Rassin, *et al.* (1978).

APPENDIX 2

Recommended International Standards for Kind and Amount of Nutrients in Formulas and Foods for Infants Under 12 Months of Age[a]

Nutrients[b]	Amount per 100 available cal	Amount per 100 available kilojoules (KJ)
Vitamin	(minimum levels unless otherwise stated)	
Vitamin A	250 IU or 75 μg expressed as retinol; maximum of 500 IU or 150 μg expressed as retinol	60 IU of 18 μg expressed as retinol; maximum of 37 μg expressed as retinol
Vitamin D	40 IU 80 IU maximum	10 IU 19 IU maximum
Ascorbic acid (vitamin C)	8 mg	1.9 mg
Thiamine (vitamin B_1)	40 μg	10 μg
Riboflavin (vitamin B_2)	60 μg	14 μg
Nicotinamide	250 μg	60 μg
Vitamin B_6	35 μg	9 μg
Folic acid	4 μg	1 μg
Pantothenic acid	300 μg	70 μg
Vitamin B_{12}	0.15 μg	0.04 μg
Vitamin K_1	4 μg	1 μg
Biotin (vitamin H)	1.5 μg	0.4 μg
Vitamin E (α-tocopherol compounds)	0.7 IU/g linoleic acid,[c] but not less than 0.7 IU/100 available cal	0.7 IU/g linoleic acid,[c] but no less than 0.15 IU/100 available kJ
Mineral		
Sodium	20 mg, 60 mg maximum	5mg, 15 mg maximum
Potassium	80 mg, 200 mg maximum	20 mg, 50 mg maximum
Chloride	55 mg, 150 mg maximum	14 mg, 35 mg maximum
Calcium[d]	50 mg	12 mg
Phosphorus[d]	25 mg	6 mg
Magnesium	6 mg	1.4 mg
Iron	1 mg[e]	0.25 mg[e]
Iron	0.15 mg	0.04 mg
Iodine	5 μg	1.2 μg
Copper	60 μg	14 μg
Zinc	0.5 mg	0.12 mg
Manganese	5 μg	1.2 μg
Choline	7 mg	1.7 mg
Protein	not less than 1.8 g[f]	not less than 0.43 g[f]
Amino acids	amount needed to improve nutritional value; only natural L forms	amount needed to improve nutritional value; only natural L forms
Fat	3.3 g, no more than 6 g	0.8 g, no more than 1.5 g
Linoleic acid[g]	300 mg	70 mg

[a]Adapted from FAO/WHO (1976).

[b]In addition to the nutrients listed, others may be added when required to provide nutrients

APPENDIX 2 *(continued)*

ordinarily found in human milk and to ensure a formulation suitable as the sole source of nutrients for the infant.

[c]Linoleic acid may be determined on a per gram basis of unsaturated fatty acids, but expressed as linoleic acid.

[d]The calcium–phosphorus ration must be not less than 1.2 nor more than 2.0.

[e]Products containing not less than 1 mg iron/100 available cal must be labeled: "Infant Formula with Iron."

[f]These quantities are required when protein is the equal or better biological quality of casein. The quality of protein may not be less than 85% that of casein. Total amount of protein may not be more than 4 g/100 available cal (or 0.96 g/100 available kJ). Quality and quantity of protein can be modified to meet requirements of individual nations or local conditions.

[g]Linoleic acid must be present as glycerides of the fatty acid.

APPENDIX 3
Vitamin Compounds Approved for Addition to Infant and Baby Food[a,b]

Vitamin	Approved form(s)[c]
Vitamin A	Retinyl acetate
	Retinyl palmitate
Provitamin A	Beta carotene
Vitamin D	
Vitamin D_2	Ergocalciferol
Vitamin D_3	Cholecalciferol
	Cholecalciferol-cholesterol
Vitamin E	d-alpha-tocopherol
	dl-alpha-tocopherol
	d-alpha-tocopherol acetate
	dl-alpha-tocopherol acetate
	d-alpha-tocopherol succinate
	dl-alpha-tocopherol succinate
Thiamine (vitamin B_1)	Thiamine chloride hydrochloride
	Thiamine mononitrate
Riboflavin (vitamin B_2)	Riboflavin
	Riboflavin 5'-phosphate sodium
Niacin	Nicotinamide
	Nicotinic acid
Vitamin B_6	Pyridoxine hydrochloride
	Pyridoxal 5'-phosphate
Biotin (vitamin H)	d-biotin
Folacin	Folic acid
Pantothenic acid	Calcium pantothenate
	Sodium pantothenate
	Pantothenol
Vitamin B_{12}	Cyanocobalamin
	Hydroxycobalamin
Vitamin K_1	Phytylmenaquinone
Vitamin C	Ascorbic acid
	Sodium ascorbate
	Calcium ascorbate
	Ascorbyl-6-palmitate
	Potassium ascorbate
Choline	Choline bitartrate
	Choline chloride
	Choline hydrogen citrate
Inositol	

[a]Dr. Robert Weik, personal communication (1979).

[b]These compounds are approved by the FAO/WHO Codex Alimentarius Commission. In addition to the compounds approved per se, purity requirements are also set.

[c]For stability and ease of handling, some vitamins must be specially prepared in suitable carrier or protective coating. Some are formulated into stabilized oily solutions, others may be coated with gelatin, still others may be embedded in fat. In whatever form the vitamin(s) is prepared, materials associated with it must also be approved as additives for this purpose. Such additives are listed in appropriate Codex Standards.

APPENDIX 4
Mineral Salts Approved for Addition to Formulas and Foods for Infants and Children[a,b]

Source of	Comment
Calcium	
Calcium carbonate	Milk substitute formulas and infant cereals
Calcium chloride	Milk-based and milk substitute formulas
Calcium citrate	Milk-based, milk substitute, protein hydrolysate, and meat-based formulas
Calcium gluconate	Protein hydrolysate formulas
Calcium glycerophosphate	
Calcium lactate	Electrolyte mixture supplement
Calcium phosphate, monobasic	Milk substitute and low sodium formulas
Calcium phosphate, dibasic	Milk substitute and protein hydrolysate formulas
Calcium phosphate, tribasic	Milk substitute, protein hydrolysate, and preterm formulas; infant cereals
Calcium oxide	Protein supplement formulas
Calcium sulfate	Infant cereals
Phosphorus	
Calcium phosphate, monobasic	Milk substitute and low sodium formulas
Calcium phosphate, dibasic	Milk substitute and protein hydrolysate formulas
Calcium phosphate, tribasic	Milk substitute, protein hydrolysate, and preterm formulas; infant cereals
Magnesium phosphate, dibasic	Milk substitute and lactose-free formulas
Magnesium phosphate, tribasic	
Potassium phosphate, monobasic	Protein hydrolysate formulas
Potassium phosphate, dibasic	Milk-based, milk substitute, and protein hydrolysate formulas
Sodium phosphate, dibasic	Electrolyte mixture supplement
Magnesium	
Magnesium carbonate	Baked products
Magnesium chloride	Milk-based, milk substitute, and lactose-free formulas
Magnesium oxide	Milk substitute, protein hydrolysate, and preterm formulas
Magnesium phosphate, dibasic	Milk substitute and lactose-free formulas
Magnesium phosphate, tribasic	
Magnesium sulphate	Electrolyte mixture supplement
Iron	
Ferrous ascorbate	
Ferrous carbonate, stabilized	
Ferrous citrate	Protein hydrolysate and lactose-free formulas
Ferrous fumarate	Vitamin plus iron supplements
Ferrous gluconate	
Ferrous glycerophosphate	
Ferrous lactate	
Ferrous succinate	
Ferrous sulfate	Milk-based, milk substitute, and protein hydrolysate formulas

(continued)

APPENDIX 4 *(continued)*

Source of	Comment
Hydrogen-reduced iron	Infant cereals
Carbonyl iron	
Ferric citrate	Not allowed in powdered formulas, cereal, or baby foods
Ferric gluconate	Not allowed in powdered formulas, cereal, or baby foods
Ferric lactate	Not allowed in powdered formulas, cereal, or baby foods
Ferric ammonium citrate	
Copper	
Cupric carbonate	Baked products and protein supplement formulas
Cupric citrate	
Cupric gluconate	
Cupric sulphate	Milk-based, milk substitute, protein hydrolysate and meat-based formulas
Iodine	
Potassium iodide	Milk-based, milk substitute, and protein hydrolysate formulas
Sodium iodide	Milk-based, milk substitute, and protein hydrolysate formulas
Sodium chloride, iodized	Milk substitute formulas
Zinc	
Zinc chloride	
Zinc lactate	
Zinc sulfate	Milk-based, milk substitute, and protein hydrolysate formulas
Zinc oxide	Protein hydrolysate formulas
Manganese	
Manganese carbonate	
Manganese chloride	Milk-based formulas
Manganese citrate	
Manganese lactate	
Manganese sulphate	Milk-based, milk substitute, and protein hydrolysate formulas
Sodium	
Sodium bicarbonate	Milk-based formulas and baked products
Sodium carbonate	Protein hydrolysate formulas
Sodium chloride	Milk substitute formulas, baby foods, and electrolyte mixture supplement
Sodium chloride, iodized	Milk substitute formulas
Sodium citrate	Milk-based, milk substitute, and protein hydrolysate formulas; electrolyte mixture supplement
Sodium gluconate	
Sodium glycerophosphate	
Sodium lactate	
Sodium malate	

APPENDIX 4 *(continued)*

Source of	Comment
Sodium phosphate, monobasic	Milk substitute formulas
Sodium phosphate, dibasic	Electrolyte mixture supplement
Sodium phosphate, tribasic	
Sodium sulfate	
Sodium tartrate	
Potassium	
Potassium bicarbonate	
Potassium carbonate	
Potassium chloride	
Potassium citrate	
Potassium gluconate	
Potassium glycerophosphate	
Potassium lactate	
Potassium phosphate, monobasic	Protein hydrolysate formulas
Potassium phosphate, dibasic	Milk-based, milk substitute, and protein hydrolysate formulas
Potassium phosphate, tribasic	
Potassium tartrate	
Chloride	
Calcium chloride	Milk-based, milk substitue, and protein supplement formulas; electrolyte mixture supplement
Choline chloride	Milk-based, milk substitute, and protein hydrolysate formulas
Manganese chloride	Milk-based formulas
Magnesium chloride	Milk-based, milk substitute, and lactose-free formulas
Potassium chloride	
Sodium chloride	Milk-substitute formulas, baby foods, and electrolyte mixture substitute
Sodium chloride, iodized	Milk substitute formulas
Zinc chloride	

[a]Dr. Robert Weik, personal communication (1979).
[b]Approved by the FAO/WHO Codex Alimentarius Commission.

APPENDIX 5

Mineral Salts Pending Approval for Addition to Formulas and Foods for Infants and Children[a,b]

Source of

Calcium	Iodine
Calcium glucuronate	Iodostearate
Calcium malate	Zinc
Calcium tartrate	Zinc acetate
Magnesium	Sodium
Magnesium acetate	Sodium glucuronate
Iron	Potassium
Ferrous glucuronate	Potassium glucuronate
Ferric tartrate	Potassium malate
Copper	
Cupric acetate	

[a]Dr. Robert Weik, personal communication (1979).

[b]These compounds will either be added to the approved Codex Alimentarius list (or dropped) pending submission of data providing evidence that the compound meets criteria for approval.

APPENDIX 6
International Allowances for Food Additives in Infant Formula[a]

Additive	Maximum level in 100 ml of ready-to-drink product
Thickening agent	
Guar gum	0.1 g, all types of infant formula
Locust bean gum[b]	0.1 g, all types of infant formula
Distarch phosphate	0.5 g singly or in combination in soy-based infant
Acetylated distarch phosphate	formula only
Phosphated distarch phosphate	2.5 g singly or in combination in hydrolyzed protein
Hydroxypropyl starch	and/or amino acid-based infant formula only
	0.3 g in regular, milk- and soy-based liquid infant
	formula only
Carrageenan	0.1 g in hydrolyzed protein and/or amino acid-based
	liquid infant formula only
Emulsifier	
Lecithin	0.5 g in all types of infant formula
Mono- and diglycerides	0.4 g in all types of infant formula
pH adjusting compound	
Sodium hydrogen carbonate	
Sodium carbonate	Limited by good manufacturing practice and within
Potassium hydrogen carbonate	limits for sodium and potassium in all types of infant
Potassium carbonate	formula
Sodium citrate	
Potassium citrate	
L (+) lactic acid	Limited by good manufacturing practice in all types
L (+) lactic acid-producing cultures	of infant formula
Citric acid	
Antioxidant	
Mixed tocopherols concentrate	1 mg in all types of infant formula
L-ascorbyl palmitate	1 mg in all types of infant formula

[a]Adapted from FAO/WHO (1976).
[b]Temporarily endorsed.

APPENDIX 7

Dietary Needs of Women, Pregnant Women, and Nursing Mothers[a]

Nutrient:	Women[b]	Pregnant women	Nursing women
Calories	2000	2300	2500
Protein (g)	44	74	64
Vitamin A (R.E.)[c]	800	1000	1200
Vitamin D (μg)[d]	5	10	10
Vitamin E (αT.E.)[e]	8	10	11
Vitamin C (mg)	60	80	100
Niacin (mg N.E.)[f]	13	15	18
Riboflavin (mg)	1.2	1.5	1.7
Thiamine (mg)	1.0	1.4	1.5
Vitamin B_6 (mg)	2.0	2.6	2.5
Vitamin B_{12} (μg)	3.0	4.0	4.0
Folacin (μg)	400	800	500
Calcium (mg)	800	1200	1200
Phosporous (mg)	800	1200	1200
Iodine (μg)	150	175	200
Iron (mg)	18	[g]	[g]
Magnesium (mg)	300	450	450
Zinc (mg)	15	20	25

[a]Adapted from National Academy of Sciences/National Research Council (1979).

[b]Needs vary to some extent by age and body size. Values given here are for women 23–50 years of age, weighing 55 kg (120 lb) and standing 103 cm (64 inches) in height.

[c]Retinol equivalents. In this case 1 retinol equivalent equals 1 μg retinol or 6 μg β-carotene.

[d]Vitamin D requirements may be partially or even totally met by exposure to sunshine. Nevertheless, values given for pregnant and lactating women are best ensured from vitamin D of food or food supplement. Micrograms (μg) of vitamin D may be converted to International Units (IU); thus, 10 μg equals 400 IU.

[e]α tocopherol equivalents. In this case 1 mg d-α-tocopherol equals 1 α T.E.

[f]Milligrams (mg) of niacin equivalents. In this case 1 N.E. of niacin equals 1 mg niacin or 60 mg dietary tryptophan.

[g]It is impossible for women to meet extra needs for iron from dietary sources alone during pregnancy. For this reason, iron supplementation is recommended at 30–60 mg daily. Though iron needs during lactation (nursing) are not much different from those of nonpregnant women, continuing supplementation for 2–3 months after delivery is recommended as a means of rebuilding iron stores lost during pregnancy.

APPENDIX 8
Recommended Nutrient Intakes for Normal Full-Term Infants, According to Various Sources

Nutrient	RDA 1979 (0–6 months)	FDA 1971 Regulations (Minimum)[b] (0–12 months)	Committee on Nutrition 1976 (Minimum)[b] (0–12 months)
Energy (kcal)	570–870	670	670
Protein (g)	13.2	12.1	12.1
Essential fatty acids (% kcal)	2[c]	2	3
Vitamin			
Vitamin A (IU)	1400 (420 μg)[d]	1675 (503 μg)[d]	1675 (503 μg)[d]
Vitamin D (IU)	400 (10 μg)[e]	268 (6.7 μg)[e]	268 (6.7 μg)[e]
Vitamin K (μg)	12[f]	—	27
Vitamin E (IU)	4.5 (3 mg αT.E.)[g]	2	2
Ascorbic acid (mg)	35	52	54
Thiamine (μg)	300	168	268
Riboflavin (μg)	400	402	402
Pyridoxine (μg)	300	235	235
Vitamin B_{12} (μg)	0.5	1	1
Niacin			
(mg)	—	—	1.68
(mg equiv)[g]	6	5.36	—
Folacin (μg)	30	27	27
Pantothenic acid			
(mg)	2[f]	2	2
Biotin (μg)	35[f]	—	10
Choline (mg)	—	—	47
Inositol (mg)	—	—	27
Mineral			
Calcium (mg)	360	335	335
Phosphorus (mg)	240	168	168
Magnesium (mg)	50	40	40
Iron (mg)	10	7	1
Iodine (μg)	40	34	34
Zinc (mg)	3	—	3
Copper μg	500–700[f]	400	400
Manganese (μg)	500–700[f]	—	34
Sodium (mg)	115–350[f]	—	134
Potassium (mg)	350–925[f]	—	536
Chloride (mg)	275–700[f]	—	369
Fluoride (μg)	100–500[f]	—	—
Chromium (μg)	10–40[f]	—	—
Selenium (μg)	10–40[f]	—	—
Molybdenum (μg)	30–60[f]	—	—

[a]From Anderson et al. (1980).

APPENDIX 8 *(continued)*

---

[b]Figures listed in these columns represent the amounts of each nutrient an infant would receive if consuming 1 liter of formula, based on energy allowances in the revised RDA's (National Research Council, 1980).

[c]As specified in the 1974 RDA's (National Research Council, 1974).

[d]Retinol equivalents. One retinol equivalent equals 3.33 IU vitamin A activity from retinol.

[e]Cholecalciferol. Ten μg cholecalciferol equals 400 IU vitamin D.

[f]Estimated safe and adequate daily dietary intakes. Because there is less information on which to base allowances, some figures were provided as ranges of recommended intakes (National Research Council, 1980).

[g]T.E. equals α-tocopherol equivalents; one mg d-α-tocopherol equals 1 α T.E. The activity of d-α-tocopherol is 1.49 IU/mg.

[h]One niacin equivalent equals 1 mg niacin or 60 mg dietary tryptophan.

References

Adinolfi, M., A. Glynn, M. Lindsay, and C. Milne (1966). Serological properties of gamma A antibodies to *Eschericia coli* present in human colostrum. *Immunology* **10**:517–526.

Ahn, C. H., and W. C. MacLean, Jr. (1980). Growth of the exclusively breast-fed infant. *Am. J. Clin. Nutr.* **33**(2):183–192.

Ambrecht, H. J., and R. Wasserman (1976). Enhancement of Ca uptake by lactose in the rat intestine. *J. Nutr.* **106**:1265–1271.

American Academy of Pediatrics, Committee on Nutrition (1972). Filled milks, imitation milks and coffee whiterners. *Pediatrics* **49**:770.

American Academy of Pediatrics, Committee on Nutrition (1976). *Pediatrics* **57**:278.

American Academy of Pediatrics, Committee on Nutrition (1978a). Calcium requirements in infancy and childhood. *Pediatrics* **62**:826–834.

American Academy of Pediatrics, Committee on Nutrition (1978b). Statement on use of milk supplies. *Pediatrics* **62**:240.

American Academy of Pediatrics, Committee on Nutrition (1979). "Pediatric Nutrition Handbook." Evanston, Illinois.

American Public Health Association (1979). Infant feeding in the United States. *The Nation's Health*, September 7, 1979.

Anderson, S. A., H. I. Chinn, and K. D. Fisher (1980). A background paper on infant formulas. Life Sciences Research Office, Federation of American Societies for Experimental Biology, Bethesda, Maryland.

Anonymous (1972). Lactase activity levels in Nigeria—genetic or acquired phenomenon? *Nutr. Rev.* **30**(7):156–158.

Anonymous (1980a). Immobilized enzyme technology commercially hydrolyzes lactose. *Food Prod. Dev.* **14**(1):50–51.

Anonymous (1980b). Vitamin B_6 enhances zinc absorption. *Agric. Res.* **29**(6):9.

Ansell, C., A. Moore, and H. Barrie (1977). Electrolyte and pH changes in human milk. *Pediatr. Res.* **11**(12):1177–1179.

Antila, P., V. Antila, and S. Kruijo (1979). The determination of vitamin D from the aqueous phase of cow's and human milk. *Meijeritieteellinen Aikakauskirja* **37**:1–22.

Aperia, A., O. Broberger, P. Herrin, and R. Zetterstrom (1979). Salt content in human breast milk during the first three weeks after delivery. *Acta Paediatr. Scand.* **68**(3):441–442.

Applebaum, R. (1976). Management of normal lactation. In Symposium on Human Lactation.

245

DHEW Pub. No. (PHS) 79-1979, National Center for Health Statistics, Hyattsville, Maryland.

Archer, D. L. (1978). Immunotoxicology of food borne substances: an overview. *J. Food Prot.* **41**(12):983–988.

Archer, D. L., and H. M. Johnson (1978). Blockage of mitogen induction of the interferon lymphokine by a phenolic food additive metabolite. *Proc. Soc. Exp. Biol. Med.* **157**:684-687.

Archer, D. L., J. Bukovic-Wess, and B. Smith (1977a). Inhibitory effect of an antioxidant, butylated hydroxyanisole, on the primary in vitro immune response. *Proc. Soc. Exp. Biol. Med.* **154**:289–294.

Archer, D. L., J. Bukovic-Wess, and B. Smith (1977b). Suppression of macrophage-dependent T-lymphocyte function(s) by gallic acid, a food additive metabolite. *Proc. Soc. Exp. Biol. Med.* **156**:465–469.

Areekul, S., and A. Utiswannakul (1978). Effect of vitamin B_{12} on lactation. *Southeast Asian J. Trop. Med. Public Health* **9**(3):446–447. (*Dairy Sci. Abstr.* **42**(7):550.)

Asquith, M. T., and J. R. Harrod (1979). Reduction of bacterial contamination in banked human milk. *J. Pediatr. (St. Louis)* **95**(6):993–994.

Atkinson, S. A. (1979). Factors affecting human milk composition. *J. Am. Diet. Assoc.* **40**(3):213–221.

Atkinson, P. J., and R. R. West (1970). Loss of skeletal calcium in lactating women. *J. Obstet. Gynaecol. Br. Commonw.* **77**:555.

Atkinson, S. A., G. H. Anderson, I. C. Radde, and M. H. Bryan (1979). Nitrogen, energy, and mineral composition of milk during early lactation from mothers giving birth prematurely and at term. *J. Can. Diet. Assoc.* **40**(4):327.

Atkinson, S A., G. H. Anderson, and M. H. Bryan (1980). Human milk: comparison of the nitrogen composition in milk from mothers of premature and full-term infants. *Am. J. Clin. Nutr.* **33**(4):811–815.

Austin, P. R., C. Brine, J. Castle, and J. Zikakis (1981). Chitin: new facets of research. *Science (Washington, D.C.)* **212**(4496):749–753.

Avery G. (1976). Human milk and the smaller premature baby. In Symposium on Human Lactation. DHEW Pub. No. (PHS) 79-1979, National Center for Health Statistics, Hyattsville, Maryland.

Bahna, S. L. 1980. Current infant feeding practices. *Dairy Counc. Dig.* **51**(1):1–5.

Bailey, P. J. and K. Shahani (1976). Inhibitory effect of acidophilus cultured colostrum and milk upon the proliferation of Ascites tumor. Proceedings of 71st Annual Meeting American Dairy Science Association, p. 41.

Baltrop, D., and N. Killala (1967). Faecal excretion of lead by children. *Lancet* **2**:1017–1019.

Barmbel, C. E., and R. E. Hunter (1958). Effect of dicumarol on the nursing infant. *Am. J. Obstet. Gynecol.* **59**:1153.

Bayless, T. M., and N. S. Rosenweig (1966). A racial difference in incidence of lactose deficiency. *JAMA* **197**:968.

Bazaral, M., H. Orgel, and R. Hamburger (1971). IgE levels in normal infants and mothers and an inheritance hypothesis. *J. Immunol.* **107**:794.

Belavady, B. (1978). Lipid and trace element composition of human milk. *Acta Paediatr. Scand.* **67**(5):566–571.

Belavady, B. (1980). Dietary supplementation and improvements in the lactation performance of Indian women. *In* "Maternal Nutrition During Pregnancy and Lactation" (H. Aebi and R. Whitehead, eds.), Hans Huber Publishers, Bern, Switzerland.

Belcheva, M., L. Vasieleva, and N. Katranushkova (1966). Breast feeding in puerperal mastitis. *Akush. Ginekol. (Sofia)* **5**(5):335–339. (*Dairy Sci. Abstr.* **31**(10):584.)

Binkiewicz, A., M. Robinson, and B. Senior (1978). Pseudo-cushing syndrome caused by alcohol in breast milk. *J. Pediatr. (St. Louis)* **93**:965–967.

Bleumink, E., and E. Young (1968). Identification of the atopic allergen in cow's milk. *Int. Arch. Allergy Appl. Immunol.* **34**:521–543.

Bongiovanni, A. M. (1965). Bile acid content of gallbladder of infants, children and adults. *J. Clin. Endocrinol.* **25**:678–685.

Borum, P. R., C. M. York, and H. P. Broquist (1979). Carnitine content of liquid formulas and special diets. *Am. J. Clin. Nutr.* **32**(11):2272–2276.

Bowie, M. (1975). Effect of lactose induced diarrhea on absorption of nitrogen and fat. *Arch. Dis. Child.* **50**:363–366.

Breneman, J. C. (1979). Food Allergy. *Contemp. Nutr.* **4**(3):1–2.

Brin, M. (1976). Drug-vitamin interrelationships. *Nutrition and the M.D.* **3**(1):1.

Brock, J. H. (1980). Lactoferrin in human milk: its role in iron absorption and protection against enteric infection in the newborn infant. *Arch. Dis. Child.* **55**(6):417–421.

Burbianka, M., I. Dluzniewska, A. Pliszka, and B. Widyga (1973). Enterotoxigenic staphylococci and enterotoxin in human milk. *Contrib. Microbiol. Immunol.* **1**:441–447.

Calkins, E. J., J. R. Garric, and M. F. Picciano (1978). Mineral intakes of breast-fed infants: Nutrition in transition. Proceedings of Western Hemisphere Nutrition Congress V, Monroe, Wisconsin.

Calloway D., and W. Chenoweth (1973). Utilization of nutrients in milk and wheat-based diets by man with adequate and reduced abilities to absorb lactose. I. Energy and nitrogen. *Am. J. Clin. Nutr.* **26**:939–951.

Cameron, M., and Y. Hofvander (1976). "Manual for Feeding Infants and Children" (2nd ed.). Protein Advisory Group of the United Nations System. New York.

Campbell, J. E., G. K. Murthy, C. P. Straub, K. H. Lewis, and J. G. Terrill (1961). Radionuclides in milk. *J. Agric. Food Chem.* **9**:117–121.

Carroll, L., M. Osman, D. Davies, and A. McNeish (1979). Bacteriological criteria for feeding raw breast-milk to babies on neonatal units. *Lancet* **2**(8145):732–733.

Catz, C. S., and G. P. Giacoia (1973). Drugs and metabolites in human milk. *In* "Dietary Lipids and Postnatal Developments," (C. Galli, ed.), Raven, New York.

Causeret, J. (1977). Vitamin value of an animal milk compared to that of human milk. *Ann. Nutr. Aliment.* **25**:A313–A334.

Cerna, M. (1979). Development of baby foods in Czechoslovakia. *Prum. Potravin* **30**(4):201–202. (*Dairy Sci. Abstr.* **42**(5):325.)

Chatranon, W., B. Chavalittamrong, S. Kritalugsana, and P. Pringsulaka (1978). Lead concentrations in breast milk at various stages of lactation. *Southeast Asian J. Trop. Med. Public Health* **9**(3):420–422. (*Dairy Sci. Abstr.* **42**(7):550.)

Chavez, A., and C. Martinez (1980). Effects of maternal undernutrition and dietary supplementation on milk production. *In* "Maternal Nutrition During Pregnancy and Lactation" (H. Aebi and R. Whitehead, eds.), Hans Huber Publishers, Bern, Switzerland.

Chordash, R. A., and N. F. Insalata (1978). Incidence and pathological significance of *Escherichia coli* and other sanitary indicator organisms in food and water. *Food Technol. (Chicago)* **32**(10):54–64.

Chumak, T. F., and Yu. A. Kozyrev (1973). Counting chamber method for microscopy estimation of cellular composition of human mammary gland secretion. *Vopr. Okhr. Materin. Det.* **18**(1):73–76. (*Dairy Sci. Abstr.* **39**(7):463.)

Clarke, T. A., M. Markarian, W. Griswold, and S. Mendoza (1979). Hypernatremic dehydration resulting from inadequate breast feeding. *Pediatrics* **63**(6):931–932.

Code of Federal Regulations (1978). Title 21, Parts 160–199, p. 58.

Codex Alimentarius Commission, Joint FAO/WHO Food Standards Programme (1976).

Recommended International Standards for Foods for Infants and Children. FAO, Rome, Italy.

Condon, J. R., J. Nassim, A. Hilbe, F. Millard, and E. Strainthorpe (1970). Calcium and phosphorus metabolism in relation to lactose tolerance. *Lancet* **2**:1027.

Conner, A. E. (1979). Elevated levels of sodium and chloride in milk from mastitic breast. *Pediatrics* **63**(6):910–911.

Cowie, A. T., and J. K. Swinburne (1977). Hormones, drugs, metals and pesticides in milk: a guide to the literature. *Dairy Sci. Abstr.* **39**(7):391–402.

Crawford, M. A., B. M. Laurance, and A. E. Munhumbo (1977). Breast feeding and human milk composition. *Lancet* **1**:99–100.

Cunningham, A. S. (1979). Morbidity in breast-fed and artificially fed infants. II. *J. Pediatr. (St. Louis)* **95**(5,I):685–689.

Cvengros, V., and A. Stadtruckerova (1978). Survey of breast feeding in Martin district. *Cesk. Pediatr.* **33**(5):302–305. (*Dairy Sci. Abstr.* **41**(5):292.)

Dairy Council Digest (1962). The nutritional significance of lactose. **33**(5):1–4.

Dairy Council Digest (1963). The nonfat composition of milk. **34**(3):1–6.

Dairy Council Digest (1971a). Composition and nutritive value of dairy foods. **42**(1)1–4.

Dairy Council Digest (1971b). Lactose intolerance. **42**(6):31–36.

Dairy Council Digest (1974). The role of lactose in the diet. **45**(5):25–28.

Dairy Council Digest (1975). Nutritive value and composition of cheese. **46**(3):13–17.

Debongnie, J., A. Newcomer, and S. Philips (1977). Small bowel function in lactase deficiency. Gastroenterology **72**:A23.

Dirks, O. B., J. Jongeling-Eijndhouen, T. Flissebaalje, and I. Gedalia (1974). Total and free ionic fluoride in human and cow's milk as determined by gas–liquid chromatography and fluoride electrode. *Caries Res.* **8**:181–186.

Dluzniewska, I. (1966). Pathogenic staphylococci in the samples from breast-feeding mothers. *Ginekol. Polska* **37**:745–755.

Dolezalek, J. (1979). Use of bifidogenic microflora in the manufacture of dried milks for feeding infants and children. *Prumy. Potravin* **30**(12):684–685. (*Dairy Sci. Abstr.* **42**(9):690.)

Donat, H. (1976). Content of total protein and immunoglobulins in human milk. *Zentralbl. Gynaekol.* **98**(26):1631–1637. (*Dairy Sci. Abstr.* **40**:248).

Droese, W., H. Stolley, and M. Kersting (1978). On additional food before the age of four months for young infants on commercially prepared milk formulae. *Monatsschr. Kinderheilk.* **126**(1):6–8. (*Dairy Sci. Abstr.* **42**(2):119).

Dubois, S., D. E. Hill, and G. H. Beaton (1979). An examination of factors believed to be associated with infantile obesity. *Am. J. Clin. Nutr.* **32**(10):1997–2004.

Edelsten, D., F. Ebbesen, and J. Hertel (1979). The removal of lactose from human milk by fermentation with *Saccharomyces fragilis. Milchwissenschaft* **34**(12):733–734. (*Dairy Sci. Abstr.* **42**(6):447).

Edozien, J. C. (1980). Dietary influences on human lactation performance. *In* "Maternal Nutrition During Pregnancy and Lactation" (H. Aebi and R. Whitehead, eds.), Hans Huber Publishers, Bern, Switzerland.

Erickson, Y. (1969). Fluoride excretion in human saliva and milk. *Caries Res.* **3**(2):159–166.

ESPGAN Committee on Nutrition (1977). Guidelines on infant nutrition. I. Recommendations for the composition of an adapted formula. *Acta Paediatr. Scand.* **262**:1–20.

Espina, F., and V.S. Packard (1979). Survival of *Lactobacillus acidophilus* in a spray drying process. *J. Food Prot.* **42**(2):149–152.

Evans, G. W., and P. Johnson (1980). Characterization and quantitation of a zinc-binding ligand in human milk. *Pediatr. Res.* **14**:876–880.

Evans, H. E., and L. Glass (1979). Breast feeding: advantages and potential problems. *Pediatr. Ann.* **8**(2):110–118.

Ewing, W. H. (1963). Isolation and identification of *Escherichia coli* serotypes associated with diarrheal diseases. U.S. Department of Health, Education, and Welfare, Atlanta, Georgia.

FAO/WHO ad hoc Expert Committee (1973). Energy and Protein Requirements. WHO Technical Report Service, No. 522.

FAO/WHO (1976). Recommended international standards for foods for infants and children. Codex Alimentarius Commission, Rome, Italy.

Federal Register (1980a). **45**(251):86362–86370.

Federal Register (1980b). **45**(97):32550–32554.

Federal Register (1980c). **45**(92):30980–30993.

Federal Register (1981). **46**(99):27614–27621.

Feeley, R. M., P. E. Criner, and H. T. Slover (1975). Major fatty acids and proximate composition of dairy products. *J. Am. Diet. Assoc.* **66**:140.

Flatz, G., C. Saengudom, and T. Sanguanbhokhai (1969). Lactose intolerance in Thailand. *J. Food Prot.* **41**(3):220–225.

Flewett, T. H., A. Bryden, H. Davies, G. Woode, J. Bridger, and J. Derrick (1974). Relation between viruses from acute gastroenteritis of children and newborn calves. *Lancet 7872*:61–63.

Foman, S. J. (1974). "Infant Nutrition," (2nd ed.). W. B. Saunders, Philadelphia.

Foman, S. J., and S. Wei (1976). Prevention of dental caries. *In* "Nutritional disorders of children," (S. J. Fomon, ed.), U.S. Department of Health, Education and Welfare, DHEW Pub. No. (HSA) 76–5612.

Food Chemical News, October 29, 1979, pp. 48–49, Washington, D.C.

Ford, J. E., B. Law, V. Marshall, and B. Reiter (1977). Influence of heat treatment of human milk on some of its protective constituents. *J. Pediatr. (St. Louis)* **90**(1):29–35.

Forsum, E. (1973). Nutritional evaluation of whey protein concentrates and their fractions. *J. Dairy Sci.* **57**(6):665–669.

Foster, D., and R. E. Harris (1960). The incidence of *Staphylococcus pyogenes* in human breast milk. *J. Obstet. Gynaecol. (Brit Commonwealth)* **67**:463–464.

Frank, K., and G. Dobias (1976). Detectability of immunoglobulins in native and heat-treated human milk. *Kiserl. Orvostud.* **28**:392–395. (*Dairy Sci. Abstr.* **42**(3):193.)

Fujita, M., and E. Takabatake (1977). Mercury levels in human maternal and neonatal blood, hair, and milk. *Bull. Environ. Cont. Toxicol.* **18**(2):205–208.

Gallagher, C. R., A. L. Molleson, and J. Caldwell (1975). Lactose intolerance and fermented dairy products. *Cul. Dairy Prod. J.* **10**(1):22.

Garza, C. (1979). Appropriateness of milk use in international supplementary feeding programs. *J. Dairy Sci.* **62**:1673–1684.

Garza, C., and N. Scrimshaw (1976). Relationship of lactose intolerance to milk intolerance in young children. *Am. J. Clin. Nutr.* **29**:192.

Gatti, G. (1975). Pesticide residues in human fat and human milk in the nine member states of the European Community (1969–1973). *Comm. Eur. Communities [Rep.] EUR* **5196**:383–424.

Gazzard, J., and C. Lee (1979). A "personalized" human milk bank. *Br. Med. J.* **1**(6160):382.

Ghitis, J. (1966). The labile folate of milk. *Am. J. Clin. Nutr.* **18**:452–457.

Glass, R. L. (1956). Ph.D. thesis, Department of Biochemistry. University of Minnesota, St. Paul.

Golden, B., and M. Golden (1981). Plasma zinc, rate of weight gain, and the energy cost of tissue deposition in children recovering from severe malnutrition on a cow's milk or soya protein based diet. *Am. J. Clin. Nutr.* **34**(5):892–899.

Golden, M., and B. Golden (1981). Effect of zinc supplementation on the dietary intake, rate of gain, and energy cost of tissue deposition in children recovering from severe malnutrition. *Am. J. Clin. Nutr.* **34**(5):900–908.

Goldman, A. S., W. A. Sellars, S. R. Halpern, D. W. Anderson, T. E. Furlow, and C. H. Johnson (1963a). Milk allergy. II. Skin testing of allergic and normal children with purified milk protein. *Pediatrics* **35**:572–579.

Goldman, A., D. Anderson, W. Sellars, S. Saperstein, W. Kniker, and S. Halpern (1963b). Milk allergy. I. Oral challenge with milk and isolated milk proteins in allergic infants. *Pediatrics* **32**:425–443.

Goldman, A. S. (1976). Immunologic aspects of human milk. Symposium on human lactation. DHEW Publication No. (HSA)79–5107, pp. 49–58.

Goldman, A. S. (1977). Human milk, leukocytes, and immunity. *J. Pediatr. (St. Louis)* **90**(1):167–168.

Goodenough, E. R., and D. H. Kleyn (1976). Influence of viable yogurt microflora on digestion of lactose by the rat. *J. Dairy Sci.* **59**(4):601.

Gorbach, S. L., and C. Khurana (1972). Toxigenic *Escherichia coli*: A cause of infantile diarrhea in Chicago. *N. Engl. J. Med.* **287**:791.

Gordon, D., J. MacRae, and D. Wheater (1957). A *Lactobacillus* preparation for use with antibiotics. *Lancet* **272**:899–901.

Grebennikov, E. P., and V. Luzhkovaya (1977). Effect of some forms of disease on the composition of human milk at the start of lactation. *Akush. Ginekol. (Sofia)* **8**:59–61. (*Dairy Sci. Abstr.* **41**(2):120.)

Gueri, M., P. Jutsum, and R. Hoyte (1978). Breast-feeding practices in Trinidad. *Bull. Pan. Am. Health. Org.* **12**(4):316–322.

Guerrant, R. L., R. Moore, P. Kirschenfeld, and M. Sande (1975). Role of toxigenic and invasive bacteria in acute diarrhea of childhood. *N. Engl. J. Med.* **293**:567.

Gyllenberg, H., and P. Roine (1957). The value of colony counts in evaluating the abundance of *Lactobacillus bifidus* in infant feces. *Acta Pathol. Microbiol. Scand.* **41**:144–150.

Gyuriscek, D., and M. Thompson (1976). Hydrolyzed lactose cultured dairy products. II. Manufacture of yogurt, buttermilk, and cottage cheese. *Cult. Dairy Prod. J.* **11**(3):12.

Haenel, H. (1970). Human normal and abnormal gastrointestinal flora. *Am. J. Clin. Nutr.* **23**:1433–1439.

Hamburger, R. N. (1976). Allergy and the immune system. *Am. Sci.* **64**(2):157–164.

Hanafy, M. M. (1980). Maternal nutrition and lactation performance in Egypt. *In* "Maternal Nutrition During Pregnancy and Lactation" H. Aebi and R. Whitehead, eds., Hans Huber Publishers, Bern, Switzerland.

Hardinge, M. G., and H. Crooks (1961). Lesser known vitamins in foods. *J. Am. Diet. Assoc.* **38**:240–245.

Hayes, A. W., P. Unger, L. Stoloff, M. Trucksess, G. Hogan, N. Ryan, B. Wray (1978). Occurrence of aflatoxin in hypoallergenic milk substitutes. *J. Food Prot.* **14**(12):974–976.

Hecht, A. (1979). Advice on breast-feeding and drugs. *FDA Consum.* **13**(9):21–22.

Hegsted, D. M. (1978). Protein-calorie malnutrition. *Am. Sci.* **65**(6):61–65.

Hemken, R. W. (1980). Milk and meat iodine content: relation to human health. *J. Am. Vet. Med. Assoc.* **176**:1119–1121.

Hide, D. W. (1979). Breast or bottle. *Br. Med. J.* **2**(6192):733.

Hill, I., and P. Porter (1974). Studies of bactericidal activity to *Eschericia coli* of porcine and colostral immunoglobulins and the role of lysozyme with secretory IgA. *Immunology* **26**:1239–1250.

Hilpert, H., H. Gerber, H. Amster, J. J. Pahud, A. Ballabriga, L. Arcalis, F. Farriaux, E. de Peyer, and D. Nussle (1975). Bovine milk immunoglobulins (Ig), their possible utilization in industrially prepared infant's milk formulae. Proceedings XIII Symposium of the Swedish Nutrition Foundation, Saltsjobaden, Sweden, pp. 182–196.

Hofvander, Y., and A. Petros-Barvazian (1978). WHO collaborative study on breast feeding. *Acta Paediatr. Scand.* **67**(5):556–560. (*Dairy Sci. Abstr.* **42**(8):602.)

Holt, P. R. (1972). The roles of bile acids during the process of normal fat and cholesterol absorption. *Arch. Intern. Med.* **130**:574–583.

Hood, R. L., and A. R. Johnson (1980). Supplementation of infant formulations with biotin. *Nutr. Rep. Int.* **21**(5):727–731.

Huffman, S. L., A. K. M. A. Chowdhury, J. Chakraborty, and N. K. Simpson (1980). Breast-feeding patterns in rural Bangladesh. *Am. J. Clin. Nutr.* **33**(1):144–154.

International Dairy Federation (1972). IDF monograph on UHT milk, Part V, Brussells, Belgium.

Ikonen, R., and K. Maki (1977). Heating human milk. *Br. Med. J.* **2**(6083):386–387.

Iyer, J. G. (1957). Trace element content of milk of Indian cattle. *Naturwissenschaften,* **44**:635.

Jacobs, F. A., M. T. Martin, J. G. Brushmiller, and K. F. Licklider (1981). Low molecular weight copper zinc binding ligands in milk ultrafiltrates. *Fed. Proc., Fed. Am. Soc. Exp. Biol.* **40**(3,II):855.

Jenness, R. (1980). Composition and characteristics of goat milk: review 1968-1979. *J. Dairy Sci.* **63**(10):1605–1630.

Jenness, R., and S. Patton (1959). Principles of Dairy Chemistry. Wiley, New York.

Jenness, R., and R. E. Sloan. (1970). The composition of milks of various species: a review. *Dairy Sci. Abstr.* **32**(10):599–612.

Johnson, A. R., R. L. Hood, and J. L. Emery (1980). Biotin and the sudden infant death syndrome. *Nature (London)* **285**(5761):159–160.

Jones, D., and M. Latham (1974). The implications of lactose intolerance in children. *Environ. Child Health*, monograph no. 36:261–271.

Jones, G. W., and J. M. Rutter (1972). Role of K88 antigen in the pathogenesis of neonatal diarrhea caused by *Escherichia coli* in piglets. *Infect. Immun.* **6**:918.

Juszkiewicz, T., T. Szprengier, and T. Radomanski (1975). Mercury content of human milk. *Pol. Tyg. Lek.* **30**(9):365–366. (*Dairy Sci. Abstr.* **39**(11):730.)

Kabara, J. J. (1980). Lipids as host-resistance factors of human milk. *Nutr. Rev.* **38**(2):65–73.

Kanao, S., T. Nakajima, and Z. Tamura (1965). Purification of a new bifidus factor from carrot root. *Chem. Pharm. Bull.* **13**:1262–1263.

Kaneko, S., T. Sato, and K. Suzuki (1979). The levels of anticonvulsants in breast milk. *Bri. J. Clin. Pharm.* **7**(6):624–627.

Kee, T. S. (1975). Breastfeeding in a rural area of Malaysia. *Med. J. Malays.* **29**(3):175–179. (*Dairy Sci. Abstr.* **42**(8):603.)

Keller, C. A., and R. A. Doherty (1980). Bone lead mobilization in lactating mice and transfer to suckling offspring. *Toxicol. Appl. Pharmacol.* **55**(2):220–228.

Kende, E., and Z. Bekesy (1977). Human milk and hospital infections from the viewpoint of immunology and hospital hygiene. *Orv. Hetil.* **118**(52):3135–3140. (*Dairy Sci. Abstr.* **42**(11):855.).

Kilara, A., and K. Shahani (1976). Lactase activity of cultured and acidified dairy products. *J. Dairy Sci.* **59**:2031–2035.

Kirksey, A., and J. A. Ernst, J. L. Roepke, and T. L. Tsia (1979). Influence of mineral intake and use of oral contraceptives before pregnancy on the mineral content of human colostrum and of more mature milk. *Am. J. Clin. Nutr.* **32**:30–39.

Kisza, J., S. Ziajka, and Z. Zbikowski (1976). Method for the production of dried humanized milk. *Polish Patent* 84 101. (*Dairy Sci. Abstr.* **41**(6):326.)

Knorr, K. (1957). Keim and resistenzbestimmungen als beitrage zur atiologie der mastitis puerperalis und der neugeboren infectionen. *Gynaecologia* **143**:112–115.

Kohler, G., and K. Amon (1974). Mastitis incidence, prevention and therapy at the University Hospital for women in Greifswald from 1957 to 1972. *Zentralb. Gynaekol.* **96**(7):207–213. (*Dairy Sci. Abstr.* **38**(5):334.)

Konishi, F., and J. Goodpasture (1981). Relationship of the fat content of breast milk to the growth patterns of infants. *Fed. Proc., Fed. Am. Soc. Exp. Biol.* **40**(3, II):897.

Kuchroo, C., and N. Ganguli (1980). Technological approaches for infant food manufacture from modified buffalo milk. *J. Food Sci.* **45**(5):1333–1335.

Kulangara, A. C. (1980). The demonstration of ingested wheat antigens in human breast milk. IRCS Medical Science. **8**(1):19. (*Dairy Sci. Abstr.* **43**(8):644.)

Kuvaeva, I. B., K. Ladodo, and S. Gribakin (1979). Natural feeding and its significance in local immunological protection of the gastro-intestinal tract during the neonatal period. *Vopr. Pitan.* **3**:25–29. (*Dairy Sci. Abstr.* **42**(5):330.)

Lackey, C. J. (1978). International symposium on infant and child feeding. *Nutr. Today* **13**(6):11–15, 31–32.

Lacroix, D. E., W. A. Mattingly, N. P. Wong, and J. A. Alford (1973). Cholesterol, fat, and protein in dairy products. *J. Am. Diet. Assoc.* **62**:275.

Larsson, B., S. A. Slorach, U. Hagman, and U. Hofvander (1981). WHO collaborative breast feeding study. II. Levels of lead and cadmium in Swedish human milk, 1978–79. *Acta Paediatr. Scand.* **70**(3):281–284.

Latham, Michael C. (1977). Public health importance of milk intolerance. *Nutr. News* **40**(4):13.

Lazarev, S. G. (1976). Composition of milk of mothers nursing overweight infants. *Pediatriya, Moscow* No. 10, pp. 60–61. (*Dairy Sci. Abstr.* **39**(6):54.)

Lebenthal, E. (1975). Cow's milk protein allergy. *Pediatr. Clin. N. Amer.* **22**:827–833.

Lee, K., and F. Clydesdale (1979). Iron sources used in food fortification and their changes due to food processing. *CRC Crit. Rev. Food Sci. Nutr.* **11**(2):117–153.

Leichtig, A., and R. E. Klein (1980). Maternal food supplementation and infant health: results of a study in rural areas of Guatemala. *In* "Maternal Nutrition During Pregnancy and Lactation" (H. Aebi and R. Whitehead, eds.), Hans Huber Publishers, Bern, Switzerland.

Lengeman, F. W. (1959). The site of action of lactose in the enhancement of calcium utilization. *J. Nutr.* **69**:23–27.

Lindblad, B. S., G. Alfven, and R. Zetterstrom (1978). Plasma free amino acid concentrations of breast-fed infants. *Acta Paediatr. Scand.* **67**(5):659–663. (*Dairy Sci. Abstr.* **42**(7):528.)

Lisker, R., B. Gonzalez, and M. Daltabuit (1975). Recessive inheritance of the adult type of intestinal lactase deficiency. *Am. J. Hum. Genet.* **27**:662–664.

Lock, F., M. Yow, M. Griffith, and M. Stout (1948). Bacteriology of the vagina in 75 normal young adults. *Surg. Gynecol. Obstet.* **87**:410–416.

Lombeck, I., K. Kasperek, B. Bonnerman, L. Feinendegen, and H. Brenner (1978). Selenium content of human milk, cow's milk, and cow's milk infant formulas. *Eur. J. Pediatr.* **129**(3):139–145.

Lonnerdal, B., E. Forsum, and L. Hambraeus. (1976). The protein content of human milk. I. A transversal study of Swedish normal material. *Nutri. Rep. Int.* **13**(2):125–134.

Lonnerdal, B., C. L. Keen, M. Ohtake, and T. Tamura (1981). Paper presented at the International Congress of Nutrition, San Diego, California, August 16–21. Reported in *Food Chem. News* **23**(26):16–17.

Lucas, A., and C. Roberts (1979). Bacteriological quality control in human milk-banking. *Br. Med. J.* **1**(6156):80–82.

Lucas, A., A. Smith, J. Baum, and D. Day (1979). Human milk banking. *Br. Med. J.* **1**(6159):343.

Luyken, R. (1972). Studies on milk intolerance. A review of literature for Latin America. *Maandschr. Kindergeneesk.* **40**:89–105.

McLaughlan, P., K. Anderson, E. Widdowson, and R. Coombs (1981). Effect of heat on the anaphylactic-sensitizing capacity of cows' milk, goats' milk, and various infant formulae fed to guinea pigs. *Arch. Dis. Child.* **56**(3):165–171.

Mahoney, A., and D. Hendricks (1978). Some effects of different phosphate compounds on iron and calcium absorption. *J. Food Sci.* **43**(5):1473–1476.

Majewski, A. (1979). Clinical picture of nicotine poisoning in breast-fed infants. *Wiad. Lek.* **32**(4):275–277. (*Dairy Sci. Abstr.* **42**(8):603.)

Mares, J., J. Hassa, O. Beer, and R. Stehlik (1975). Present state of puerperal mastitis in a metropolis. Cesk. Gynekol. **40**(1):47–48. (*Dairy Sci. Abstr.* **38**(7):477.)

Marshall, B. R., J. Hepper, and C. Zirbel (1975). Sporadic puerpural mastitis. An infection that need not interrupt lactation. *J. Am. Med. Assoc.* **233**(13):1377–1379.

Martinez-Suarez, H., and V. Packard (1981). In-bottle pasteurizer for small lots of milk. Integrating paper for Master of Agriculture degree. University of Minnesota, St. Paul.

Mata, L. J., and R. Wyatt (1971). Host resistance to infection in the uniqueness of human milk. *Am. J. Clin. Nutr.* **24**:976.

Mathias, M. M., D. E. Hogue, and J. K. Loosli (1967). The biological value of selenium in bovine milk for the rat and chick. *J. Nutr.* **93**:14.

Mellies, M. J., T. Ishikawa, P. Gartside, K. Burton, J. MacGee, K. Allen, P. M. Steiner, D. Brady, and C. J. Glueck (1978). Effects of varying maternal dietary cholesterol and phytosterol in lactating women and their infants. *Am. J. Clin. Nutr.* **31**(8):1347–1354.

Mendez, A., and A. Olano (1979). Lactulose. A review of some chemical properties and applications in infant nutrition and medicine. *Dairy Sci. Abstr.* **41**(9):531–535.

Mes, J., D. Davies, and W. Miles (1978). Traces of Mirex in some Canadian human milk supplies. *Bull. Environ. Contam. Toxicol.* **19**(5):564–570.

Meyer, F., G. Erhardt, and B. Senft (1981). Environmental and genetic aspects of lysozyme in cow's milk. *Zuchtungskunde* **53**(1):17–27.

Midulla, M., G. Russo, and G. Sabatino (1976). Bacteriostatic effect of biologically acidified milk on some salmonella strains. *Boll. Soc. Ital. Biol. Sper.* **52**(20):1751–1757. (*Dairy Sci. Abstr.* **42**(7):512.)

Miller, R. W. (1977). Pollutants in breast milk. *J. Pediatr.* **90**:3, 510.

Miller, W. J. (1970). Zinc nutrition of cattle: a review. *J. Dairy Sci.* **53**(8):1123–1135.

Minneapolis Tribune, June 18, 1981, p. 8A.

Mizrahi, A., R. D. London, and D. Gribetz (1968). Neonatal hypocalcemia: its causes and treatment. *N. Engl. J. Med.* **278**:1163–1165.

Montgomery, T. L., M. Wise, W. Lang, R. Mandle, and M. Fritz (1959). A study of staphylococci colonization of postpartum mothers and newborn infants. *Am. J. Obstet. Gynecol.* **66**:1227–1233.

Moore, K. (1978). Status report on the enzyme industry. *Food Prod. Dev.* **12**(6):41–42.

Morris, M., W. Featherston, P. Phillips, and S. McNult (1963). Influence of lactose and dried skimmilk upon the magnesium deficiency syndrome in the dog. *J. Nutr.* **79**:437–44.

Mulchandani, R. P., R. V. Josephson, and W. J. Harper (1979b). Effects of processing on liquid infant milk formulas. II. Products stored six months. *J. Dairy Sci.* **62**(10):1537–1545.

Muller, B., and H. Schroder (1978). Biocides in human fatty tissue and human milk— a contribution to the problem of infant feeding. *Ernaehr.-Umsch.* **25**(7):205–209. (*Dairy Sci. Abstr.* **42**(6):414.)

Mutai, M., M. Mada, and K. Shimada (1980). Method of producing foods and drinks containing bifidobacteria. U.S. Patent 4, 187, 321.

Myeres, A. W. (1979). A retrospective look at infant feeding practices in Canada: 1965–1978. *J. Can. Diet. Assoc.* **40**(3):200–209.

Nagasawa, T., M. Tomita, T. Watanabe, and T. Ubayashi (1975). *United States Patent* 3 901 979.

Naismith, D. J., and K. N. Cashel (1979). Taurine in breast milk: a role in fat utilization. *Proc. Nutr. Soc.* **38**(3):105A.

Nath, M., and P. Geervani (1978). Diet and nutrition of pregnant and lactating women and infants of urban slums of Hyderabad. *Indian J. Nutr. Diet.* **15**(12):422–428.

National Academy of Sciences/National Research Council (1972). Background information on lactose and milk intolerance. *Nutr. Rev.* **30**(8):175–176.

National Academy of Sciences/National Research Council (1979), Food and Nutrition Board, Recommended Daily Allowances, 9th revision, Washington, D.C.

National Academy of Sciences/National Research Council (1980). Recommended Dietary Allowances. National Academy of Sciences. Washington, D.C.

Naude, S., J. Prinsloo, and C. Haupt (1979). Comparison between a humanized cow's milk and a soy product for premature infants. *South Afr. Med. J.* **55**(24):982–986.

Nelson, K., and N. Potter (1979). Iron binding by wheat gluten, soy isolate, zein, albumen and casein. *J. Food Sci.* **44**(1):104–107.

Nestel, P. J., A. Poyser, and T. J. C. Boulton (1979). Changes in cholesterol metabolism in infants in response to dietary cholesterol and fat. *Am. J. Clin. Nutr.* **32**(11):2177–2182.

Nestlé Products Technical Assistance Co. Ltd. (1975). *Nestle Research News* 1974/75, Lausanne, Switzerland.

Newcomer, A. D. (1979). Lactase deficiency. *Contemp. Nutri.* **4**(4):1–2.

Nishikawa, I., N. Murata, E. Deya, G. Kawanishi, and E. Furuichi (1976). Nitrogen distribution and non-protein nitrogenous compounds in human and bovine milk. *J. Jpn. Soc. Food. Nutr.* **29**(2):77–83. (*Dairy Sci. Abstr.* **39**(1):67.)

Niskanen, A., L. Koiranen, and K. Roine (1978). Staphylococcal enterotoxin and thermonuclease production during induced bovine mastitis and the clinical reaction of enterotoxin in udders. *Infect. Immun.* **19**(2):493–498.

Niv, M., W. Levy, and N. Greenstein (1963). Yogurt in the treatment of infantile diarrhea. *Clin. Pediatr.* **2**:407.

Norman, A., B. Strandvik, and O. Ojamae (1972). Bile acids and pancreatic enzymes during absorption in the newborn. *Acta Paediatr. Scand.* **61**:571–576.

North–South Institute (1979). Handle with care. Ottawa, Canada, KIN 064.

Nowakowski, W., M. Trzesniowska, Z. Zientek, and P. Heczko (1976). Biochemical and toxic properties of staphylococci isolated from milk of puerperae. *Med. Dosw. Mikrobiol.* **28**(4):329–332. (*Dairy Sci. Abstr.* **40**(10):633.)

Nyahn, W. L. (1978). Infant nutrition and vegetarian mothers. *Parents* **53**(12):29.

O'Brien, T. E. (1974). Excretion of drugs in human milk. *Am. J. Hosp. Pharm.* **31**:844–854.

O'Brien, T. E. (1975). Excretion of diphenylhydantoin in human milk. *Am. J. Hosp. Pharm.* **32**:14.

O'Connor, P. (1978). Failure to thrive with breast feeding. *Clin. Pediatr.* **17**(11):833–835.

Ogasa, K. (1980). Powder composition comprising viable bifidobacteria cells containing powder and lactulose. *British Patent* 1 582 068. (*Dairy Sci. Abstr.* **43**(8):602.)

Ogra, S., D. Weintraub, and P. Ogra (1977). Immunologic aspects of human colostrum and milk. III. Fate and absorption of cellular and soluble components in the gastrointestinal tract of the newborn. *J. Immunol.* **119**:245–248.

Olano, V. A. (1979). Simultaneous production of lactulose and β lactulose from α lactose hydrate. *Rev. Inst. Lacticinios Candido Tostes* **34**(202):3–7 (*Dairy Sci. Abstr.* **42**(1):144.)

Olszyna-Marzys, A. E. (1978). Contaminants of human milk. *Acta Paediatr. Scand.* **67**(5):571–576. (*Dairy Sci. Abstr.* **42**(8):603.)

Oosthuizen, J. C. 1962. The kinetics of the rennin-casein reaction in abnormal cow's milk and milk of some other species and of the action of rennet substitutes on normal cow's milk. *J. Dairy Res.* **29**:297–305.

Orme, M. L'E. P. Lewis, M. de Swiet, M. Serlin, R. Sibeon, J. Baty, and A. Breckenridge (1977). May mothers given warfarin breast feed their infants? *Br. Med. J.* **1**:1564.

Otnaess, A. B., and I. Orstavik (1980). The effect of human milk fractions on rotavirus in relation to the secretory IgA content. *Acta Pathol. Microbiol. Scand.* **88**(1):15–21. (*Dairy Sci. Abstr.* **42**(9):684.)

Owen, D. F., and J. M. McIntire (1976). Technology of fortification of foods. Proc. of NAS Workshop, Washington, D.C., pp. 44–65.

Pao, E. (1979). Nutrient consumption patterns of individuals in 1977 and 1965. News release of a presentation made at Agricultural Outlook Conference, Washington, D.C., November 6.

Parkash, S., and R. Jenness (1967). Status of zinc in cow's milk. *J. Dairy Sci.* **50**:127–134.

Parkash, S., and R. Jenness (1968). The composition and characteristics of goat's milk: a review. *Dairy Sci. Abstr.* **30**(2):67–87.

Pearson, M. (1980). New weapon in an old war. *Agenda* **3**(10):11–13.

Picciano, M. F., and H. A. Guthrie (1976). Copper, iron, and zinc contents of mature human milk. *Am. J. Clin. Nutr.* **29**:242–254.

Picciano, M. F., H. A. Guthrie, and D. M. Sheehe (1978). The cholesterol content of human milk. A variable constituent among women and within the same woman. *Clin. Pediatr.* **17**(4):359–362.

Picciano, M. F., and R. H. Deering (1980). The influence of feeding regimens on iron status during infancy. *Am. J. Clin. Nutr.* **33**(4):746–753.

Pillinger, S., and K. Langley (1978). Fractionation of whey proteins. In XX International Dairy Congress, Vol. E. pp. 922–923.

Pinkerton, C., D. Hammer, K. Bridbord, J. Creason, J. Kent, and G. Murthy (1972). Human milk as a dietary source of cadmium and lead. Trace Substances in Environmental Health—VI. Proceedings of University of Missouri's 6th Annual Conference, Columbia, Missouri.

Polishuk, Z. W., M. Ron, M. Wasserman, S. Cucos, D. Wasserman, and C. Lemesch (1977). Organochlorine compounds in human blood plasma and milk. *Pest. Monit. J.* **10**:121.

Posati, L. P., J. E. Kinsella, and B. K. Watt (1974). The fatty acid composition of milk and eggs. Paper presented at the 57th annual meeting, American Dietetic Association, Philadelphia.

Prema, K. (1978). Pregnancy and lactation: some nutritional aspects. *Indian J. Med. Res.* **78**:70–79 (supplement). (*Dairy Sci. Abstr.* **42**(8):602.)

Prentice, A. M. (1980). Variations in maternal dietary intake, birthweight and breast-milk output in the Gambia. *In* "Maternal Nutrition During Pregnancy and Lactation" (H. Aebi and R. Whitehead, eds.), Hans Huber Publishers, Bern, Switzerland.

Protein Advisory Group of the United Nations (1972). PAG statement 17 on low lactase activity and milk intake. *PAG Bull.* Vol. II, No. 2, New York, pp. 9–11.

Rafsky, H. A., and J. Rafsky (1955). Clinical and bacteriological studies on a new *Lactobacillus acidophilus* concentrate in functional gastrointestinal disturbances. *Am. J. Gastroenterol.* **24**:87–92.

Rajalakshmi, R. (1980). Gestation and lactation performance in relation to the plane of maternal nutrition. *In* "Maternal Nutrition During Pregnancy and Lactation" (H. Aebi and R. Whitehead, eds.), Hans Huber Publishers, Bern, Switzerland.

Rajalakshmi, K., and S. G. Srikantia (1980). Copper, zinc, and magnesium content of breast milk of Indian women. *Am. J. Clin. Nutr.* **33**(3):664–669.

Rantasalo, J., and M. Kauppinen (1959). The occurrence of *Staphylococcus aureus* in mother's milk. *Ann. Cir. Gyn. Fenn.* **48**:246–258.

Rassin, D. K., J. A. Sturman, and G. E. Gaull (1978). Taurine and other free amino acids in milk of man and other mammals. *Early Hum. Dev.* **2**(1):1–13.

Reddy, V., and J. Pershad (1972). Lactase deficiency in Indians. *Am J. Clin. Nutr.* **25**:114–119.

Reiter, B. (1978). Review of the progress of dairy science: antimicrobial systems in milk. *J. Dairy Res.* **45**:131–147.

Reiter, B., and J. Oram (1968). Iron and vanadium requirements of lactic acid streptococci. *J. Dairy Res.* **35**:67–69.

Renterghem, R. van, and L. Devlaminck (1980). Polychlorinated biphenyl compounds in milk and dairy products. *Z. Lebensm. Unters. Forsch.* **170**(5):346–348.

Ripp, J. A. (1961). Soybean-induced goiter. *Am. J. Dis. Child.* **102**:106.

Roepke, J. L. B., and A. Kirksey. (1979a) Vitamin B_6 nutriture during pregnancy and lactation. I. Vitamin B_6 intake, levels of the vitamin in biological fluids, and condition of the infant at birth. *Am. J. Clin. Nutr.* **32**(11):2249–2256.

Roepke, J. L. B.,and A. Kirksey (1979b). Vitamin B_6 nutriture during pregnancy and lactation II. The effect of long-term use of oral contraceptives. *Am. J. Clin. Nutr.* **32**(11): 2257–2264.

Roten, H., W. Minder, and R. P. Zurbrugg (1978). Quality control and keeping quality of human milk. *Ther. Umsch.* **35**(8):619–622. (*Dairy Sci. Abstr.* **42**(4):246.)

Rowe, J. C., D. H. Wood, D. Rowe, and L. G. Raisz (1979). Nutritional hypo-phosphatemic rickets in a premature infant fed breast milk. *N. Engl. J. Med.* **300**(6):293–296.

Roy, S., and B. S. Arant (1979). Alkalosis from chloride-deficient Neo-Mull-Soy. *N. Engl. J. Med.* **301**:615.

Ryder, R. W., A. Crosby-Ritchie, B. McDonough, and W. Hall (1977). Human milk contaminated with Salmonella kottbus. A cause of nosocomial illness in infants. *J. Am. Med. Assoc.* **238**(14):1533–1534.

Ryu, J., E. Ziegler, and S. J. Foman (1978). Maternal lead exposure and blood lead concentration in infancy. *J. Pediatr.* **93**(3):476–478.

Saarinen, U. M., and M. A. Siimes (1979). Iron absorption from breast milk, cow's milk, and iron-supplemented formula: an opportunistic use of changes in total body iron determined by hemoglobin, ferritin and body weight in 132 infants. *Pediatr. Res.* **13**(3):143–147.

Sagy, M., E. Birenbaum, A. Balin, S. Orda, Z. Barzilay, and M. Brish (1980). Phosphate-depletion syndrome in a premature infant fed human milk. *J. Pediatr.* **96**(4):683–685.

Sahi, T. (1974). The inheritance of selective adult-type lactose malabsorption. *Scand. J. Gastroenterol.* **9**:(30):1–13.

Sakazaki, R., K. Tamura, and A. Nakamura (1974). Further studies on enteropathogenic *Escherichia Coli* associated with diarrheal diseases in children and adults. *Jpn J. Med. Sci. Biol.* **27**:7.

Salata, A. (1979). Feeding infants in Slovakia. *Cesk. Pediatr.* **34**(1):16–17. (*Dairy Sci. Abstr.* **42**(2):117.)

Sandine, W. E. (1979). Roles of lactobacillus in the intestinal tract. *J. Food Prot.* **42**(3):259–262.

Sandine, W., and M. Daly (1979). Milk intolerance. *J. Food Prot.* **42**(5):435–437.

Sandine, W., K. S. Muralidhara, P. R. Elliker and D. C. England (1972). Lactic acid bacteria in food and health: A review with special references to enteropathogenic *Escherichia coli* as well as certain enteric diseases and their treatment with antibiotics and lactobacilli. *J. Milk Food Technol.* **35**(12):691–702.

Sarzhanova, K., and D. Kudayarov (1978). Use of enriched Biolakt in complex treatment of young children simultaneously suffering from anaemia and pneumonia. *Zdravookhr. Kirg.* **3**:42–44. (*Dairy Sci. Abstr.* **42**(2):43.)

Schupbach, M. R., and H. Egli (1979). Oranochlorine pesticides and polychlorinated biphenyls in human milk. *Mitt. Lebensmittelunters. Hyg.* **70**(4):451–463. (*Dairy Sci. Abstr.* **42**(8):595.)

Scrimshaw, N., C. Taylor, and J. Gordon (1968). Interaction of nutrition and infection. World Health Organization, Geneva, Switzerland.

Selikoff, I. (1979). Quoted in *Food Chem. News,* October 29, 1979, p. 48.

Shahani, K. M. (1974). Presentation made at the 69th Annual Meeting of the American Dairy Science Association, June 23–26, Guelph, Ontario, Canada.

Shahani, K. M., and R. C. Chandan (1979). Nutritional and healthful aspects of cultured and culture-containing dairy foods. *J. Dairy Sci.* **62**:1685–1694.

Shapiro, S. (1960). Control of antibiotic-induced gastrointestinal symptoms with yogurt. *Clin. Med.* **7**:295.

Sharmanov, T. Sh., and P. V. Fedotov (1979). The new enriched cultured milk product Baldyrgan. *Vopr. Pitan.* **6**:38–41.

Shearer, T. R., and D. Hadjimarkos (1975). Geographic distribution of selenium in human milk. *Arch. Environ. Health* **30**(5):230–233.

Sheibak, M., L. Evets, and A. Pal'tseva (1978). Di- and monosaccharide composition of human milk and mixtures intended as substitutes for human milk. *Vopr. Pitan.* **4**:82–83. (*Dairy Sci. Abstr.* **41**(2):120.)

Shukla, T. P. (1975). Beta-galactosidase technology: A solution to the lactose problem. *CRC Crit. Rev. Food Technol.* **5**(3):325–356.

Siimes, M., and N. Hallman (1978). A perspective on human milk banking. *J. Pediatr.* **94**(1):173–174.

Simoons, F. J. (1978). The geographic hypothesis and lactose malabsorption. A weighing of the evidence. *Am. J. Dig. Dis.* **23**:963–980.

Sinatra, F. R., and R. J. Merritt. (1981). Latrogenic kwashiorkor in infants. *Am. J. Dis. Child.* **135**:21–23.

Singh, R. S., Sukhbir Singh, V. K. Batish, and R. Ranganathan (1980). Bacteriological quality of infant milk foods. *J. Food Prot.* **43**(5):340–342.

Smialek, J. E., J. Monforte, R. Aronow, and W. Spitz (1977). Methadone deaths in children. *JAMA* **238**:2516.

Smith, A., M. Picciano, and R. Deering (1981). Folate studies during infancy as influenced by feeding practice. *Fed. Proc., Fed. Am. Soc. Exp. Biol.* **40**(3, II):865.

Smoczynski, S. (1979). Occurrence of chlorinated hydrocarbons and other foreign substances in human, cow's and mares' milk. *Zesz. Nauk. Akad. Roln. Tech. Olsztynie Technol. Zywn.* **14**:315–359. (*Dairy Sci. Abstr.* **42**(9):671–672.)

Sneed, S. M., C. Zane, M. R. Thomas, and B. B. Alford (1979). The effects of ascorbic acid, vitamin B_{12}, vitamin B_6, and folate supplementation in low socio-economic lactating women. *Fed. Proc.* **38**:(3,I):557 (Abstract).

Sorenson, I. (1978). Baby food powder. Technical Information Bulletin, Niro Atomizer Ltd., Copenhagen, Denmark.

Speck, M. L. (1975). Contributions of microorganisms to foods and nutrition. *Nutr. News* **38**(4):13.

Speck, M. (1976). Interactions among lactobacilli and man. *J. Dairy Sci.* **59**:338–343.

Stadhouders, J., L. A. Jansen, and G. Hup (1969). Preservation of starters and mass production of starter bacteria. *Neth. Milk Dairy J.* **23**:193–198.

Stanway, P. (1978). Drugs and breastfeeding. *Chem. Drug.* **210**:601,603,605–606.

Stoliar, O., R. Pelley, E. Kaniecki-Green, M. Klaus, and C. Carpenter (1976). Secretory IgA against enterotoxins in breast-milk. *Lancet* **7972**:1258–1261.

Szokolay, A., L. Rosival, J. Uhnak, and A. Madaric (1977). Dynamics of benzene hexa-chloride (BHC) isomers and other chlorinated pesticides in the food chain and in human fat. *Ecotoxicol. Environ. Saf.* **1**(3):349–359.

Takase, M., Y. Fukuwatari, K. Kawase, I. Kiyosawa, K. Ogasa, S. Suzuki, and T. Kuroume (1979). Antigenicity of casein enzymatic hydrolysate *J. Dairy Sci.* **62**(10):1570–1576.

Tashkin, D. P. (1980). Quoted in Land O'Lakes Mirror, May 1980, Minneapolis, Minnesota.

Taylor, S. (1980). Food allergy—the enigma and some potential solutions. *J. Food Prot.* **43**(4):300–306.

Thomas, J. W. (1970). Metabolism of iron and manganese. *J. Dairy Sci.* **53**(8):1107–1123.

Thomas, M. R., S. M. Sneed, C. Wei, P. Nail, and M. Wilson (1979). The effects of vitamin supplements on the breast milk and maternal status of well-nourished women at six months post-partum. *Fed. Proc.* **38**(3,I):610 (Abstract).

Thompson, A. W., A. R., Wilson, W. J. Cruickshank, and A. H. Jeffries (1976). Evidence for a selective cytotoxic effect of carrageenan on cells of the immune system *in vivo* and *in vitro*. *Experientia* **32**:525–526.

Tinanoff, N., and B. Mueller (1978). Fluoride content in milk and formula for infants. *J. Dent. Child.* **45**(1):53–55.

Tomana, M., J. Mestecky, and W. Niedermeier. (1972). Studies of human secretory immuno-globulin A. IV. Carbohydrate composition. *J Immunol.* **108**(6):1631–1636.

U.S. Department of Agriculture (1976). Agricultural Research Service, Agricultural Handbook No. 8-1 (revised), Washington, D.C.

U.S. Department of Health, Education, and Welfare (1976). "Symposium on Human Lactation," (L. R. Waletzky, ed.), DHEW Publication No. (HSA) 79–5107, Rockville, Maryland.

U.S. Department of Health, Education, and Welfare (1979). "Trends in breast-feeding among American mothers." DHEW Publication No. (PHS) 79-1979. National Center for Health Statistics. Hyattsville, Maryland.

U.S.A. Human Lactation Center (1978). Breast feeding and weaning among the poor. *Lactation Rev.* **3**(1):1–6.

Vakil, J., R. Chandan, R. Parry, and K. Shahani (1969). Susceptibility of several micro-organisms to milk lysozymes. *J. Dairy Sci.* **52**:1192–1197.

Valjak, B., B. Stampar-Plasaj, and Z. Jezerinac (1978). Development of some kidney functions in premature infants fed with concentrated humanized cow's milk. *Lijec. Vjesn.* **100**(7):417–420. (*Dairy Sci. Abstr.* **42**(10):766.)

Vaughan, L. A., C. W. Weber, and S. Kemberling (1978). Trace minerals in human milk. *In* "Nutrition in Transition." Proceedings, Western Hemisphere Nutrition Congress V., Monroe, Wisconsin.

Vicek, A., and J. Kneifl (1964). On experiments on normalization of disordered intestinal flora in infants. II. Clinical experiments I. Omniflora in premature infants. *Z. Kinderheilkd.* **89**:155–159.

Vobecky, J., J. S. Vobecky, D. Shapcott, P. Demers, D. Reid, C. Fisch, R. Blanchard, D. Cloutier, and R. Black (1979). Food intake patterns of infants with high serum cholesterol level at six months. *Int. J. Vitam. Nutr. Res.* **49**(2):189–198.

Vuori, E. (1979a). Intake of copper, iron, manganese and zinc by healthy, exclusively-breast-fed infants during the first three months of life. *Br. J. Nutr.* **42**(3):407–411.

Vuori, E. (1979b). A longitudinal study of manganese in human milk. *Acta Paediatr. Scand.* **68**(4):571–573. (*Dairy Sci. Abstr.* **42**(4):256.)

Vuori E., S. M. Makinen, R. Kara, and P. Kuitunen (1980). The effects of the dietary intakes of copper, iron, manganese, and zinc on the trace element content of human milk. *Am. J. Clin. Nutr.* **33**(2):227–231.

Walker, B., Jr. (1980). Lead Content of Milk and Infant Formula. *J. Food Prot.* **43**(3):178–179.

Walravens, P. A., and K. M. Hambidge (1976). Growth of infants fed a zinc-supplemented formula. *Am. J. Clin. Nutr.* **29**:1114–1121.

Walravens, P. A. (1980). Nutritional importance of copper and zinc in neonates and infants. *Clin. Chem.* **26**(2)185–189.

Walton, J., and L. Messer (1981). Dental caries and fluorosis in breast-fed and bottle-fed children. *Caries Res.* **15**(2):129–137.

Waterlow, J. C., and A. M. Thompson (1979). Observations on the adequacy of breast-feeding. *Lancet* **2**(8136):328–341.

Watson, R. R. (1981). Nutrition and immunity. *Contemp. Nutr.* **6**(5):1–2.

Watson, R. R., and D. N. McMurray (1979). The effects of malnutrition on secretory and cellular immune process. *CRC Crit. Rev. Food Sci. Nutr.* **12**(2)113–159.

Webb, B. H., and A. H. Johnson, (1965). Fundamentals of Dairy Chemistry, AI Publ. Co., Westport, Connecticut.

Webb, B. H., and E. O. Whittier (1970). By-Products from Milk. AI Publ. Co., Westport, Connecticut.

West, P. A., J. Hewitt, and O. Murphy (1979). The influence of methods of collection and storage on the bacteriology of human milk. *J. Appl. Bacteriol.* **46**(2):269–277.

Whitehead, R. (1976). The infant-food industry. *Lancet* **2**(7996):1192–1194.

Wiatrowski, E., L. Kramer, D. Osis, and H. Spencer (1975). Dietary fluoride intake of infants. *Pediatrics* **55**:517–522.

Winkelstein, A. (1956). *Lactobacillus acidophilus* tablets in the therapy of functional intestinal disorders. *Am. Pract.* **1**:1637–1639.

Woidich, H., and W. Pfannhauser (1980). Trace elements in nutrition of babies: arsenic, lead, cadmium. *Z. Lebensm. Unters. Forsch.* **170**(2):95–98. (*Dairy Sci. Abstr.* **42**(7):549.)

Woodward, D. R. (1976). The chemistry of mammalian caseins: a review. *Dairy Sci. Abstr.* **38**(3):137–150.

Wyoming Agricultural Experiment Station (1965). Vitamin E Content of Food and Feeds, Bulletin 435.

Yaffe, S. J., and L. Waletzky (1976). Drugs and chemicals in breast milk. *In* "Symposium on Human Lactation" (L. R. Waletzky, ed.), DHEW Pub. No. (PHS) 79–1979, National Center for Health Statistics, Hyattsville, Maryland.

Yeh, C., P. Kuo, S. Tsai, G. Wang, and Y. Wang (1976). A study on pesticide residues in umbilical cord blood and maternal milk. *J. Formosan Med. Assoc.* **75**(8):463–470.

Yelton, D., and M. Scharff (1980). Monoclonal antibodies. *Am. Sci.* **68**:510–516.

Zimmerman, A. W., and K. M. Hambidge (1980). Low zinc in mother's milk and zinc deficiency syndrome in breast-fed premature infants (Abstract). *Am. J. Clin. Nutr.* **33**(4):951.

General References

Anonymous (1973). Factors of whey affecting lactose metabolism. *Nutr. Rev.* **31**(1):30–31.

Anonymous (1976a) Lactose intolerance deemed no cause for school feeding alarm. *Dairy and Ice Cream Field* **159**(5):20.

Anonymous (1976b) The lactose intolerance test and milk consumption. *Nutr. Rev.* **34**(10): 302–304.

Anonymous (1979). Drugs and breast-feeding. *Br. Med. J.* **1**(6164):642.

Antila, P. (1979). The determination of vitamin D from the aqueous phase of cow's and human milk. *Kemia-Kemi* **6**(12):760.

Asako, K., and Y. Yamushiro (1977). A case of intractable diarrhea. *Japan J. Pediatr.* **30**:653.

Baum, J. (1979). Raw breast milk for babies on neonatal units. *Lancet* **2**(8148):898.

Collins-Thompson, D. L., K. F. Weiss, G. W. Riedel, and S. Charbonneau (1980). Microbiological guidelines and sampling plans for dried infant cereals and powdered infant formula from a Canadian national microbiological survey. *J. Food Prot.* **43**(8):613–616.

Dairy Council Digest (1976). Current concepts in infant nutrition. **47**(2):7–12.

Dairy Council Digest (1977). The role of dairy foods in the diet. **48**(3):16.

Dairy Council Digest (1977). Utilization of milk components by the food industry. **48**(5):27.

Dairy Council Digest (1979). Perspective on milk intolerance. **49**(6):31–36.

Dairy Council Digest (1980). Current Infant Feeding Practices. **51**(1):1–5.

Davis, J. G. and F. J. MacDonald (1953). Richmond's Dairy Chemistry, Charles Griffin and Co. Limited, London England. pp. 88–93.

Ferrier, L. K., D. Bird, L. S. Wei, and A. I. Nelson (1975). Weaning food prepared from whole soy beans and bananas by drum drying: Proceedings of a meeting held in Ribeirao Preto, Brazil. *Arch. Latinoam. Nutr.* pp. 281–295.

Foman, S. J. (1975). What are infants fed in the United States? *Pediatrics* **56**:350.

Fransson, G. B. and B. Tonnerdal (1980). Iron in human milk. *J. Pediatr. (St. Louis)* **96**(3,I):380–384.

Gross, S. J., R. David, L. Bauman, and R. M. Temarelli (1980). Nutritional composition of milk produced by mothers delivering preterm. *J. Pediatr. (St. Louis)* **96**(4):641–644.

Holsinger, V. H. (1976). New products from lactose hydrolyzed milk. *Dairy and Ice Cream Field* **159**(3):30–32.

260

Institute of Food Technologists (1972). Expert Panel on Food Safety and Nutrition and the Committee on Public Information. Botulism. *Food Technol.* **26**(10):insert.

Jelliffe, D. B. and E. F. P. Jelliffe (1976). Nutrition and human milk. *Postgrad. Med.* **60**(1):154–156.

Jelliffe, D. B., and E. F. P. Jelliffe (1979). Adequacy of breast-feeding. *Lancet* **2**(8144):691–692.

Katz, R., and E. Speckman (1978). A perspective on lactose intolerance. *J. Food Prot.* **41**(3):220–225.

Kretchmer, N. (1972). Lactose and Lactase. *Sci. Am.* **227**(10):71–78.

Kroger, M. (1976). How do you want your yogurt: with or without bacteria? *Dairy and Ice Cream Field* **159**(4):59–64.

Kuromiya, M. (1960). The study on the effect of cinder-like substances, especially carrot powder, in dyspeptic infants. *Ochanomizu Igaku Zasshi* **8**:88–102.

Lee, V. A. and K. Lorenz (1978). The nutritional and physiological impact of milk in human nutrition. *CRC Crit. Rev. Food Sci. Nutr.* **11**(1):41–116.

Lockhart, M. D. (1979). Breast milk. *Contemp. Nutr.* **4**(1):1–2.

Manus, L. (1979). Liquid cultured dairy products. *Cult. Dairy Prod. J.* **14**(1):9–14.

Mathur, B. N., and K. M. Shahani (1979). Use of total whey constituents for human food. *J. Dairy Sci.* **62**(1):99–105.

Miller, H. R., and M. Secretin. 1980. Infant milk formula and process for its manufacture. *United States Patent* 4 216 236.

Mossel, D. A. A., and J. H. P. Jonxis (1978). Medical, especially microbiological, aspects of the supply of milk products to healthy infants in developing countries. *Ned. Tijdschr. Geneeskd.* **122**(41):1573–1578. (*Dairy Sci. Abstr.* **42**(5):324.)

Mulchandani, R. P., R. V. Josephson, and W. J. Harper (1979a). Effects of processing on liquid infant milk formulas. I. Freshly processed products. *J. Dairy Sci.* **62**(10):1527–1536.

Nelson, A. I., M. P. Steinberg, and L. S. Wei (1978). INTSOY Series, Number 14, International Agricultural Publications, College of Agriculture, University of Illinois, Urbana, Illinois.

Ogra, P. L., and D. H. Dayton (editors) (1979). Immunology of breast milk. Raven Press, New York.

Perraudin, M. L., and M. Sorin (1978). Probable poisoning of a newborn infant by nicotine present in maternal milk. *Ann. Pediatr.* **25**(1):41–44. (*Dairy Sci. Abstr.* **42**(6):420.)

Phillips, M. C., and George Briggs (1975). Milk and dairy products for the American diet. *J. Dairy Sci.,* **58**(11):1751–1763.

Saarinen, U. M., P. Pelkonen, and M. A. Siimes (1979). Serum immunoglobulin A in healthy infants; an accelerated postnatal increase in formula-fed compared to breast-fed infants. *J. Pediatr.* **95**(3):410–412.

Sadauskas, V. M., and A. M. Morkunas (1978). Some problems of breast feeding of newborns and of lactational function of the mammary gland in women with pulmonar tuberculosis. *Probl. Tuberk.* No. 3: 81–82. (*Dairy Sci. Abstr.* **42**(9):679.)

Sampson, R. R., and D. B. L. McClelland (1980). Vitamin B_{12} in human colostrum and milk. Quantitation of the vitamin and its binder and the uptake of bound vitamin B_{12} by intestinal bacteria. *Acta Paediatr. Scand.* **69**(1):93–99.

Schanler, R. J., and W. Oh (1980). Composition of breast milk obtained from mothers of premature infants as compared to breast milk obtained from donors. *J. Pediatr.* **96**(4):679–681.

Schramel, P. (1979). Determination of boron in milk and milk products by ICP-analysis. *Z. Lebensm.-Unters. Forsch.* **169**(4):255–258. (*Dairy Sci. Abstr.* **42**(6):460.)

Sekine, K., K. Maeda, T. Nakayama, and T. Nemoto (1978). Successful treatments of two cases of intractable diarrhea. *Pediatr. Jpn.* **19**:321.

Stintzing, G., and R. Zetterstrom (1979). Cow's milk allergy, incidence and pathogenic role of early exposure to cow's milk formula. *Acta Paediatr. Scand.* **68**(3):383–387. (*Dairy Sci. Abstr.* **42**(5):331.)

Sroufe, L. A. (1981). Quoted in the Minneapolis Tribune, September 13, 1981.

Timonen, E., H. K. Akerblom, K. Hasunen, and K. Kouvalainen (1979). Effect of diet on the fatty acid composition in human milk. (Abstract). *Pediatr. Res.* **13**(1):82.

Walker, W. A. (1976). Host defense mechanisms in the gastrointestinal tract. *Pediatrics* **57**:901–916.

Waterlow, J. C. (1979a). Adequacy of breast-feeding. *Lancet* **2**(8148):897–898.

Waterlow, J. C. (1979b). Observations on the protein and energy requirements of pre-school children. *Indian J. Nutr. Diet.* **16**(5)175–188.

Weller, S. D. V. (1980). Aspects of breast feeding. *J. R. Soc. Med.* **73**(1):3–4.

Widdowson, E. M. (1979). Vitamin D in human milk. *Nutr. Food Sci.* **58**:4–5.

Woodruff, C. W. (1981). Supplementary foods for infants. *Contemp. Nutr.* **6**(1):1–2.

Index

263

FOOD SCIENCE AND TECHNOLOGY

A SERIES OF MONOGRAPHS

Maynard A. Amerine, Rose Marie Pangborn, and Edward B. Roessler, PRINCIPLES OF SENSORY EVALUATION OF FOOD. 1965.

S. M. Herschdoerfer, QUALITY CONTROL IN THE FOOD INDUSTRY. Volume I — 1967. Volume II — 1968. Volume III — 1972.

Hans Reimann, FOOD-BORNE INFECTIONS AND INTOXICATIONS. 1969.

Irvin E. Leiner, TOXIC CONSTITUENTS OF PLANT FOODSTUFFS. 1969.

Martin Glicksman, GUM TECHNOLOGY IN THE FOOD INDUSTRY. 1970.

L. A. Goldblatt, AFLATOXIN. 1970.

Maynard A. Joslyn, METHODS IN FOOD ANALYSIS, second edition. 1970.

A. C. Hulme (ed.), THE BIOCHEMISTRY OF FRUITS AND THEIR PRODUCTS. Volume 1 — 1970. Volume 2 — 1971.

G. Ohloff and A. F. Thomas, GUSTATION AND OLFACTION. 1971.

George F. Stewart and Maynard A. Amerine, INTRODUCTION TO FOOD SCIENCE AND TECHNOLOGY. 1973.

C. R. Stumbo, THERMOBACTERIOLOGY IN FOOD PROCESSING, second edition. 1973.

Irvin E. Liener (ed.), TOXIC CONSTITUENTS OF ANIMAL FOODSTUFFS. 1974.

Aaron M. Altschul (ed.), NEW PROTEIN FOODS: Volume 1, TECHNOLOGY, PART A — 1974. Volume 2, TECHNOLOGY, PART B — 1976. Volume 3, ANIMAL PROTEIN SUPPLIES, PART A — 1978. Volume 4, ANIMAL PROTEIN SUPPLIES, PART B — 1981.

S. A. Goldblith, L. Rey, and W. W. Rothmayr, FREEZE DRYING AND ADVANCED FOOD TECHNOLOGY. 1975.

R. B. Duckworth (ed.), WATER RELATIONS OF FOOD. 1975.

Gerald Reed (ed.), ENZYMES IN FOOD PROCESSING, second edition. 1975.

A. G. Ward and A. Courts (eds.), THE SCIENCE AND TECHNOLOGY OF GELATIN. 1976.

John A. Troller and J. H. B. Christian, WATER ACTIVITY AND FOOD. 1978.

A. E. Bender, FOOD PROCESSING AND NUTRITION. 1978.

D. R. Osborne and P. Voogt, THE ANALYSIS OF NUTRIENTS IN FOODS. 1978.

Marcel Loncin and R. L. Merson, FOOD ENGINEERING: PRINCIPLES AND SELECTED APPLICATIONS. 1979.

Hans Reimann and Frank L. Bryan (eds.), FOOD-BORNE INFECTIONS AND INTOXICATIONS, second edition. 1979.

N. A. Michael Eskin, PLANT PIGMENTS, FLAVORS AND TEXTURES: THE CHEMISTRY AND BIOCHEMISTRY OF SELECTED COMPOUNDS. 1979.

J. G. Vaughan (ed.), FOOD MICROSCOPY. 1979.

J. R. A. Pollock (ed.), BREWING SCIENCE, Volume 1 — 1979. Volume 2 — 1980.

Irvin E. Liener (ed.), TOXIC CONSTITUENTS OF PLANT FOODSTUFFS, second edition. 1980.

J. Christopher Bauernfeind (ed.), CAROTENOIDS AS COLORANTS AND VITAMIN A PRECURSORS: TECHNOLOGICAL AND NUTRITIONAL APPLICATIONS. 1981.

Pericles Markakis (ed.), ANTHOCYANINS AS FOOD COLORS. 1982.

Vernal S. Packard, HUMAN MILK AND INFANT FORMULA. 1982.

In preparation

George F. Stewart and Maynard A. Amerine, INTRODUCTION TO FOOD SCIENCE AND TECHNOLOGY, SECOND EDITION. 1982.

Malcolm C. Bourne (ed.), FOOD TEXTURE AND VISCOSITY: CONCEPT AND MEASUREMENT. 1982.

Héctor A. Iglesias and Jorge Chirife, HANDBOOK OF FOOD ISOTHERMS: WATER SORPTION PARAMETERS FOR FOOD AND FOOD COMPONENTS. 1982.

John A. Troller, SANITATION IN FOOD PROCESSING AND SERVICE. 1983.